The Poisoned Patient:
the role of the laboratory

The Ciba Foundation for the promotion of international cooperation in medical and chemical research is a scientific and educational charity established by CIBA Limited – now CIBA-GEIGY Limited – of Basle. The Foundation operates independently in London under English trust law.

Ciba Foundation Symposia are published in collaboration with Associated Scientific Publishers (Elsevier Scientific Publishing Company, Excerpta Medica, North-Holland Publishing Company) in Amsterdam.

Associated Scientific Publishers, P.O. Box 211, Amsterdam

The Poisoned Patient: the role of the laboratory

Ciba Foundation Symposium 26 (new series)

1974

Elsevier · Excerpta Medica · North-Holland

Associated Scientific Publishers · Amsterdam · Oxford · New York

ISBN Excerpta Medica 90 219 4028 0
ISBN American Elsevier 0-444-15144-3

Published in 1974 by Associated Scientific Publishers, P.O. Box 211, Amsterdam, and American Elsevier, 52 Vanderbilt Avenue, New York, N.Y. 10017.

Suggested series entry for library catalogues: Ciba Foundation Symposia.
Suggested publisher's entry for library catalogues: Associated Scientific Publishers.

Ciba Foundation Symposium 26 (new series)

Printed in The Netherlands by Mouton & Co, The Hague

Contents

Participants

Symposium on The Poisoned Patient: the role of the laboratory held at the Ciba Foundation, London, 19th–21st February, 1974

A. S. CURRY (*Chairman*) Home Office Central Research Establishment, Aldermaston, Reading, Berkshire RG7 4PN

S. AGURELL Faculty of Pharmacy, Department of Pharmacognosy, Lindhagensgatan 128, S–112 51 Stockholm, Sweden

A. H. BECKETT Department of Pharmacy, Chelsea College, University of London, Manresa Road, London SW3 6LX

J. W. BRIDGES Department of Biochemistry, University of Surrey, Guildford, Surrey GU2 5XH

S. S. BROWN MRC Clinical Research Centre, Division of Clinical Chemistry, Watford Road, Harrow, Middlesex HA1 3UJ

V. P. DOLE The Rockefeller University, New York, NY 10021, USA

D. J. GEE Department of Forensic Medicine, The University of Leeds, 30 Hyde Terrace, Leeds LS2 9LN

J. R. GILLETTE Laboratory of Chemical Pharmacology, National Heart & Lung Institute, National Institutes of Health, Bethesda, Maryland 20014, USA

R. GOULDING Poisons Unit, Guy's Hospital, New Cross Hospital, Avonley Road, London SE14 5ER

B. HOLMSTEDT Department of Toxicology, Swedish Medical Research Council, Karolinska Institutet, 10401 Stockholm 60, Sweden

J. V. JACKSON Drugs and Toxicology Section, The Metropolitan Police Forensic Science Laboratory, 2 Richbell Place, Holborn, London WC1N 3LA

H. LEACH Group Pathology Laboratory, Caernarvonshire and Anglesey General Hospital, Bangor, Caernarvonshire

G. MACHATA Universitäts-Institut für Gerichtliche Medizin, Sensengasse 2, 1090 Vienna 9, Austria

A. C. MOFFAT Home Office Central Research Establishment, Aldermaston, Reading, Berkshire RG7 4PN

*R. W. NEWTON Regional Poisoning Treatment Centre, Ward 3, The Royal Infirmary, Edinburgh EH3 9YW

C. W. PARKER Department of Internal Medicine, Washington University School of Medicine, Barnes and Wohl Hospitals, 660 S. Euclid Avenue, St Louis, Mo. 63110, USA

A. R. PATEL Department of Medicine, University of Glasgow, Western Infirmary, Glasgow G11 6NT

L. F. PRESCOTT University Department of Therapeutics, The Royal Infirmary, Edinburgh EH3 9YW

W. RIESS Department of Pharmacological Chemistry, CIBA–GEIGY Ltd, CH–4002 Basle, Switzerland

R. P. W. SCOTT Hoffmann-La Roche Inc., Nutley, New Jersey 07110, USA

I. SUNSHINE Institute of Pathology, Case Western Reserve University, Cleveland, Ohio 44106, USA

B. WIDDOP Poisons Unit, Guy's Hospital, New Cross Hospital, Avonley Road, London SE14 5ER

Editors: RUTH PORTER and MAEVE O'CONNOR

* Present address: Ninewells Hospital, Ninewells, Dundee

Chairman's introduction

ALAN S. CURRY

Home Office Central Research Establishment, Aldermaston, Reading, Berkshire

From our programme it seems that clinicians, laboratory workers and pathologists in turn will discuss the role of the laboratory in the treatment of patients who have poisoned themselves with barbiturates. In fact, the 'patient' we intend to discuss is the person who is ill as a result of the use or abuse of 'drugs'. Clearly this definition includes those who have taken overdoses and we will indeed have to debate the role of the laboratory with great care, since opinions differ so greatly. However, my definition also brings in the habitual user of drugs and the addict. Obviously, alcoholics would come under this definition too, but at this meeting we would probably do better to refer to alcoholism for comparative purposes only, and concentrate instead on the person who abuses barbiturates, tranquillizers, amphetamines, cannabis, LSD (lysergide), heroin and so on.

What *is* the role of the laboratory in dealing with such cases? Has it a major or a minor part to play in the treatment or control, or both, of those who habitually take these drugs? What techniques can be used? Are large centralized laboratories essential? What hope is there that a 'dipstick' will soon be developed with which general practitioners can test drug concentrations in their patients?

At this symposium we ought to be able to examine first what the laboratory can do to discover drug-induced biochemical lesions, and then the possible implications of this work for the clinician. I hope that we will also find time to discuss which techniques are specific enough to justify society in imprisoning anyone for being a drug addict.

As well as the addict and the patient who has taken an overdose, we must consider the person who may be receiving too much or too little medication. Anti-epileptic drugs and cardiac glycosides are two obvious instances in which the regimen of therapy needs to be monitored in the laboratory, but I am sure we shall hear other decided views on what a modern hospital laboratory should be expected to do, both now and in the future. Are toxicologists going to drift into a situation where people admitted to hospital will be tested not only for electrolytes, sugar and urea (to the limit of how many automated machines the hospital possesses) but also for aspirin, barbiturates and numerous other common drugs? Should such tests be extended to include the measurement of lead in blood and perhaps the trace elements that may play a part in deficiencies in healing and in coronary artery disease? And just how much monitoring of drugs is necessary in the practice of psychiatric medicine?

Another type of patient we must consider is the person with iatrogenic disease after drug therapy—surely he has been poisoned? The laboratory clearly has a role to play in discovering the side effects of drugs and reporting drug interactions, especially now that undesirable effects seem to be becoming more common. Can the laboratory of the future do anything to prevent vaginal carcinoma from developing twenty years later in the offspring of oestrogen-treated mothers? I do not think we should discuss the implications of teratology for the toxicologist here, but simply by mentioning this aspect I hope I am re-emphasizing that we are not here just to discuss overdoses of barbiturates.

I do not want even to attempt a complete definition of the role of the laboratory. As a chemist I naturally think of the laboratory as a place that used to have a characteristic smell but where now one trips over wires or bumps into gas cylinders. But there must be no limit to what can be discussed at this symposium—if anyone specializing in botany, for example, has found that when a certain weed is fed on LSD it gyrates in the reverse direction to the sun, we want to hear about it! However, the programme will probably take us more often into the chemical laboratory and we shall have to examine in detail direct or indirect (i.e. extraction first) procedures, methods for specific and general toxicology, and qualitative and quantitative procedures. All of us know that many modern analytical instruments are massively expensive not only in money but also in manpower. Is the laboratory in danger of getting caught up in a heart-transplant versus varicose veins type of argument? Has enough effort been put into the techniques that the smaller hospital laboratory can use? And is sufficient time spent on teaching analytical toxicology? The really dramatic advances in technique are leading to analyses that are sensitive to the order of 1 part in 10^{12}, or about 10^7 times better than was possible in post-mortem toxicology 20 years ago. Then we have to ask what the figures mean. This question leads us on to others about metabolic processes, metabolic blocks, antimetabolites, and—for the clinician—the value of laboratory results in deciding on a course of treatment. Does a person die because his metabolism cannot cope with the amount of drug ingested? If so, how can increased metabolism be induced? Do toxic metabolites affect the patient? And how much should the toxicology laboratory do towards initiating and coordinating these investigations?

Unfortunately the poisoned arrow of the Greeks—which incidentally gave us our name as toxicologists—has not transformed itself into Ehrlich's silver bullet: many patients still die from drugs and in the final part of this symposium we shall discuss post-mortem chemistry and pathology. What does the distribution of drugs in the tissues of a dead body tell us? Are the results reliable? Can macroscopic and microscopic lesions be definitive? More questions, I am afraid, but I hope they are ones we can try to answer during this meeting.

In mentioning so many aspects of toxicology I am not trying to change the title of the symposium but rather emphasizing that the laboratory can often help the clinician. I shall leave it to members of the symposium to debate where and how the laboratory can be most useful. I also want to stress that as well as learning about the current state of the art from our speakers we should think about what might be done in the future.

The clinician's requirements from the laboratory in the treatment of the acutely poisoned patient

R. W. NEWTON

*The Regional Poisoning Treatment Centre, Royal Infirmary, Edinburgh**

Abstract Emergency treatment of acutely poisoned patients consists of the application of basic therapeutic principles. Adequate respiration must be ensured, and hypothermia and adverse effects on the cardiovascular system must be promptly dealt with. Effective support from the laboratory at this stage therefore lies in the provision of results of blood gas and electrolyte analysis on an emergency basis.

The further management of the patient does not rest on the provision of the appropriate antidote, for such is available in less than 1% of instances. After the initial phase, with some important exceptions, the management is intensive supportive therapy irrespective of the poison ingested. The exceptions are salicylates, opiates, paracetamol, iron and long-acting barbiturates. Salicylates can be determined with accuracy by the clinician, opiate poisoning can usually be diagnosed clinically and confirmed by a therapeutic test; however the laboratory must provide urgent support in iron and paracetamol poisoning if rational therapy is to be applied. In poisoning by long-acting barbiturates, laboratory results are not needed on an emergency basis.

Thus, in the current routine management of poisoned patients the laboratory has a limited role. The situation is entirely different when research and forensic aspects of acute poisoning are considered. In the future, if safe haemoperfusion procedures or antidotes (specific pharmacological antagonists), or both, become available, the requirements of the physician may increase.

Acutely poisoned patients account for an increasing proportion of emergency medical admissions of adults to hospitals and for some 10% of the total medical admissions. Baird *et al.* (1972) reported that in 129 days 216 patients had to be urgently resuscitated in the Accident and Emergency Department of the Royal Infirmary, Edinburgh. Poisoning accounted for 75 (38%) of these.

Initially, these patients were treated according to basic therapeutic principles, irrespective of the substance ingested. Since ventilatory failure is a common complication of overdoses with central nervous system depressants the practice

* Present address: Ninewells Hospital, Ninewells, Dundee

is to ensure an adequate airway by clearing debris such as vomitus or saliva and, if necessary, inserting an oropharyngeal or cuffed endotracheal tube. A rough but practical guide to adequate ventilation can then be obtained by measuring the volume of expired air—the minute volume—with a Wright's spirometer. Respiratory depression, however, can be accurately assessed only by measuring the arterial P_{O_2}, P_{CO_2} and pH (Matthew & Lawson 1972, p. 19).

'Shock' may be treated by raising the foot of the bed or, if that does not work, by cautiously giving vasopressors or infusing a plasma expander. However, if drugs such as metaraminol are used uncritically they may cause renal failure, while in patients poisoned with tricyclic antidepressants they may induce ventricular dysrhythmia. Further, plasma expanders may lead to pulmonary oedema in patients intoxicated with barbiturates or methaqualone. The clinical state of these patients may be aggravated by associated hypoxia or acidaemia. Again analysis of arterial P_{O_2}, P_{CO_2} and pH is essential.

Thus, in the initial phase of emergency care the laboratory should provide information about blood gases and, if the patient has been unconscious for a long time before admission, about plasma electrolytes, rather than about the narrow field of toxicological analysis (Matthew *et al.* 1969).

If the further management of poisoned patients rested on giving specific pharmacological antagonists, a full 'coma screen' would always be necessary for identification of the drug taken. But since appropriate antidotes are very few, the coma screens of our American colleagues are an expensive luxury. An antidote is, however, available for the relatively common cases of poisoning with opiates. This type of poisoning is particularly dangerous because severe respiratory depression is a constant feature, often associated with coma and pinpoint pupils. The clinical diagnosis is usually straightforward, for there are few other situations, if any, in which severe hypoxia is associated with constricted pupils. Opiate poisoning can now be treated and confirmed by giving naloxone, a new and potent narcotic antagonist with virtually no agonist activity. It can safely be given to comatose patients when the diagnosis is in doubt, since it will not cause respiratory depression in those poisoned with non-narcotics (Evans *et al.* 1973). Hence laboratory confirmation is no longer needed in the immediate treatment of opiate poisoning.

In patients who have taken overdoses of tricyclic antidepressants, the atropine-like effects on the central and peripheral nervous systems can be consistently reversed with physostigmine salicylate, a cholinesterase inhibitor which is lipid-soluble enough to cross the blood–brain barrier; rapid arousal, slowing of the pulse rate and conversion of the plantar response from extensor to flexor after therapy are dramatic. The undesirable cholinergic effects that may be produced by physostigmine, however, preclude its use as an antidote in routine management (Newton 1974). On the other hand in some circumstances it may be indicated and should be given after a clinical diagnosis has been made. Laboratory confirmation of the poison taken is not required.

Likewise, the phenothiazines may produce severe extrapyramidal effects such as torticollis, oculogyric crises and other muscular spasms. These episodes may need immediate treatment with benzatropine (benzatropine methanesulphonate). Again there is no question of waiting for laboratory confirmation.

The folly of delaying treatment until after laboratory confirmation of cyanide poisoning is all too obvious.

After the initial phase, the management of the poisoned patient continues to consist of intensive supportive therapy, irrespective of the drug ingested. In 1967 Marks noted that 'in sedative drug poisoning, therapeutic emphasis has shifted from desperate efforts at arousal to an orderly if unspectacular regimen of supportive therapy'. In addition to intensive supportive therapy, attempts to eliminate the poison actively may be justified in a small minority of cases—less than 5%; in this event qualitative and quantitative analyses are essential and indeed it would be wrong to use any form of dialysis or forced diuresis without toxicological evidence.

The commonest poison for which active measures for promoting excretion are available is salicylate. Whereas elaborate laboratory equipment and specialized techniques are needed for the chemical analysis of most poisons, plasma salicylate can be measured rapidly and accurately in the ward side-room by a modification of the Trinder method (Trinder 1954; Brown & Smith 1968). The decision about whether forced alkaline diuresis should be instituted is based on the concentration of salicylate in serum and can be made with the minimum of delay. In severely poisoned patients the laboratory may be called upon to assist in assessing acid–base status and hypokalaemia on an emergency basis but this is quite exceptional in adults.

Similarly, in patients who have ingested Paraquat (1,1′-dimethyl-4,4′-bipyridinium dichloride), a simple but sensitive urine test is available that indicates whether systemic absorption has taken place, whether organ damage is likely to occur, and whether any kind of therapy is indicated (Matthew *et al.* 1968).

In Edinburgh what we need most urgently from the laboratory is help in assessing and treating patients who have taken large overdoses of paracetamol. Hepatic damage in such patients has in the past resulted from paracetamol being converted by microsomal enzymes into a highly reactive intermediate metabolite which binds covalently with liver macromolecules. At therapeutic doses of paracetamol the small quantities of active metabolites are preferentially conjugated with hepatic glutathione. When stores of glutathione are reduced to less than 30% of normal, the excess metabolite alkylates vital cell constituents and causes necrosis. Administered glutathione does not enter cells readily but precursors such as cysteine and other nucleophilic thiol compounds such as cysteamine (mercaptamine) can prevent paracetamol-induced hepatic necrosis. Prescott *et al.* (1974) have now shown that cysteamine is strikingly effective in protecting the liver from such necrosis. Although liver damage occurs early, cysteamine has been effective even when given up to 10 hours after ingestion of paracetamol. However, not all patients claiming to have taken paracetamol should be treated this way, as cysteamine has temporary but distressing side effects on the gastrointestinal tract and the central nervous system. The decision about treatment depends on the concentration of the drug being determined rapidly and accurately: if the concentration indicates that severe liver damage is a strong probability, therapy must be begun immediately.

In adults iron poisoning is rarely severe and the chelating agent desferrioxamine (deferoxamine) can usually be given orally before the serum iron estimation is available. Further parenteral therapy may be indicated if the clinical state of the patient deteriorates or if the serum concentration is extremely high. Thus in these circumstances rational therapy largely depends on prompt laboratory aid.

Apart from the instances of salicylate, paracetamol and iron poisoning, widespread confusion exists as to the requirements of the clinician from the laboratory in the management of the acutely poisoned patient. The confusion over what information is needed about the concentrations of drugs in serum is typified by misconceptions concerning the assessment and treatment of patients who have taken overdoses of barbiturates, glutethimide or methaqualone. Clinicians would like to be able to use drug concentrations as indications for action, as they do in salicylate poisoning, but with overdoses of hypnotic drugs the concentrations are not a reliable indication of severity of poisoning and may indeed be misleading. In barbiturate poisoning the depth of coma depends on the concentration of barbiturate in the brain rather than in the serum (Clowes *et al.* 1940). The lack of consistency in the response of animals, and even more of humans, to barbiturates is well known, with the response to barbiturates in experimental animals often varying by as much as 50%; in addition individual animals are known to respond in different ways to the same dose on repeated occasions (Richards & Taylor 1956).

In a review of 776 patients from the Regional Poisoning Treatment Centre in Edinburgh, Matthew & Lawson (1966) stated that serum concentrations of barbiturates were often not closely related to the clinical state. Berman *et al.* (1956) found that more than half of their patients with 'potentially fatal levels' did not need active methods of treatment to increase the removal of poison but recovered with supportive therapy alone. Baker (1969) has shown that intensive supportive therapy alone can produce results as good as when combined with active elimination. In 553 patients unconscious from overdoses of a variety of drugs he reported a mortality of 0.74% and a low morbidity. In no case was any attempt made to speed up elimination. In Edinburgh, where we strongly favour intensive supportive therapy without active elimination except where it is clearly indicated, our results are similar, the mortality being 0.48%. Thus, the use of serum concentrations of barbiturate as the strict criterion for instituting methods of increasing elimination (Lee & Ames 1965) is unfounded. This is particularly true for epileptics and other patients habituated to these drugs.

The toxicological analysis may be helpful in the assessment of a patient with barbiturate poisoning, but the clinical condition is more important. The real significance of the analysis for the clinician is whether a long-acting barbiturate (such as barbitone or phenobarbitone) is implicated.

Mawer & Lee (1968) observed that short-acting and medium-acting barbiturates were eliminated mainly by biotransformation and the excretion of inactive metabolites. Their results supported conclusions of Bloomer (1967). Excretion of unchanged active drug, however, is of great importance with phenobarbitone. Therefore, before deciding to use forced alkaline diuresis or dialysis to increase the elimination of a drug, the clinician must obtain qualitative and quantitative estimations of barbiturates from the laboratory. Of course, when adequate facilities for supportive therapy exist, such estimates are not necessarily urgent. The same remarks apply to glutethimide and methaqualone.

There are, of course, less common problems in this country for which laboratory assistance may be sought. In organophosphate poisoning, for example, the availability of information about serum and red cell concentrations of cholinesterase is a comforting diagnostic guide when massive doses of atropine are being infused into an unfortunate patient. Similarly, in methaemoglobinaemia, which is becoming rare since phenacetin stopped being used therapeutically, specific therapy is more confidently controlled with the help of laboratory estimates.

In the immediate management of the acutely poisoned patient it would therefore appear that the laboratory has a limited role.

The usefulness of the laboratory lies more in its ability to make retrospective comparisons of patients and to confirm diagnoses, as well as in dealing with medico-legal aspects. Some indication of which poison was used may of course be apparent on clinical examination. For example in glutethimide poisoning (Doriden), a fluctuating level of consciousness, associated with papilloedema and sudden apnoea, may be a marked feature. In methaqualone overdosage, severe depression of consciousness may be associated with exaggerated limb reflexes and the plantar response may be extensor. These features, together with spontaneous muscle twitching, dilated pupils and tachycardia, are characteristic of poisoning with tricyclic antidepressants. Bullae occur in 8% of patients poisoned with barbiturates and may occur in those poisoned with glutethimide, tricyclic antidepressants or carbon monoxide.

Difficulties in distinguishing between overdosage and other conditions will inevitably occur. Although unconsciousness in a patient between the ages of 15 and 55 years who has no head injury is almost certainly due to drug overdosage, in rare circumstances the clinician must ensure that no other neurological abnormalities are present. In this event the laboratory may be helpful. Again, there are few objective differences between patients with delirium tremens and those recovering from overdoses of tricyclic antidepressants. Visual hallucination, speech disorder, disorientation and tachycardia are to be expected in both types of case.

A positive diagnosis of poisoning, although not essential in management, is desirable in the severely poisoned patient and is achieved ultimately only when the agent or agents involved are identified in the blood, urine or gastric aspirate.

The role of the laboratory is of the utmost importance in research on acute poisoning. Many anecdotal reports attribute dramatic recoveries from overdoses of central nervous system depressants to some plainly futile method of treatment, although toxicological screening is not mentioned and alcohol must have been the agent responsible. Even worse are the countless instances of patients being reported as 'severely intoxicated' after overdoses of benzodiazepines, with almost inevitably no estimation being made of serum concentrations of barbiturates or methaqualone. The efficacy of treatment or the condemnation of drugs previously thought to be safe can only be validly assessed after adequate laboratory screening has been done for other drugs that might be implicated.

In the future haemoperfusion may become safer and technically more simple; at the same time specific pharmacological antagonists, free from dangerous side effects, may gradually become available. In these circumstances the clinician's requirements from the laboratory will probably increase, since the emphasis will shift to rapid identification of all drugs involved in overdosage, so that the appropriate antidote can be administered or the patient connected to a charcoal column or ion-exchange resin column. At that time the clinician may be a clinician in the true sense no longer.

References

BAIRD, R. N., NOBLE, J. & McLEAN, D. (1972) *Br. Med. J. 4*, 90
BAKER, A. B. (1969) *Med. J. Aust. 1*, 497
BERMAN, L. B., JEGHERS, H. J., SCHREINER, G. E. & PALLOTTA, A. J. (1956) *J. Am. Med. Assoc. 161*, 820
BLOOMER, H. A. (1967) *Lancet 2*, 986
BROWN, S. S. & SMITH, A. C. A. (1968) *Br. Med. J. 4*, 327
CLOWES, G. H. A., KELTER, A. K. & KRAHL, M. E. (1940) *J. Pharmacol. Exp. Ther. 68*, 312
EVANS, L. E. J., ROSCOE, P., SWAINSON, C. P. & PRESCOTT, L. F. (1973) *Lancet 4*, 452–455
LEE, H. A. & AMES, A. C. (1965) *Br. Med. J. 1*, 1217
MARKS, L. C. (1964) *Am. J. Med. Sci. 254*, 296
MATTHEW, H. & LAWSON, A. A. H. (1966) *Q. J. Med. 35*, 539–552
MATTHEW, H. & LAWSON, A. A. H. (1972) *Treatment of Common Acute Poisonings*, 2nd edn., Churchill Livingstone, Edinburgh
MATTHEW, H., LOGAN, A., WOODRUFF, M. F. A. & HEARD, B. (1968) *Br. Med. J. 3*, 759–763
MATTHEW, H., PROUDFOOT, A. T., BROWN, S. S. & AITKEN, R. C. B. (1969) *Br. Med. J. 3*, 489
MAWER, G. E. & LEE, H. A. (1968) *Br. Med. J. 2*, 790
NEWTON, R. W. (1974) *J. Am. Med. Assoc.* in press
PRESCOTT, L. F., NEWTON, R. W., SWAINSON, C. P., WRIGHT, N., FORREST, A. R. W. & MATTHEW, H. (1974) *Lancet 1*, 588–592
RICHARDS, A. K. & TAYLOR, J. D. (1956) *Anesthesiology 17*, 3, 414
TRINDER, P. (1954) *Biochem. J. 57*, 301

Discussion

Holmstedt: Why did you use physostigmine as an antidote to the effects of tricyclic antidepressants on the central nervous system, Dr Newton?

Newton: At therapeutic doses tricyclic antidepressants are thought to change the ratio of acetylcholine and amines acting as neurotransmitters. The tricyclic antidepressants produce unconsciousness, which can in practice be reversed by physostigmine salicylate.

Holmstedt: Physostigmine is a general central stimulant.

Newton: Yes, but the action of tricyclic antidepressants is mainly through the anticholinergic effects in overdosage and therefore physostigmine would be expected to reverse these effects.

Holmstedt: Not everybody will agree with that. The pharmacodynamics of the tricyclic antidepressants are not really known.

Did you say that cholinesterase determinations in blood may be useful as a guide for atropine treatment in acute cases of poisoning with the organophosphates?

Newton: No, I said that it was comforting for the clinician to know, when giving large doses of atropine, that the diagnosis is organophosphate poisoning.

Holmstedt: I agree with you, because one wouldn't see any change in cholinesterase activity after atropine.

Scott: For proper treatment it is probably more important for the clinician to know what the drug is than to know how much of it is present.

Newton: I agree.

Gillette: Plasma concentrations of a drug don't mean much if one doesn't know what the drug is. A meaningful quantitative analysis has to be based on knowing what the drug is.

Curry: One also needs to know whether metabolites are being measured, as well as the parent drug.

Sunshine: You said that barbiturate concentrations do not correlate with the clinical condition of the patient, Dr Newton. Our experience is that essentially most of them do (Parker *et al.* 1970; Sunshine 1971). You went on to indicate that these concentrations are of value in estimating whether haemodialysis or some other heroic type of therapy ought to be used. That is quite different from correlating the condition of the patient with the barbiturate concentration in his blood or plasma. The barbiturate concentration is a good indication of the state of depression of the central nervous system, if one makes allowances for the tolerance that develops in people who have been using the drugs for a long time.

Newton: In barbiturate poisoning, irrespective of the concentration, it is the clinical state of the patients that determines the therapy.

Sunshine: If the patient has 14 or 18 mg phenobarbitone in 100 ml plasma he is going to be severely depressed and possibly eligible for heroic therapy.

Newton: Yes, but the clinician does not have to know whether the figure is 12 or 18 mg/100 ml before he decides how to treat the patient. Eventually he must know the concentration but treatment does not depend on the concentration alone.

Sunshine: Obviously not, but if the patient is severely depressed yet has a phenobarbitone concentration of 6 mg/100 ml plasma, the clinician should not consider heroic therapy. The probability there is that other substances are present, as well as phenobarbitone, or that some other process may be present that contributes to depression of the central nervous system.

Newton: I agree, but I must stress again that the clinical circumstances decide the treatment.

Widdop: I accept your conservative views about active elimination measures, but can you really describe haemodialysis as heroic therapy these days?

Newton: It is perhaps less heroic than it was but it is not without dangers even now. Amongst other things, platelet numbers change significantly, with the inevitable risk of haemorrhage; infection is a constant threat; and haemolysis is inevitable.

Goulding: What constitutes a significant change in the number of platelets?

Newton: The *average* decrease in platelet numbers during dialysis is not large, according to the published figures, but this means that in some patients the number must fall by 40 or 50%, which is a significant drop.

Patel: When you told us that the level of consciousness and the concentration of barbiturate were not necessarily correlated you did not mention the role of alcohol. In Glasgow a high percentage of our patients have taken excessive amounts of alcohol before poisoning themselves (Patel *et al.* 1972).

Newton: Irrespective of whether alcohol is present, in my opinion there is no correlation between the level of consciousness and the drug concentration (Matthew & Lawson 1966) [and see this volume, pp. 302–305].

Prescott: People who say there is such a correlation should provide evidence to support their statements. The variation is so striking that intensive investigation is needed to determine the causes.

Leach: I agree with much of what Dr Newton has said, but there is a vast difference between a specialized regional treatment centre and the ordinary general district hospital, where patients admitted as emergency cases are often treated by junior members of staff. In a general hospital the laboratory plays another role—that of providing reassurance. The analogy here is with the consultant who would not ask for much laboratory investigation and the junior registrar or house surgeon who would need it before he was prepared to do anything.

Newton: I agree. Our unit doesn't really need reassurance about these unconscious patients but my colleagues in peripheral hospitals may be happier when they know why a patient is unconscious.

Goulding: How many patients are admitted to your unit from other wards in the hospital after having been admitted with another diagnosis and then found to be poisoned? And how many patients do you get in your ward who are ultimately found not to be suffering from poisoning?

Newton: Very few.

Sunshine: Do poisoned patients in Edinburgh come in with a tag saying 'I am poisoned'? In our experience a lot of patients are admitted to the emergency room without a diagnosis and the laboratory can help in establishing whether or not a chemical agent is responsible. How do you sift them out?

Newton: One should assume that the unconscious patient under 50 years of age who has no obvious neurological abnormalities is poisoned.

Parker: Can the simple bedside tests for salicylate or Paraquat intoxication be done by a house officer without any special training?

Newton: I could teach you to estimate the salicylate concentration by Dr Brown's method (Brown & Smith 1968) in about 30 seconds. The test for

Paraquat (Matthew *et al.* 1968) is also very simple and sensitive. Sodium carbonate and sodium dithionate turn blue, indicating reliably whether Paraquat has been absorbed.

Beckett: No one has argued against your main contention that in urgent cases the laboratory generally has only a very small role to play, initially. Surely we must concentrate on removing foreign compounds, most of which are lipid-soluble, so giving the laboratory time to help in the second phase of treatment?

Newton: It depends on whether identification is useful in the second phase. If the use of barbiturates, methaqualone and so on, continues to go down, as we hope it will, the identification of benzodiazepines and other safe hypnotics and tranquillizers might be of limited value for clinicians treating poisoned patients. For research and publication identification is of course important.

Beckett: How much emphasis has there been on removing foreign molecules when we don't know what those molecules are? Surely the logic of what you are saying is that not many drugs can be identified quickly enough to help the patient, therefore we have to be able to get rid of them by some technique even though we know nothing about their structures. There are techniques which remove most of the compounds which are producing toxicity, and most problems arise with lipid-soluble materials.

Newton: What advantage would it be to know what the drugs are?

Beckett: Then you could get rid of them by haemodialysis or preferably by filtration of blood through coated charcoal.

Newton: Why use haemodialysis when the patients, properly treated, get better without it?

Widdop: They would get better more quickly with haemodialysis.

Newton: I don't think anybody can prove that.

Brown: Is there any difficulty in differentiating between diabetic coma and *severe* salicylate poisoning in which there is acidaemia? The textbooks say that the ferric chloride reagent, as used in the side-room test for salicylate (Brown & Smith 1968), gives a violet colour with ketone bodies, notably acetoacetate. Could staff in district hospitals be misled by this?

Newton: That should not be a problem for the clinician unless the patient is particularly obstructive. Usually patients will eventually tell you whether they have taken tablets, even if they don't accurately state the number ingested.

Curry: Does that test give you false positive results, Dr Brown?

Prescott: Not in the blood, surely!

Brown: Unconscious patients with salicylate poisoning can't tell you how many tablets they have taken.

Newton: Such cases are rare. It is also rare for diabetic ketoacidosis to produce unconsciousness.

Scott: Either there are a limited number of substances with which people get poisoned or there are a limited number of substances that something can be done about if they have been taken as poisons. Even a wonderful machine—which we haven't got—which told us exactly what a poison was, and its concentration, would not help at all if no treatment was known. The two problems are to improve the general treatment for poisons, and to learn more about how to handle the different specific poisons that have been taken. At present it would appear that there are only a few substances which the clinician needs to have identified.

Gee: Usually treatment does not depend on identification of the poison, but if there is any possibility that the doctor will be sued for negligence, it may be very important to identify a poison or establish its concentration.

Goulding: The question is not whether the laboratory has any role, but what is the extent of that role. I don't think Dr Newton is saying that the laboratory has no role at all.

Curry: What Dr Scott said crystallizes the present situation. More facts are needed for assessing treatment and we must look to the future. As Professor Beckett said, how are we going to get rid of the poisons? Somewhere we need figures, and I hope you all agree that in future the laboratory will play a larger role.

References

BROWN, S. S. & SMITH, A. C. A. (1968) Salicylate estimation in the side-room. *Br. Med. J. 4*, 327

MATTHEW, H. & LAWSON, A. A. H. (1966) Acute barbiturate poisoning—a review of 2 years' experience. *Q. J. Med. 35*, 539–552

MATTHEW, H., LOGAN, A., WOODRUFF, M. F. A. & HEARD, B. (1968) Paraquat poisoning—lung transplantation. *Br. Med. J. 3*, 759–763

PARKER, K. D., ELLIOTT, H. W., WRIGHT, J. A., NOMOF, N. & HINE, C. H. (1970) Blood and urine concentrations of subjects receiving barbiturates, meprobamate, glutethimide or diphenylhydantoin. *Clin. Toxicol. 3*, 131–145

PATEL, A. R., ROY, M. & WILSON, G. M. (1972) Self poisoning and alcohol. *Lancet 2*, 1099

SUNSHINE, I. (ed.) (1971) in *Manual of Analytical Toxicology*, p. 42, CRC Press, Cleveland, Ohio

The role of the laboratory in the treatment of narcotic poisoning

VINCENT P. DOLE

Rockefeller University, New York

Abstract The toxicologist is of central importance in forensic problems, of secondary value to the clinician in treatment of acute poisoning, and an uncertain factor in rehabilitation programmes.

Determining the cause of death can be difficult. Sophisticated analytical techniques are needed to measure the amounts of potent drugs in tissues, and the range of tests must be broad enough to include all possible lethal agents. On the other hand, the detection of a commonly used drug such as methadone does not in itself prove poisoning. In this area the clinician must rely on the judgement of an experimental toxicologist.

However, in acute narcotic poisoning, treatment cannot be delayed for laboratory diagnosis. Hypoxia must be dealt with immediately, by artificial respiration and an antidote. The ideal antidote, naloxone, specifically reverses respiratory depression due to narcotic poisoning and does no harm if the depression is due to some other cause. Of course samples of urine and blood taken during the acute episode will permit review of the case, but in general the issue of survival will have been decided before the laboratory data are available.

In rehabilitation programmes the danger is that test data can be used to incriminate or alienate patients. Objective data are needed to evaluate the success of narcotic treatment programmes, but they must be used sensitively if they are not to hamper the rehabilitation process.

Clinical chemists can usually limit their concern to the quality of their tests. In most areas of toxicology there is no reason to question the value of accurate laboratory data. But in work on narcotics the situation is not so clear.

Results of urine tests for narcotics can be used to incriminate people as well as to help them. In the United States a positive urine test for narcotics can be used to send a man to prison (either by revocation of parole or by civil commitment), or cause him to be fired from a job when he is being considered for promotion, or—incredibly—may lead to his dismissal from some programmes that purport to be treating him for addiction. In many such programmes urine testing hampers rehabilitation by setting up an adversary relation between staff and patients on the inquisitor–sinner model. At best, routine monitoring is expensive: for example, it costs about $10 million a year in the US to meet the Federal requirements for weekly testing of all patients receiving methadone maintenance treatment. The cost of laboratory work in a clinical programme would be unimportant if funds were unlimited, but they are not: urine testing and rehabilitation services have to compete for the money available. Speaking as a clinician, I would like to see less money spent in the laboratory and more on job training and placement.

Obviously the analyst is not to be blamed for the excessive number of tests that are done, or for any misuse of his data: the demand comes from clinicians and administrators. The chemist has done his job when he provides a reliable report, regardless of how it is used afterwards. But a toxicologist must be more than an analytical technician. His responsibility extends to the interpretation of results, and thus both to the indications for the test and to the weight the results carry in clinical judgements. Subject, then, to challenge in a controversial field, let me offer my opinions on the proper function of the toxicologist in narcotics work, and on the dangers arising from misuse of his data.

WHEN ARE LABORATORY DATA NEEDED?

First (and unarguably), comprehensive analyses are needed to identify the lethal agents in cases of fatal poisoning. The problems here come mainly from over-interpretation of data. Those of us who have spent much time at the laboratory bench are aware of the limitations of laboratory data: for some chemicals the threshold of detection may be quite high in relation to the quantity that can cause severe poisoning, so a negative result may not exclude a suspected agent. Conversely, the detection of a single drug is not conclusive evidence about the cause of death, because drug abusers commonly take more than one drug, and tests for the offending drug may have been omitted.

Until recently the tests available for measuring narcotic drugs in tissues were not sufficiently sensitive or specific to define the role of narcotics in causing the so-called 'acute narcotic reaction' or 'acute overdose' syndrome. Because these acute episodes of pulmonary oedema and coma tend to occur capriciously, sometimes affecting only one person in a group using what had appeared to be the same batch of narcotic, there has been much speculation about the possible role of allergens or other poisons in the mixture. The question is still not settled, although the evidence to date strongly suggests that this acute syndrome is in fact caused by narcotics. The problem is now being actively studied in a number of clinical centres. With the availability of greatly improved methods (especially immunochemical techniques) for quantitative analysis of narcotic drugs at the nanogram level, and with correlated physiological studies, the pathogenesis of this syndrome should soon be clarified.

A more subtle problem has been a tendency of some pathologists to accept the first drug detected as the cause of death or disability. With the now extensive use of methadone for maintenance treatment of former heroin addicts, many thousands of people are excreting this drug in their urine. In the general population of individuals taking no drugs at all a certain number die of obscure causes; if such a death occurs in a methadone patient the cause of death might be assigned to this drug since it is easily detected. In some cases reported as 'methadone-related deaths' in New York City no search for other drugs was made, even when the person was known to have been taking several drugs. In cases such as these the toxicologist can contribute by calling the attention of the clinicians to the need for comprehensive analyses and for a careful review of all the clinical data.

As already discussed by Dr Newton (this volume, p. 6), the laboratory is of only secondary value when the clinician is confronted with cases of probable narcotic overdosage. An acute case of narcotic poisoning needs immediate symptomatic treatment. Death after an overdose of a narcotic is produced by anoxia, caused by depression of the respiratory centre and pulmonary congestion. The apnoeic subject needs artificial respiration, whatever the diagnosis. If narcotic poisoning is suspected, the patient should also be given an intravenous injection of naloxone. This antidote is specifically effective in reversing respiratory depression if this is due to an overdose of a narcotic, and does no harm if the respiratory depression is due to some other cause. Administration of the antidote is therefore both diagnostic and therapeutic, and in any suspected case of narcotic poisoning naloxone should be given immediately, without waiting for laboratory confirmation. A further problem in acute emergencies is that special skills and equipment are needed for reliable identification of drugs, whereas cases of narcotic poisoning typically appear in emergency rooms in the middle of the night. Samples of blood and urine should of course be taken for later analysis, but until analytical techniques have been radically simplified the primary treatment of narcotic poisoning will continue to be guided by clinical judgement.

Much more controversial is the role of urine testing in the treatment of narcotic addiction, which for the present discussion might be considered to be a sort of chronic poisoning. Unlike the comatose subject with an acute overdose, the addict could tell us (if he were willing) what drugs he took or thinks he took. The issue here is more one of human relations than of toxicological diagnosis, and there is room for differences of opinion over the best way to proceed. If the objective of a clinical examination is to detect misbehaviour, then urine analysis can be a powerful tool; if the objective is to rehabilitate patients, this procedure must be used more gently.

When we began research on maintenance treatment for addiction ten years ago we made urine testing a routine, and it continues to be an integral part of our programmes. But we use it to document the results of the treatment, not to detect wrongdoing. Indeed, we feel quite strongly that if a therapist needs a urine test to discover that his patient has taken an illicit drug, he should look at himself before punishing the culprit. A relation of trust, in which a patient feels secure enough to discuss his problems with his physician, is fundamental to rehabilitation. In our opinion the best way to use urine testing in a therapeutic programme is to have the laboratory send the results to a central office for statistical evaluation, not to the clinics where their effect is apt to be divisive.

TECHNOLOGY

The methods now being used for routine qualitative analysis of drugs in urine and tissues can be classified into three groups: chromatographic, fluorometric and immunological. Of these, the oldest and most versatile methods are those employing thin-layer chromatography (TLC); almost all drug laboratories use this technique as an adjunct even when more specialized methods are available. However, the pressing demand for large numbers of tests, rapid answers and high sensitivity has led to new and sophisticated procedures being developed during the past decade.

Tables 1 and 2 summarize the capabilities of the various methods now available. The sensitivities and costs shown in these tables are of course only approximate indices, since both the state of the art and the cost of reagents are changing rapidly. To be accurate, summary tables of these data would have to be revised at least twice a year, and they would need to be corrected for the special conditions of each laboratory (the volume of work done, the equipment available, the allocation of expenses, and the technical skill of the staff). Recent reviews provide more detailed evaluations of these methods (Catlin 1973; Mulé *et al.* 1974).

UNMET NEEDS

What clinicians need most from the laboratory, and do not obtain at present, are objective measures of narcotic tolerance and physical dependence. No laboratory tests are available for defining these physiological changes. Surely biochemical changes must be induced in addicts who repeatedly use narcotics,

TABLE 1
Sensitivity and costs of seven methods for detection of drugs in urine (data of B. Davidow, unpublished)

	Chromatographic		*Fluoro-metric*	*Immunological*			
	TLC	*GLC*		*FRAT*	*EMIT*	*RIA*	*HI*
Sensitivity (μg/ml)							
Morphine	0.5–1[a]	0.5–1[a]	0.2[a]	0.25–0.5[b]	0.25–0.5[b]	0.03[b]	0.03[b]
Barbiturates	1–5	1	–	1–2	1–2	–	–
Amphetamine	2–5	1	–	1	1	–	–
Methadone	2–5	1	–	0.25–0.5	0.25–0.5	–	–
Cocaine metab.	2–5	1	–	1	1	–	–
Quinine	0.1	1	–	–	–	–	–
Tests/technician (per day)	50–100	25–35	200	250[c]	250[c]	250	250
Reagent cost ($)	0.40–0.75	0.10	0.10	0.50[c]	0.75[c]	0.50	0.20
Equipment ($)[d]	500	10 000	6000 to 20 000	23 000	6000	15 000	100
Processing	Extensive	Moderate	Moderate	None	None	Little	Little

[a] Free
[b] Free and combined
[c] Per test (separate test required for morphine, amphetamine, methadone, barbiturates)
[d] Special laboratory equipment (does not include centrifuge, ovens, etc.)
TLC: thin-layer chromatography; GLC: gas-liquid chromatography;
FRAT: free radical assay technique; EMIT: enzyme-mediated immunoassay technique;
RIA: radioimmunoassay; HI: haemagglutination inhibition

TABLE 2
Probability of detecting morphine in urine (data of B. Davidow, unpublished)

Method	*Hours after last dose of heroin*			
	24	*48*	*72*	*96*
Chromatographic				
TLC	+++	++	—	—
GLC	+++	++	—	—
Fluorometric	++++	+++	±	—
Immunological				
FRAT	++++	+++	+	—
EMIT	++++	++++	+	—
RIA	++++	++++	+++	++
HI	++++	++++	+++	++

since the pharmacological response of both man and animals is consistently altered by exposure to narcotic drugs? An objective test of tolerance, apart from challenge with a dose of a narcotic (usually contraindicated), would be of value in diagnosis and treatment. It would enable clinicians to define addiction in physiological terms, distinguish psychological from pharmacological symptoms, and measure the reversibility of physical dependence after detoxification. Here is an important frontier for research by pharmacologists and toxicologists.

ACKNOWLEDGEMENTS

This article is based on research activities supported through a grant from the New York State Narcotic Addiction Control Commission. Conclusions stated here are not necessarily those of the Commission.

References

CATLIN, D. H. (1973) Urine testing: A comparison of five current methods for detecting morphine. *Am. J. Clin. Pathol. 60*, 719

MULÉ, S. J., BASTOS, M. L. & JUKOFSKY, D. (1974) Evaluation of immunoassay methods for the detection of drugs subject to abuse in urine. *Clin. Chem.* in press

Discussion

Sunshine: It is the clinician who has to determine what tests should be done and how often. The toxicologists are only the hands of the clinician when they test for narcotics, and I agree with you that the demands are unreasonable, Dr Dole. However, because a lot of money has been made available for drug testing, a lot of second-rate laboratories have got into the act. Some deplorable chemistry has resulted. We must see to it that this deficiency is somehow remedied and that only reliable work comes out of the laboratories. This certainly poses a challenge to the profession as a whole.

Techniques are already available by which the drug taken by a patient can be identified in a matter of minutes. But is that laboratory service of real value to the clinician in his counselling of a patient?

Dole: The toxicologist should be more than the servant, or the hands, of the clinician. There must be enough interaction between the two disciplines for the clinician to have to prove that a test is really needed.

Immediate testing of the urine is not only of no value to the clinician in treating the patient; it may even be of negative value because it substitutes a laboratory report for the clinical interaction. In our own research clinic, the patients are seen mostly by my wife, Dr M. E. Nyswander. The routine laboratory results are sent to my desk, not to her clinic or to her. She and the physicians or counsellors working with her should know when a person has taken a drug because the person will tell them. If a person tries to deceive his counsellor, a more important question than whether he took the drug is why he is deceiving the counsellor. Tests are important for showing how well a rehabilitation programme is progressing, and for raising the question of why a patient is so alienated as to try to deceive his clinic. Rehabilitation programmes should first give the patient a sense of security. If tests are used punitively, they alienate the patient. We should not need a $25000 machine to tell us that a patient is cheating.

Leach: With radioimmunoassay, a person who has taken codeine could easily be accused of having taken morphine. In screening programmes might someone be accused of being addicted just because they had a splitting headache?

Dole: Screening can be misused. The whole concept of using this to incriminate people is bad. I try to avoid this possibility by having another urine sample tested independently if a positive sample comes in. If the second sample is positive, we have to arrange a careful evaluation. Codeine of course can be distinguished from morphine in urine, but in New York things are so bad that some organizations discharge employees if only quinine is found in the urine—quinine tests being part of the screening procedure.

Leach: But if you use radioimmunoassay or a specific fluorometric method you will obtain incontrovertible evidence of the presence of morphine in a person who has taken codeine. Once that accusation has been made, it is very difficult for it to be refuted.

Dole: I agree. We must insist strongly that decisions be made on the basis of comprehensive evidence, not automatically after any laboratory test.

Sunshine: One should never report a test on the basis of one presumptive result. All these tests should be confirmed, particularly when they are potentially punitive. In the type of case Mr Leach mentioned, where a person had taken codeine, morphine would have been detected but the confirmatory test would have indicated that codeine was also present and that it might be the reason for the positive morphine test. This type of confirmation is part of the quality control we should demand from the laboratories.

Beckett: In sport, some competitors are sophisticated enough to use a lot of morphine with just a little bit of codeine.

Holmstedt: If morphine can be methylated and codeine demethylated, how does one discover what the patient has taken?

Is it true, Dr Dole, that some government agencies and private companies in the USA require a negative test for narcotics in the urine before they employ a person?

Dole: In some places it is a routine part of the medical examination for employment. The prejudice is so great that in some cases, if the test is positive, the man will be denied a job. What is more, this can happen to even a genuine patient on a treatment programme if a urine test is positive for the methadone that is prescribed for him. I am glad to report that this practice is becoming less common, although it is not yet extinct. We have had many useful talks with people in government and industry. Leading corporations in New York are now actively cooperating with us in finding employment opportunities for our patients. They are beginning to understand their social responsibilities better.

Scott: What you are saying implies that the tests are being asked for and interpreted irresponsibly, not that the tests themselves are a bad thing, Dr Dole. That depends on how they are used. We should not go anti-test all of a sudden, even if tests have been used badly in the past.

You emphasized the expense of some of these tests. If they have no real advantages, there is no point in spending either $1 or $50000. But if tests can help to save a patient, more money can be spent, since we cannot put a mercenary value on human life. If we want to tackle a different analytical problem, we are almost certainly going to have to put a lot of effort, both physical and economic, into it. We should not really place too much stress on either the cost of the equipment or the fact that tests may be used irresponsibly.

Dole: I am not anti-test. Curiously enough, I am asking toxicologists not to be too humble. If the clinical chemist and the clinician are both involved in evaluating the use of test data, the patient will benefit.

Beckett: It is not enough to depend on an assessment by a physician of what is happening in such complex situations. We must have objective tests. The same problems arise in sport: we cannot go by someone's subjective feelings—we need objective tests. However, perhaps we are all at fault in not bringing the physician and the scientist closer together in decision-making and its legal aspects. Primarily we are criticizing not the physician or the scientist, but the action taken after objective results.

We have done some work on the lipid solubility and the distribution of methadone and similar drugs. From the rate processes I suspect that they clear rapidly from blood. Do you think that the drugs themselves produce pulmonary oedema because the rate of absorption to the site is so fast, or could that effect be due to metabolites?

Dole: It could be the drug. Alkaloids in the narcotic family release histamine from mast cells, so the potential for producing oedema is there. Certainly after an intravenous injection there is a large and immediate impact on the lungs. Beyond that it is just a guess.

Parker: In your Table 1 (p. 21) you showed that the spin-label assay and the standard radioimmunoassay differed in their sensitivity by about one order of magnitude. Is this based on your personal experience with the assays, Dr Dole? My impression, from the published papers, and from talking to Carleton Hsia, who has done developmental work on the spin-label technique (Hsia & Piette 1969), is that the difference in sensitivity is as much as three or even four orders of magnitude.

Dole: The table is based on the work of two laboratories—that of Dr B. Davidow, who runs the City Health Department Laboratory in New York, and that of Dr S. J. Mulé, who runs the State Narcotics Commission Laboratory. Both of them use a variety of techniques and both have emphasized that these comparisons are only approximations. The results in any case depend on details of the techniques, the skills of the laboratory, and so on. The table gives only a general framework.

Machata: I think the most reliable information about drug concentrations comes from use of a nitrogen-specific detector in gas chromatography. This gives a thousandfold increase in sensitivity compared with flame ionization detector and it is only moderately expensive.

Curry: You are beginning to look forward to testing drug concentrations in blood rather than urine?

Parker: I presume that the costs you quoted, Dr Dole, were based on commercially available reagents and an immunological procedure standardized by the suppliers. Costs would be much lower in a laboratory which made its own immunogens and antisera; alternatively the reagents could be prepared in a central research laboratory and made available on a national scale. Since a technician can measure 500 samples a day by immunoassay, even without automated equipment, if the reagent cost were controlled the overall cost would be closer to $0.05 or $0.10 than to $0.50 a test.

Dole: Many years ago, when I went to work in Dr D. D. Van Slyke's laboratory, my first job as a 'new fellow' was to blow my own pipettes. I took very good care of those and that kept the cost down. Today we buy pipettes at many times the cost. This is the trend, and of course it inflates the cost of laboratory work. The main justification for using commercial reagents in drug testing is that it helps to standardize the results.

Brown: I strongly support the view that the laboratory must play an active, not a passive, role in liaising with the clinician. In the UK, the laboratory's role is often that of an active 'counsellor' of the physician.

You commented on the proficiency testing of laboratories, Dr Dole. In clinical biochemistry generally, proficiency testing is not so much a weapon against the laboratory as one designed to reveal bad methods or bad means of practice. If a laboratory's performance is bad, do you try to find out why?

Dole: Yes, there is some feedback from the testing centre. Two testing services have been developed in our area. One is for the New York City area, run by the New York City Health Department. The other is a nationally organized test, operated by the Center for Disease Control, Atlanta, Georgia. At least in the New York area, we have tried to set up a consultation service for laboratories which are having difficulties with their tests. Their problems were not due to using the wrong kinds of tests but to misuse of standard tests. Thin-layer chromatography can be treacherous if the stains are poor and are interpreted by inexperienced people. At least for narcotics, the problems lay in ineptness in applying what would otherwise be a reliable test. Things have become simpler since standardized plates were developed commercially. In early work with thin-layer chromatography, of course we made our own plates, and that requires much expertise.

Bridges: How often are interlaboratory comparisons made and what range of compounds are used?

Dole: Test packets are sent out about four times a year. In some cases in the city the inspector takes the packet to a laboratory himself, to make sure it will be processed by the normal laboratory routine and not by some superior technician. The drugs tested for include morphine, methadone, barbiturates, amphetamines, tranquillizers, quinine and occasionally odd drugs that are put in to confuse them. The laboratories are judged in comparison with each other. We argue endlessly about the scoring technique.

Curry: The Air Force testing system at Washington is computer controlled.

Holmstedt: The President's Special Action Office has published a very thorough evaluation of the techniques for testing dependence-producing drugs (Catlin 1973).

The Professor of Forensic Psychiatry in Stockholm tried to obtain urine from prisoners for an evaluation of screening tests for narcotics but this was not permissible under Swedish law. Urine samples may be taken from people who are involved in drunken driving and similar things, but prisoners cannot be screened in this way.

Prescott: Has anybody shown whether the results of treatment are better, the same, or worse, when urine is tested routinely by clinics using these expensive methods, compared with the conventional relationship between the patient and a doctor, psychiatrist or social worker who does not depend on figures from the laboratory? This is the crucial question: is the expense justified by the results?

Dole: You can judge effectiveness either according to whether the programme has more success or less success in rehabilitating patients, or whether the clinician feels more comfortable about it.

Prescott: Many tests are done for the benefit of the clinician, not for the patient, which is an important distinction.

Dole: We are limited in what we can do about this, because the Federal Government requires us to test all patients in the methadone programmes. In our own clinic, where the laboratory findings are not given to the clinicians, our results are generally much better than those from other clinics. A larger-scale evaluation was done by Gordon *et al.* (1974) who reported on a complex of programmes treating over 1000 patients in Westchester County, New York. The director asked the laboratory to send all the data to his office, and not to the clinicians in the various clinics. He also asked the clinicians to report to him whenever they were aware that a man was using drugs. There was a high correlation between the laboratory data and the clinical reports. It was unusual for a clinician not to have already identified a man with a positive test. Dr Gordon's clinics had far better results than the national average. He forced the clinicians to act as clinicians but at the same time the programme was still being monitored.

Programmes such as therapeutic communities which do not do urine testing have such limited clinical data that their effectiveness cannot be evaluated.

Scott: If you have 1000 tests which cost $1000 each, and only one test saves somebody's life, how can anyone decide whether it is worth it or not? The costs of drug analysis are also difficult to determine. There are two kinds of costs, capital and running costs, and the emphasis you can give to these depends on the country you are in. A request for $100000 in capital may be turned down, whereas authorization to spend $1000 a week for two years may be comparatively easy to obtain in England, for example. Yet an initial investment of $100000 capital may in the end produce a much less expensive series of tests.

Dole: Another consideration is whether such expenditure has to compete with other types of health expenditure. If you consider the question in isolation, you can easily say it is worth $1 million to cure one person.

Goulding: We have moved from proficiency testing, or quality control, of the laboratory to cost–benefit. This raises moral issues on the clinical scene. Some people might ask why any money at all should be spent on drug addicts rather than on the hernias of the working man, or the varicose veins of the working woman. In hospital we accept that we must try to save them all.

Clinicians claim that one series of treatments, or one system of management, is better than another, but they seldom undertake any quality control of their own operations and I don't think that they will ever be able adequately to do so. They are always ready to criticize the laboratory for getting a wrong result, but they object strongly if anyone slings an arrow in the other direction, namely at the demerits of clinical care.

We must also draw a distinction between the prevailing method of working with drug addicts in the States and what is done in England. Here we do no tests at all on drug-dependent patients unless the clinicians ask us, and they do that only for selected patients. One good reason for a test is so that the clinician himself is not deluded into thinking that the patient is doing splendidly on a particular drug when the patient is really taking something else altogether. If we find anomalous results, then normally there is a two-way enquiry by both the analyst and the clinician.

Sunshine: I want to support what Dr Goulding has just said very strongly. In the States, as Dr Dole said, each addict is tested once a week for morphine and once a month for other drugs that are abused. This is mandatory for all programmes that receive federal subsidies for the treatment and rehabilitation of drug addicts. But who made that decision and what was it based on? As Dr Goulding pointed out, in many instances these tests have minimal value. Very few toxicologists were involved in that decision-making process in the States or we would have protested vehemently.

Dole: It was a political matter. There was a widespread and mistaken fear that methadone given to patients for maintenance would cause a new epidemic of methadone addiction. This became a very popular theme and it was amplified by Congressmen who were responding to the public hysteria. The requirements for testing were imposed by the Food and Drug Administration with almost minimal review by anybody with experience in any treatment programmes. I myself am appalled at the political process that has dominated professional decisions.

Sunshine: As a group of professionals, what have we tried to do to stem this tide? It is basically our responsibility, and we haven't lived up to it.

Dole: I objected. That may have contributed to the fact that testing is required only once a week and not even more often!

Leach: Isn't there really very little that one can do about political decisions, which develop a sort of awesome momentum of their own? An analogous area is cervical screening. There seems to be no evidence that this enormously costly and widespread screening programme has done anything to reduce the death rate from carcinoma of the cervix. But nobody has the remotest chance of halting this programme even at its present level. It will continue to expand, and I really don't think that the professionals can do anything about this any longer.

References

CATLIN, D. H. (1973) A guide to urine testing for drugs of abuse (Special Action Office Monograph, Ser. B, No. 2), Executive Office of the President, Washington, D.C.

GORDON, E., EPPS, A. & ROGERS, S. (1974) Methadone treatment in Westchester County: 1971. *N.Y. State J. Med. 74*, 551

HSIA, J. C. & PIETTE, L. H. (1969) Spin-labelling as a general method in studying antibody active site. *Arch. Biochem. Biophys. 129*, 296–307

Formation of reactive metabolites as a cause of drug toxicity

JAMES R. GILLETTE

Laboratory of Chemical Pharmacology, National Heart and Lung Institute, National Institutes of Health, Bethesda, Maryland

Abstract The principles of pharmacokinetics of reactive metabolites are used to explain how various inducers and inhibitors of drug-metabolizing enzymes and various doses can affect the covalent binding of reactive metabolites of bromobenzene, acetaminophen (paracetamol) and furosemide to tissue macromolecules such as protein. Correlations between changes in the amount of covalent binding of these reactive metabolites to liver protein and changes in the incidence and severity of liver necrosis indicate that the toxic effects are mediated by chemically reactive metabolites.

It is well known that metabolites of various foreign compounds may have pharmacological and toxicological effects in addition to those caused by the parent drugs, and that inducers and inhibitors of enzymes that metabolize drugs may alter the magnitude and duration of these effects. When the metabolites are chemically inert and exert their effects by combining reversibly with action sites, the magnitude of the effects may often be predicted by identifying the metabolites and measuring their concentrations in blood plasma.

However, it has become evident that chemically inert foreign compounds can be converted in the body into chemically reactive metabolites that combine with tissue macromolecules and thereby cause cancer (Miller & Miller 1966; Miller 1970; Magee & Barnes 1967; Weisburger & Weisburger 1973) and mutations. Brodie (1967) and others (Judah *et al.* 1970; Recknagel 1967; Slater 1966) have suggested that drugs and environmental toxicants may also evoke serious kinds of toxic effects, including cellular necrosis, hypersensitivity reactions, blood dyscrasias and damage to fetuses, through the formation of reactive metabolites. Because of the seriousness of these effects, it has become important to develop rapid test systems for elucidating which kinds of reactive metabolites mediate toxicity and which are innocuous. Clearly, the severity of such toxic effects would not be related to the concentrations of the toxicants in plasma.

Our laboratory has approached the problem by identifying the toxic effects of various drugs and other foreign compounds and determining whether those effects are related to the covalent binding of reactive metabolites. Here I shall describe the assumptions on which our approach is based and ways in which measurements of the biological half-life of drugs and determinations of the pattern of their urinary metabolites have proved invaluable in elucidating various aspects of toxicity.

In previous studies of the mechanisms of different kinds of toxicity mediated by chemically reactive metabolites, other laboratories assumed that toxicity resulted from covalent binding of the metabolite with a single kind of target substance. They therefore put much effort into attempts to identify the target substance that mediates the toxicity. However, in the development of a general test system that would be useful in studies of different kinds of toxicity, this approach seemed fruitless, for a number of reasons. It seemed obvious to us that the target substance would depend on the effect being studied: some toxic effects may be mediated by covalent binding of the reactive metabolite to nuclear DNA, others by covalent binding to lipids or to certain enzymes. Moreover, in some kinds of toxicity, such as tissue necrosis and hypersensitivity reactions, the target substance may be any one of several different intracellular components, and indeed may differ with the reactive metabolite. For example, many investigators believe that the chemically reactive metabolite of carbon tetrachloride causes liver necrosis by combining with phospholipids in the endoplasmic reticulum, thereby promoting lipid peroxidation (Judah *et al.* 1970; Recknagel 1967; Slater 1966). But many other substances that also cause centrilobular liver necrosis, such as bromobenzene, do not promote lipid peroxidation (Reynolds 1972) and therefore cannot cause liver necrosis in this way. Furthermore, we realized that the specificity of covalent binding of different reactive metabolites to macromolecules can vary markedly. At one end of the spectrum, some reactive metabolites, particularly those of low chemical reactivity, may become preferentially bound to certain macromolecules in tissues by first combining reversibly with active centres on a specific macromolecule, so forming a complex that rearranges to become a covalently bound conjugate. Indeed, this mechanism is the basis of affinity labelling of receptor sites by chemically reactive analogues of endogenous chemical mediators (Singer 1970); it is also the basis of the preferential inhibition of choline esterases by organophosphate insecticides and their precursors (O'Brien 1960). In these situations, where few macromolecules are covalently bound to the metabolite or where the toxicity mimics well-characterized pharmacological actions, identification of the target substance is at least plausible if not relatively easy. At the other extreme, however, highly reactive metabolites of foreign compounds combine indiscriminately with many different kinds of intracellular components, including protein, lipids, glycogen, DNA and RNA (Miller & Miller 1966; Miller 1970; Magee & Barnes 1967; Weisburger & Weisburger 1973). But the relative rates of covalent binding to different kinds of macromolecules frequently vary with the reactive metabolite and the tissue. Thus identification of the target substance would be very difficult. Indeed, when a reactive metabolite interacts with several biochemical systems at once, it is difficult to determine whether changes in cell function result from a sequence of changes originating from a single biochemical alteration or from the concerted action of several different initial biochemical alterations.

Because highly reactive metabolites can react with so many different kinds of macromolecules in tissues, and because we know so little about the mechanisms by which a given metabolite–macromolecular conjugate might lead to diverse toxic effects and even less about how combinations of metabolite–macromolecular conjugates might evoke toxicity, there seemed to be little reason for selecting any particular type of macromolecule as the basis of a general test system for determining whether toxicity caused by a given foreign compound is mediated by a reactive metabolite. It also seemed clear that finding a radiolabel covalently bound to tissue macromolecules after a radiolabelled foreign compound had been given would not be sufficient proof that a reactive metabolite mediated either the toxic effect under investigation or any other toxic effect.

Nevertheless, it seemed likely that the incidence and severity of any toxic effect mediated by a chemically reactive metabolite would be roughly proportional to the number of target macromolecule–metabolite conjugates formed in the tissue after the foreign compound had been given. It also seemed likely that changes in the concentration of the reactive metabolite within a given tissue would alter not only the rate of covalent binding of the reactive metabolite to the target macromolecule but also its rate of covalent binding to other macromolecules. Thus, treatments that alter the pattern of metabolism of the toxicant in animals should cause parallel *changes* in the amount of covalent binding to both the target macromolecules and other macromolecules, and in the incidence and severity of toxicity. According to this view, it would not be necessary to identify either the reactive metabolite or the target macromolecule before determining whether toxicity was mediated by a chemically reactive metabolite, an inert drug, or inert metabolites. Indeed, with highly reactive metabolites it may not even be necessary for the target substance to be present in the sample being assayed for covalent binding.

THEORETICAL PHARMACOKINETICS OF COVALENT BINDING

In our approach, we pretreated animals with various inducers and inhibitors of drug-metabolizing enzymes and determined the effects of these agents on the covalent binding of reactive metabolites to tissue macromolecules. Some of the effects, however, may seem unusual to those familiar only with the pharmacokinetics of reversibly acting drugs. To learn what might be expected after a given treatment, it is perhaps useful to review the basic principles of the kinetics of covalent binding of reactive metabolites to macromolecules in the body (Gillette 1973). The pharmacokinetic equations shown in Fig. 1 were derived on

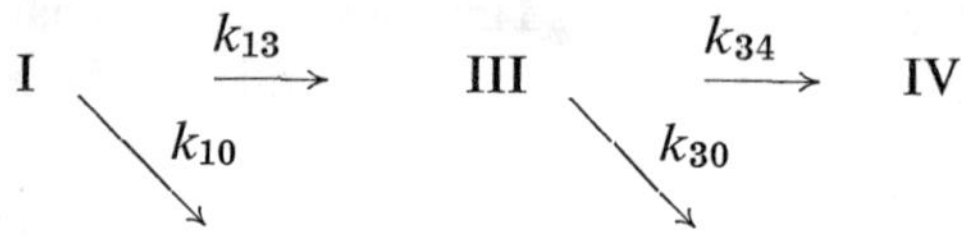

$$IV = Q_0 \left(\frac{k_{13}}{a}\right) \left(\frac{k_{34}}{c}\right) \left(1 - E\,e^{-at} + F\,e^{-ct}\right)$$

At $t = \infty$

$$IV_\infty = Q_0 \left(\frac{k_{13}}{a}\right) \left(\frac{k_{34}}{c}\right)$$

$$\text{Let } A = \frac{k_{13}}{a} = \frac{k_{13}}{k_{10} + k_{13}}; \quad B = \frac{k_{34}}{c} = \frac{k_{34}}{k_{30} + k_{34}}$$

$$IV_\infty = Q_0\,A\,B$$

FIG. 1. One-compartment model for covalent binding of reactive metabolites to macromolecules.

Definitions:

Q_0 = Dose of foreign compound.

I = Amount of unchanged foreign compound at any given time.

III = Amount of reactive metabolite at any given time.

IV = Total amount of covalently bound reactive metabolite including that bound to target macromolecules at any given time.

k_{13} = Rate constant for the formation of the reactive metabolite.

k_{10} = Sum of the rate constants for the reactions by which the foreign compound is converted into non-reactive metabolites and for its excretion by the lungs and kidneys.

k_{34} = Sum of the rate constants for the reactions by which the reactive metabolite covalently combines with the different kinds of macromolecules in a given tissue.

k_{30} = Sum of the rate constants for the reactions by which the reactive metabolite is converted to inactive metabolites. When the reactive metabolite is so stable that it is excreted into urine the rate constant of excreted metabolite is also included.

a = $k_{10} + k_{13}$

c = $k_{30} + k_{34}$

the following assumptions: (1) All processes, including elimination of the parent compound, formation of the reactive metabolite, covalent binding of the reactive metabolite to various macromolecules and conversion of the reactive metabolite to inactive secondary metabolites, follow first-order kinetics. (2) The rate of elimination of the parent compound approaches that predicted by a one-compartment model; that is, the rate constant of elimination is very small compared with the rate constants for tissue distribution. (3) The metabolism of the macromolecules with which the reactive metabolite combines is negligible compared with the rate of metabolism of the foreign compound. Under these conditions, the amount of covalently bound metabolite in any given tissue will accumulate until all the foreign compound is metabolized. But as time approaches infinity, both the exponential terms ($\exp^{-at}$ and $\exp^{-ct}$) shown in Fig. 1 become zero and the total amount of foreign compound that eventually becomes covalently bound equals the dose × the product of the two ratios, A and B. Although expressed in terms of rate constants, ratio A is the proportion of the dose of foreign compound that is converted to the reactive metabolite, and ratio B is the proportion of the reactive metabolite that becomes covalently bound to tissue macromolecules.

It is noteworthy that changes in the rate of absorption of a foreign compound or in the rate of its distribution to tissues could affect the *rate* of covalent binding to tissue macromolecules, but would not be expected to affect the *maximum amount* of covalently bound metabolite in rapidly perfused tissues except when the rate of metabolism of the drug in poorly perfused tissues is significant (Fig. 2). Notice that when all the foreign compound is metabolized ($t = \infty$), the equation in Fig. 2 for covalent binding does not contain the rate constant for absorption (k_a) and that when there is negligible metabolism in the deep compartment (compartment II), the equation for covalent binding is identical to that shown in Fig. 1.

From these equations, it is evident that any drug or other treatment that changes the activities of drug-metabolizing enzymes will alter the ultimate amount of covalent binding of highly reactive metabolites to macromolecules in any given tissue only when the drug or treatment alters either ratio A or ratio B, or both, in that tissue. Since ratio A may be altered by changing either its numerator or its denominator, the magnitude of the alteration depends on the importance of the activation reaction compared to that of the other reactions

←

$E = c/(c - a)$
$F = a/(c - a)$
A = The proportion of the dose that is converted to the reactive metabolite.
B = The proportion of the reactive metabolite that becomes covalently bound by the different kinds of macromolecules.

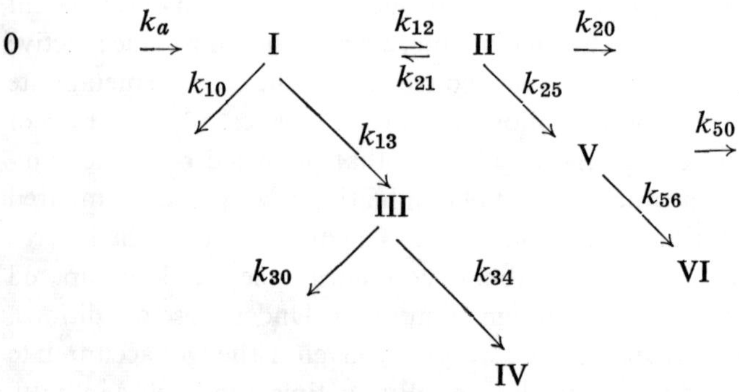

$$IV = Q_0 \left(\frac{k_{13}\, b}{\alpha\beta}\right) \left(\frac{k_{34}}{c}\right) \left[1 - Re^{-kat} + Se^{-\alpha t} - Te^{-\beta t} + Ue^{-ct}\right]$$

$$VI = Q_0 \left(\frac{k_{12} k_{25}}{\alpha\beta}\right) \left(\frac{k_{56}}{f}\right) \left[1 - We^{-kat} + Xe^{-\alpha t} - Ye^{-\beta t} + Ze^{-ft}\right]$$

At $t = \infty$

$$IV_{\infty} = Q_0 \left(\frac{k_{13}\, b}{\alpha\beta}\right) \left(\frac{k_{34}}{c}\right) = Q_0\, A'\, B'$$

$$VI_{\infty} = Q_0 \left(\frac{k_{12} k_{25}}{\alpha\beta}\right) \left(\frac{k_{56}}{f}\right) = Q_0\, C'\, D'$$

When k_{20} and k_{25} are 0, i.e. negligible amounts of the foreign compound are metabolized in the deep compartment (II, V, VI), then

$$IV'_{\infty} = Q_0 \left(\frac{k_{13}}{k_{10} + k_{13}}\right) \left(\frac{k_{34}}{c}\right) = Q_0\, A\, B$$

Fig. 2. Two-compartment model for covalent binding of reactive metabolites to macromolecules with first order absorption.

Definitions:

Q_0 = Dose of foreign compound.
0 = Compartment into which the foreign compound is introduced (e.g. intestine).
I = Rapidly perfused compartment. It usually includes liver, heart, lung, kidneys and other vital organs.
II = Deep or poorly perfused compartment. It usually includes muscle and fat.
III = Amount of reactive metabolite in compartment I at any given time.
IV = Total amount of covalently bound reactive metabolite in compartment I at any given time including that bound to target macromolecules.
V = Amount of reactive metabolite in compartment II at any given time.
VI = Total amount of covalently bound reactive metabolite in compartment II at any given time including that bound to target macromolecules.

(See Appendix, p. 48, for further definitions.)

that help to eliminate the foreign compound. When nearly all of the parent compound is converted into its reactive metabolite, an increase or decrease in the activity of the enzyme system that catalyses the formation of the reactive metabolite would not be expected to markedly change the proportion of the dose converted into the reactive metabolite, because changes in the numerator would parallel changes in the denominator of A. Even when a small proportion of the parent compound is converted into its reactive metabolite, inducers and inhibitors of the enzyme that catalyses the formation of the reactive metabolite may not markedly change the magnitude of the covalent binding when they also cause parallel changes in the rates at which the foreign compound is eliminated along the major pathways. Indeed, inducers and inhibitors of drug-metabolizing enzymes would be expected to exert their greatest effect on A by changing the activity of an enzyme that catalyses the formation of the reactive metabolite along a relatively minor pathway without affecting the rate of formation of metabolites along the major pathways of elimination. Hence inducers and inhibitors may greatly affect A without markedly affecting the biological half-life of the parent compound, whereas inducers and inhibitors that greatly change the biological half-life of the parent compound may not always cause marked changes in A.

If covalent binding of the reactive metabolite to macromolecules in tissues occurs non-enzymically, it seems unlikely that ratio B can be markedly altered by changing its numerator unless the treatment causes marked changes in the concentrations of the macromolecules. It seems likely, therefore, that most treatments that alter B act by changing the denominator of B, that is they change the rate of elimination of the reactive metabolite. If only a little of the reactive metabolite were covalently bound to macromolecules, and if the rest of the reactive metabolite were inactivated by only one reaction, then an inducer that specifically increased the activity of the enzyme which catalysed that reaction would be expected to decrease the covalent binding of the reactive metabolite without markedly changing either the biological half-life of the parent compound or the pattern of its urinary metabolites. In most instances, however, the reactive metabolite is inactivated by several reactions, and alterations in the activity of an enzyme that catalyses the inactivation of the reactive metabolite can usually be detected from measurements of changes in the amounts of the inactive metabolites excreted into urine. Nevertheless, these considerations indicate that a foreign compound may be toxic in one animal species and not in another, even though the metabolism of the foreign compound may appear to be virtually identical in the two species.

In some instances a primary metabolite of a foreign compound is not sufficiently reactive to combine rapidly with tissue macromolecules, but is converted

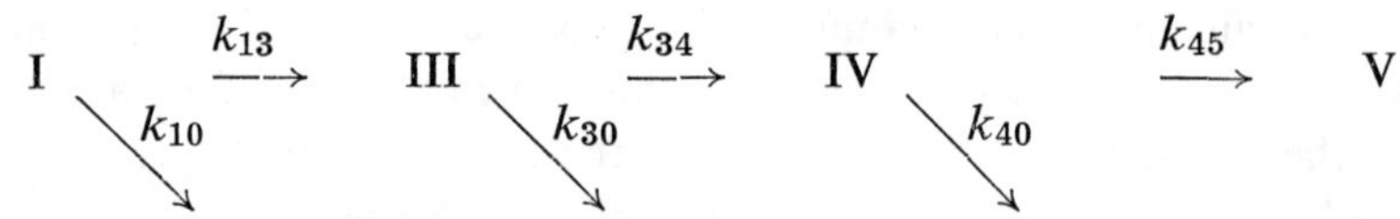

$$V = Q_0 \left(\frac{k_{13}}{a}\right) \left(\frac{k_{34}}{b}\right) \left(\frac{k_{45}}{c}\right) \left[1 - Ee^{-at} + Fe^{-kt} - Ge^{-ct}\right]$$

At $t = \infty$

$$V_\infty = Q_0 \left(\frac{k_{13}}{a}\right) \left(\frac{k_{34}}{b}\right) \left(\frac{k_{45}}{c}\right)$$

$$A = \frac{k_{13}}{a} = \frac{k_{13}}{k_{10} + k_{13}}; \quad B = \frac{k_{34}}{b} = \frac{k_{34}}{k_{30} + k_{34}}$$

$$C = \frac{k_{45}}{c} = \frac{k_{45}}{k_{40} + k_{45}}$$

$$V_0 = Q_0\, A\, B\, C$$

FIG. 3. One-compartment model for covalent binding when an inert metabolite is converted to a reactive metabolite.

Definitions:
Q_0 = Dose of foreign compound.
I = Amount of unchanged foreign compound at any given time.
III = Amount of the intermediate inert metabolite at any given time.
IV = Amount of reactive metabolite at any given time.
V = Total amount of covalently bound reactive metabolite including that bound to target macromolecules at any given time.

(See Appendix, p. 49, for further definitions.)

in the body into metabolites that are even more chemically reactive. For example, 2-fluorenylacetamide is first converted into its *N*-hydroxylamine derivative, *N*-hydroxy-2-fluorenylacetamide; a portion of this is then converted into its highly reactive sulphate ester and another portion into its relatively stable glucuronide, which is rapidly excreted into urine (Miller 1970; Weisburger & Weisburger 1973). Thus, the pharmacokinetic equation for the covalent binding of this substance and perhaps certain other acetylated aromatic amines can be quite complex (Fig. 3). However, the proportion of the dose that ultimately becomes covalently bound depends on the product of three ratios, i.e. the proportion of the dose that is converted into the *N*-hydroxylamine derivative (ratio A), the proportion of the *N*-hydroxylamine derivative that is converted into the sulphate ester (ratio B), and the proportion of the sulphate ester that becomes covalently bound to tissue macromolecules (ratio C). With the increase in complexity of the pharmacokinetics, it becomes even more difficult to predict changes in the magnitude of covalent binding from changes in the biological half-life of the drug and in the pattern of urinary metabolites. For example, suppose that a treatment increased the proportion of the dose that was converted into the hydroxylamine but also either increased the activity of UDP glucuronyl transferase or decreased the activity of the aryl sulphotransferase. The treatment then would have decreased the covalent binding even though it increased the proportion of the dose excreted as the glucuronide of the acetylated *N*-hydroxylamine metabolite. Thus, the effects of treatment on the amount of covalent binding of such secondary metabolites can be very difficult to predict with accuracy.

The equations shown in Figs. 1, 2 and 3 were derived on the assumption that the metabolite was so chemically reactive that it never left the tissue in which it was formed. Since foreign compounds may be converted into chemically reactive metabolites in several different tissues, however, the degree of covalent binding in the various tissues would depend not only on the rates of formation and inactivation of the reactive metabolite in the given tissue but also on the rate constant for elimination of the unchanged foreign compound. Thus, ratio A for one tissue may differ markedly from that for another tissue because the numerators of all A ratios for the various tissues would differ even if the denominators were identical. In this situation, any treatment that specifically altered the activity of the enzyme catalysing the formation of the major metabolite in the tissue that metabolized most of the drug in the body would alter the denominator of the A ratios in all the other tissues, even if that treatment did not affect enzyme activities in the other tissues. For example, when the major pathway of elimination of a foreign compound is through the formation of its reactive metabolite in the liver, a substance that induces only the liver enzyme may tend to increase the covalent binding of the reactive metabolite in the liver and decrease it in other tissues, whereas a substance that inhibits the enzyme only in the liver would tend to decrease the covalent binding in the liver but increase it in the other tissues. For this reason, inhibitors that decrease toxic effects in one organ may enhance them in others.

By contrast, when the reactive metabolite is sufficiently stable to leave the organ in which it is formed, the rate of covalent binding of the reactive metabolite will depend on many interrelated factors: (1) the chemical reactivity of the metabolite, (2) the diffusibility of the metabolite, (3) the rate of blood flow to the various tissues, and (4) the activities of the enzymes that catalyse the formation and inactivation of the reactive metabolites in the various tissues. Obviously, pharmacokinetic equations that included these interrelationships would be very complex. But even in these situations, the concept of ratios A and B is useful in elucidating the main factors that determine the covalent binding of reactive metabolites in various tissues.

The kinetics of covalent binding become even more complex when the reactive metabolite inactivates the enzyme that catalyses its formation. For example, carbon tetrachloride (Smuckler *et al.* 1967; Castro *et al.* 1968; Greene *et al.* 1969) and dimethylnitrosamine (Smuckler *et al.* 1967) rapidly destroy cytochrome *P*-450 in liver microsomes. Covalent binding under these conditions would be expected to be self-limiting. Indeed, Glende (1972) has reported that the administration of sublethal doses of carbon tetrachloride to animals protects them from the lethal effects of high doses of the toxicant. The kinetics described in Figs. 1, 2 and 3 will not be valid in these situations, although the general concept of ratios A and B is still useful in elucidating mechanisms of covalent binding.

There are other situations in which the kinetics of covalent binding of reactive metabolites to tissue macromolecules *in vivo* do not fit the idealized models described in Figs. 1, 2 and 3. But studies of why the kinetics do not fit them have led to a better understanding of the biochemistry of the reactive metabolites.

EXAMPLES OF REACTIVE METABOLITES THAT CAUSE LIVER NECROSIS

The validity of correlating *changes* in the incidence and severity of toxic effects with changes in the maximum amount of covalent binding was tested in studies of the mechanism of liver necrosis induced by large doses of bromobenzene. Although the urinary metabolites of bromobenzene were identified many years ago (Baumann & Preusse 1879; Azouz *et al.* 1953; Knight & Young 1958), a recent series of *in vivo* and *in vitro* experiments revealed that nearly all the bromobenzene administered to animals was converted into its chemically reactive arene oxide, bromobenzene-3,4-epoxide (Zampaglione *et al.* 1973; Jollow *et al.* 1974) by a cytochrome *P*-450 enzyme system located mainly in liver microsomes (Jollow *et al.* 1974; Brodie *et al.* 1971) (Fig. 4). Some epoxide rearranges non-enzymically to form 4-bromophenol and some is converted to a dihydrodiol, presumably by an epoxide hydrase in liver microsomes; the dihydrodiol in turn is dehydrogenated to 4-bromocatechol (4-bromo-1,2-benzenediol), presumably by an enzyme in the soluble fraction of liver. But about 70% of the epoxide formed in rats receiving a non-toxic dose of bromobenzene is converted into a glutathione conjugate by a glutathione transferase in the liver-soluble fraction; the conjugate is hydrolysed to the cysteinyl derivative, which is then acetylated to the mercapturic acid and excreted into urine (Zampaglione *et al.* 1973). The steady-state concentration of the epoxide in

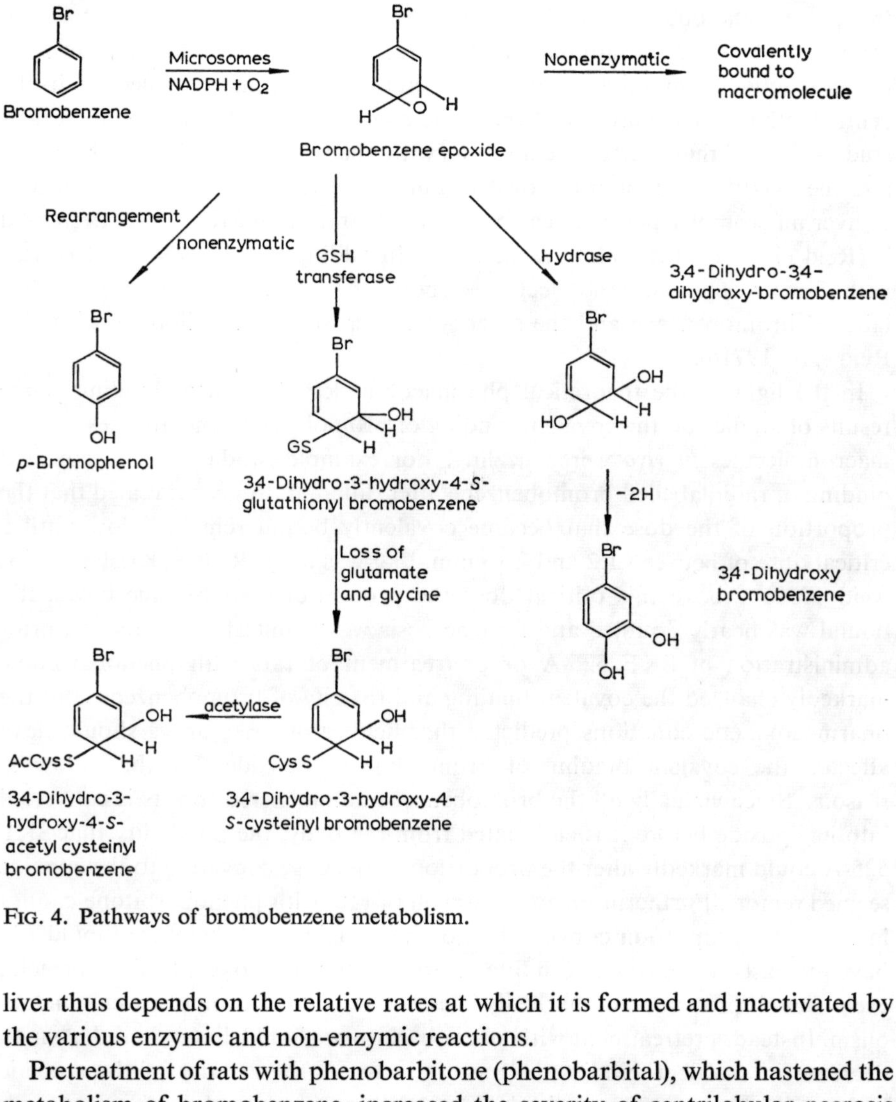

FIG. 4. Pathways of bromobenzene metabolism.

liver thus depends on the relative rates at which it is formed and inactivated by the various enzymic and non-enzymic reactions.

Pretreatment of rats with phenobarbitone (phenobarbital), which hastened the metabolism of bromobenzene, increased the severity of centrilobular necrosis caused by large doses of the toxicant (Brodie *et al.* 1971; Reid *et al.* 1971*a*). In contrast, SKF 525-A (proadifen: 2-diethylaminoethyl 2,2-diphenylvalerate), which slowed the metabolism of bromobenzene, decreased the severity of necrosis. Moreover, the incidence of necrosis caused by bromobenzene in various animal species paralleled the rates of metabolism of the toxicant in these species (Mitchell *et al.* 1971). Although these first studies indicated that the toxicity was not mediated by bromobenzene but by one of its metabolites, they did not indicate whether the active metabolite was chemically reactive or inert. Nevertheless, autoradiographic studies after the administration of radiolabelled bromobenzene revealed that a reactive metabolite combined preferentially with macromolecules in the centrilobular necrotic areas of liver (Brodie *et al.* 1971). Moreover, subsequent studies showed that pretreatment of rats with phenobarbitone increased the rate and the maximum amount of covalent binding of radiolabelled bromobenzene to liver macromolecules, whereas prior administration of SKF 525-A decreased it (Reid *et al.* 1971*a*; Jollow *et al.* 1972). In addition, prior treatment of rats with 3-methylcholanthrene decreased both the covalent binding of radiolabelled bromobenzene and the severity of necrosis (Zampaglione *et al.* 1973; Reid *et al.* 1971*b*).

In the light of the theoretical pharmacokinetics of covalent binding, some results of studies on the covalent binding of bromobenzene metabolites to liver macromolecules *in vivo* were puzzling. For example, studies on the covalent binding of radiolabelled bromobenzene after different dosages revealed that the proportion of the dose that became covalently bound remained low until a critical dose of between 1.2 and 2.15 mmol/kg was used (Reid & Krishna 1973; Reid 1973). Above this critical dose the proportion that became covalently bound was nearly doubled and liver necrosis was manifested. Moreover, prior administration of SKF 525-A or pretreatment of rats with phenobarbitone markedly changed the covalent binding and toxicity of bromobenzene. But the pharmacokinetic equations predicted that neither of these drugs should have affected the covalent binding of bromobenzene epoxide, for the following reasons. Since virtually all the bromobenzene administered to rats is converted into its epoxide before it is eliminated from the body, the possibility that SKF 525-A could markedly alter the proportion of the dose converted to the epoxide seemed remote. Furthermore, pretreatment of rats with phenobarbitone cannot increase the proportion converted into the epoxide and therefore should not have increased the covalent binding of bromobenzene epoxide to liver protein, even though pretreatment markedly increases the rate of bromobenzene metabolism. Instead, pretreatment with phenobarbitone should have caused a small decrease in covalent binding because it increases the activity of the epoxide hydrase (Daly *et al.* 1972). Indeed, phenobarbitone decreased the covalent binding of bromobenzene when low non-toxic doses of the toxicant were administered (Reid 1973; Reid & Krishna 1973).

The explanation of the threshold dose effect became clear when we realized that glutathione concentrations in liver decrease after toxic doses of bromobenzene until the rate of formation of the glutathione conjugate is limited by the availability of this co-substrate. Under these conditions ratio B in Fig. 1 would be increased as the dose of bromobenzene was increased. This view was confirmed by Jollow *et al.* (1974), who showed that the rate of covalent binding of bromobenzene metabolites to liver macromolecules was markedly increased after the glutathione concentrations were depleted. Although the decrease in glutathione might by itself lead to the liver necrosis caused by bromobenzene, other substances such as diethyl maleate bring glutathione concentrations in liver (Boyland & Chasseaud 1970) down to about the same extent as does bromobenzene, but do not cause necrosis. However, the severity of necrosis and the magnitude of the covalent binding can be markedly increased by the prior administration of diethyl maleate (Reid & Krishna 1973; Reid 1973), which depletes liver glutathione without causing necrosis. Thus, glutathione protects the liver against the toxic effects of bromobenzene epoxide by combining with it to form the glutathione conjugate.

The way in which SKF 525-A administration and phenobarbitone pretreatment affect the covalent binding of bromobenzene metabolites is more subtle. If glutathione synthesis were negligible during the metabolism of bromobenzene, then the amount of bromobenzene epoxide that would be converted into mercapturic acid after bromobenzene administration should not be changed by changes in the rate of epoxide formation. But glutathione is rapidly synthesized in liver and thus much of the bromobenzene epoxide is still inactivated by its conjugation with glutathione (about 50% in rats), even after the concentrations of glutathione in liver have decreased to very low levels (Zampaglione *et al.* 1973). However, the rate of synthesis of the glutathione conjugate is now limited by the rate of synthesis of glutathione, and therefore is no longer directly proportional to the bromobenzene epoxide concentration; thus the proportion of the bromobenzene epoxide that is inactivated by formation of the glutathione conjugate can be altered by changing the rate of formation of the epoxide. Hence, because phenobarbitone pretreatment accelerates epoxide formation, it decreases the proportion of the epoxide inactivated by the glutathione conjugate pathway and thereby increases covalent binding to tissue macromolecules.

In contrast to the effects of phenobarbitone, pretreatment of rats with 3-methylcholanthrene decreases both the covalent binding of bromobenzene to liver protein and the severity of liver necrosis (Zampaglione *et al.* 1973; Reid *et al.* 1971*b*) by a number of interdependent mechanisms. Since the pretreatment does not alter the biological half-life of bromobenzene in rats, and actually increases the rate of bromobenzene metabolism by liver microsomes, the protective effect must have been due to a marked alteration in the pattern of metabolism of bromobenzene. Studies of the pattern of urinary metabolites in rats receiving a toxic dose of bromobenzene revealed that treatment with 3-methylcholanthrene resulted in a decrease in the mercapturic acid and 4-bromophenol but an increase in the bromocatechol, bromocyclohexadienediol and 2-bromophenol (Zampaglione *et al.* 1973). Since 2-bromophenol cannot be formed from the non-enzymic rearrangement of bromobenzene 3,4-epoxide it seems likely that 3-methylcholanthrene induces the formation of a different epoxide, presumably bromobenzene 2,3-epoxide. Moreover, the increase in the bromocatechol and the bromocyclohexadienediol fractions at the expense of mercapturic acids in the urine of 3-methylcholanthrene-treated rats implies that the epoxide hydrase, as well as the cytochrome *P*-450 enzyme, was induced (Zampaglione *et al.* 1973; Daly *et al.* 1972). Increasing the formation of the bromobenzene 2,3-epoxide thus decreases the proportion of the dose of bromobenzene that is converted into bromobenzene 3,4-epoxide, which may be the more reactive arylating intermediate. At the same time, increasing the activity of epoxide hydrase decreases the dependence of hepatic cells on the glutathione transferase in the inactivation of the epoxides and hence decreases the rate of utilization of glutathione. When the rate of formation of glutathione conjugates is decreased, the concentration of glutathione in liver cells can be maintained at high levels by the synthesis of glutathione and the mobilization of nucleophilic substances, such as cysteine, from body stores. The net effect is thus a decrease in both ratio A and ratio B in the pharmacokinetic equation shown in Fig. 1.

In another series of studies, the centrilobular necrosis caused by large overdoses of the commonly used analgesic, acetaminophen (paracetamol) (Prescott *et al.* 1971), was shown to be mediated by a chemically reactive metabolite (Mitchell *et al.* 1973*a*, *b*; Jollow *et al.* 1973*a*; Potter *et al.* 1973). As with bromobenzene, the severity of necrosis parallels the magnitude of the covalent binding of radiolabelled paracetamol to liver macromolecules. For example, pretreatment of mice with phenobarbitone increases both the severity of the centrilobular necrosis and the covalent binding to liver macromolecules, whereas pretreatment of mice with cobalt (II) chloride, piperonyl butoxide (Mitchell *et al.* 1973*a*; Jollow *et al.* 1973*a*) or 1-naphthyl isocyanate (J. R. Mitchell, W. Z. Potter & D. J. Jollow, unpublished) decreases both of these effects. Dose–response studies revealed that the amount of covalent binding per dose was negligible until a critical threshold dose was reached (about 300 mg/kg in mice). Below this critical threshold dose, not only is covalent binding to protein negligible but there is also no necrosis, which presumably accounts for the remarkable safety of the drug when used at the usual therapeutic dosage.

In addition to its conversion into glucuronide and sulphate conjugates, paracetamol is also metabolized by a minor pathway to a mercapturic acid (Jagenburg & Toczko 1964) $< 15\%$ in untreated hamsters (Jollow *et al.* 1973*b*) (Fig. 5). Since it seemed unlikely that paracetamol itself would react with glutathione, the presence of the mercapturic acid in urine suggested that a small proportion of the paracetamol might be converted into a reactive metabolite which reacts

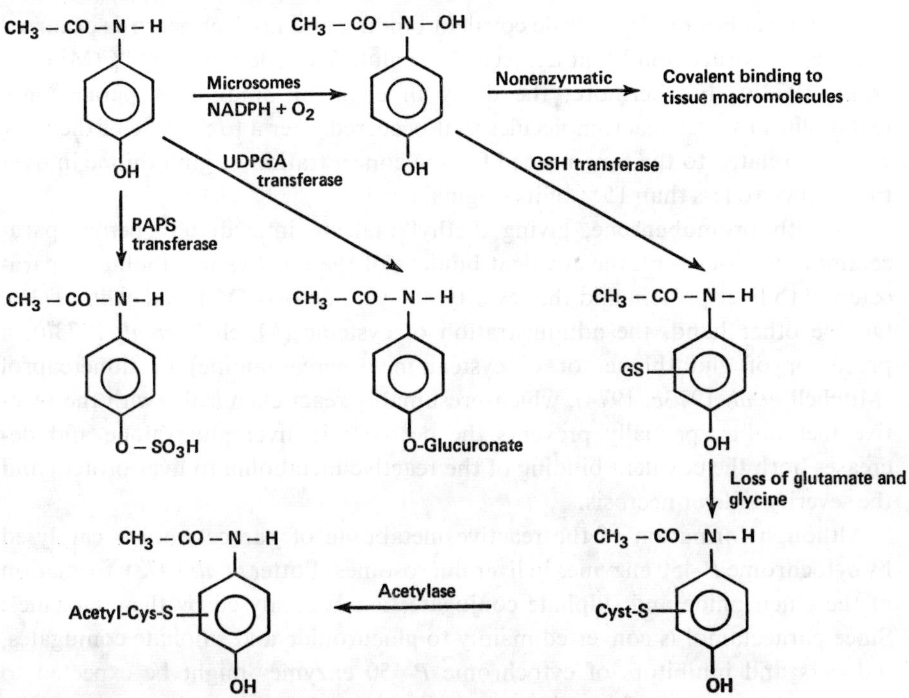

FIG. 5. Pathways of paracetamol (acetaminophen) metabolism.
UDPGA transferase: UDP glucuronyltransferase
PAPS transferase: aryl sulphotransferase
Acetylase: *S*-acetyltransferase

with glutathione. It also seemed possible that as the dose of paracetamol was increased, the concentrations of glutathione in liver would decrease until the rate of inactivation of the reactive metabolite would be limited by the rate of glutathione synthesis or the rate of mobilization of cysteine from proteins in the body tissues. Under these conditions ratio B would be increased, because the concentration of the reactive metabolite in liver would increase and thereby result in an increase in its covalent binding to liver macromolecules. In accord with this view, the proportion of paracetamol excreted as mercapturic acid in hamsters was smaller after a toxic dose than after a non-toxic dose (Jollow *et al.* 1973*b*), presumably because the reactive metabolite was channelled not only towards covalent binding but also to an unknown metabolite. Moreover, in mice the level of glutathione in liver decreased as the dose of the drug was increased (Mitchell *et al.* 1973*b*). In addition, the severity of liver necrosis paralleled not only the magnitude of the covalent binding of radiolabelled paracetamol to liver protein but also the decrease in glutathione concentrations in liver. For example, little covalent binding and no liver necrosis occurred at doses of paracetamol that depleted liver glutathione less than 85% (Mitchell *et al.* 1973*b*). Furthermore, the delay in covalent binding of paracetamol metabolites to liver macromolecules that occurred after a toxic dose of the drug was also related to the time needed for the concentration of glutathione in liver to go down to less than 15% of its original level.

As with bromobenzene, giving diethyl maleate immediately before paracetamol increases both the covalent binding of the reactive metabolite of paracetamol to liver protein and the severity of liver necrosis (Mitchell *et al.* 1973*b*). On the other hand, the administration of cysteine (Mitchell *et al.* 1973*b*), a precursor of glutathione, or of cysteamine (mercaptamine) or dimercaprol (Mitchell *et al.* 1973*c*, 1974), which presumably react chemically with the reactive metabolite, partially prevents the decrease in liver glutathione and decreases both the covalent binding of the reactive metabolite to liver protein and the severity of liver necrosis.

Although formation of the reactive metabolite of paracetamol is catalysed by cytochrome *P*-450 enzymes in liver microsomes (Potter *et al.* 1973), formation of the glucuronide and sulphate conjugates is not catalysed by these enzymes. Since paracetamol is converted mainly to glucuronide and sulphate conjugates, inducers and inhibitors of cytochrome *P*-450 enzymes might be expected to increase the amount of reactive metabolite formed but would not necessarily alter the biological half-life of the parent drug. In fact, pretreatment of mice with either phenobarbitone or cobalt (II) chloride did not appreciably alter the biological half-life of paracetamol, even though these substances markedly changed its covalent binding to liver macromolecules and the severity of liver necrosis (Mitchell *et al.* 1973*a*; Jollow *et al.* 1973*a*). These findings thus illustrate that such treatment can markedly change the toxicity of drugs without markedly changing the total body clearance of the drugs. They also illustrate the difficulty of finding an animal in which both the metabolism and toxicity of drugs are similar to those in man, when toxicity is mediated by metabolites formed along minor pathways.

Large doses of another commonly used drug, furosemide, cause midzonal and centrilobular necrosis in male mice, apparently through the formation of a chemically reactive metabolite (Mitchell *et al.* 1973*c*; Weihe *et al.* 1974). In support of this conclusion is the finding that administration of piperonyl butoxide, cobalt (II) chloride or 1-naphthyl isocyanate prevented the necrosis caused by furosemide and markedly decreased the covalent binding of radiolabelled furosemide metabolites to liver protein. As with the necrosis caused by paracetamol, that caused by furosemide occurs only at high doses. Below a critical dose of 150 mg/kg there is little covalent binding and no necrosis in mice (Mitchell *et al.* 1973*d*).

Unlike bromobenzene and paracetamol, furosemide does not deplete the liver of glutathione (Weihe *et al.* 1974). Moreover, it seems unlikely that the threshold is due to the liver being depleted of other nucleophilic substances or co-substrates, because there is no delay in covalent binding to liver macromolecules after a toxic dose of furosemide. Thus, as the dose of furosemide is increased, there must be an increase in ratio A rather than in ratio B of the equation shown in Fig. 1; that is, the clearance of the drug by the enzyme that catalyses the formation of the reactive metabolite relative to the total body clearance of the drug increases as the dose is increased. In accord with this view, at subtoxic doses of furosemide most of the drug is excreted unchanged into the urine, but as the dose is increased to above the threshold amount, the proportion of the dose that is metabolized increases (Weihe *et al.* 1974).

Since it seems unlikely that the drug activates the enzyme that catalyses the formation of the reactive metabolite, the increase in ratio A may be due to a decrease in the clearance of the drug by the kidney or perhaps by biliary excretion. A possible mechanism for this is indicated by the finding that threshold toxic doses result in plasma concentrations of the drug at which reversible binding sites of the plasma proteins become saturated, and that higher doses result in disproportionate increases in concentration of the unbound drug in plasma and in its concentration in the liver (Weihe *et al.* 1974). Although an increase in the proportion of unbound drug in plasma should not decrease clearance of the drug (rate of excretion/concentration of unbound drug) by glomerular filtration, it could decrease the urinary or biliary clearance by active transport systems in kidney or liver. For example, the clearance of highly bound drugs by active transport systems in kidney may exceed the blood flow rate through the kidney because the reversible drug–protein complexes dissociate as the concentration of unbound drug in plasma is decreased by the transport system. Thus, the clearance of drug would tend to decrease as the percentage of bound drug in plasma decreases. Alternatively, the transport systems in kidney or liver may become saturated as the concentration of unbound drug is increased, and thereby cause a decrease in the clearance into urine or bile.

As pointed out in the theoretical section of this paper (p. 33) and Fig. 2, changes in the rate of absorption of the drug from the gastrointestinal tract would not ordinarily be expected to change the proportion of the dose that becomes covalently bound to tissue macromolecules. But when the clearance of the drug is decreased as the concentration of unbound drug is increased, the total body clearance of the drug would depend on the plasma concentration of the drug and therefore on the rate of absorption of the drug. Thus, the rate of absorption would affect the proportion of the dose that is converted into the reactive metabolite and covalently bound to tissue macromolecules. With certain kinds of foreign compounds, therefore, the magnitude of covalent binding may depend on the rates of absorption and excretion of the drug as well as on the activity of enzyme systems that catalyse the formation of reactive metabolites.

GENERAL COMMENTS

The use of ratios A and B in studies of covalent binding of reactive metabolites of foreign compounds to tissue macromolecules has clarified the mechanisms by which chemically reactive metabolites are formed, distributed and eliminated. It has also helped to explain why seemingly contradictory or inconsistent results may be obtained. The finding that a proportion of the dose of a foreign compound that becomes covalently bound can increase with increasing doses has led to the idea that there may be dose-thresholds in the toxicity of certain compounds. Moreover, these studies, together with those on the distribution of urinary metabolites, have provided estimates of the relative importance of the metabolic pathways that lead to reactive and inert metabolites. These studies in turn have led to an understanding of why opposite effects on the covalent binding of reactive metabolites may be seen after low and high doses of foreign compounds.

The use of ratios A and B has also provided reasons for species differences in the toxicity of foreign compounds even when both the biological half-life and the pattern of urinary metabolites are similar in the various species. In addition, the concept illustrates how various drugs that seemingly have little effect on the metabolism of a foreign compound may markedly affect its toxicity, whereas those that markedly change the half-life of a foreign compound may have little effect on the toxicity.

The pharmacokinetic equations for covalent binding reveal how various drugs may increase the toxic effects in some tissues but decrease them in others. It further shows how a toxic effect in a given tissue may be decreased by either an inducer or an inhibitor of drug-metabolizing enzymes.

From these considerations, it becomes obvious that it is difficult to predict with accuracy whether a given drug will increase or decrease the covalent binding of reactive metabolites to macromolecules in any given tissue. Nevertheless, studies of covalent binding can be used to determine whether a toxic effect caused by a foreign compound is mediated through the formation of a reactive metabolite. When a drug alters the incidence or severity of toxicity by changing the metabolism of the toxicant, changes in the magnitude of covalent binding should parallel changes in toxicity, whether the drug increases or decreases the covalent binding of the reactive metabolite.

References

AZOUZ, W. M., PARKE, D. V. & WILLIAMS, R. T. (1953) *Biochem. J. 55*, 146–151

BAUMANN, E. & PREUSSE, C. (1879) *Ber. Dtsch. Chem. Ges. 12*, 806–810

BOYLAND, E. & CHASSEAUD, L. F. (1970) *Biochem. Pharmacol. 19*, 1526–1528

BRODIE, B. B. (1967) in *Drug Responses in Man (Ciba Found. Symp.)*, pp. 188–213, Churchill, London

BRODIE, B. B., REID, W. D., CHO, A. K., SIPES, G., KRISHNA, G. & GILLETTE, J. R. (1971) *Proc. Natl. Acad. Sci. 68*, 160–164

CASTRO, J. A., SASAME, H., SUSSMAN, H. & GILLETTE, J. R. (1968) *Life Sci. 7*, 129–136

DALY, J. W., JERINA, D. M. & WITKOP, B. (1972) *Experientia (Basel) 28*, 1129–1149

GILLETTE, J. R. (1973) in *Toxicological Problems* (Loomis, T. A., ed.), (*Proc. V Int. Congr. Pharmacol.*, vol. 2), pp. 187–202, Phiebig, White Plains, N.Y.

GLENDE, E. A., JR. (1972) *Biochem. Pharmacol. 21*, 169–172

GREENE, F. E., STRIPP, B. & GILLETTE, J. R. (1969) *Biochem. Pharmacol. 18*, 1531–1533

JAGENBURG, O. R. & TOCZKO, K. (1964) *Biochem. J. 92*, 639–643

JOLLOW, D., MITCHELL, J. R., ZAMPAGLIONE, N. & GILLETTE, J. R. (1972) *V Int. Congr. Pharmacol.* Abs. Vol. Papers 117, Karger, Basel

JOLLOW, D. J., MITCHELL, J. R., POTTER, W. Z., DAVIS, D. C., GILLETTE, J. R. & BRODIE, B. B. (1973*a*) *J. Pharmacol. Exp. Ther. 187*, 195–202

JOLLOW, D. J., THORGEIRSSON, S. S., POTTER, W. Z., MITCHELL, J. R., GILLETTE, J. R. & BRODIE, B. B. (1973*b*) *Fed. Proc. 32*, 305

JOLLOW, D. J., MITCHELL, J. R., ZAMPAGLIONE, N. & GILLETTE, J. R. (1974) *Pharmacology (Basel)*, *11*, 151–169

JUDAH, J. D., MCLEAN, A. E. M. & MCLEAN, E. K. (1970) *Am. J. Med. 49*, 609–617

KNIGHT, R. H. & YOUNG, L. (1958) *Biochem. J. 70*, 111–119

MAGEE, P. N. & BARNES, J. M. (1967) *Adv. Cancer Res. 10*, 163–256

MILLER, E. C. & MILLER, J. A. (1966) *Pharmacol. Rev. 18*, 805–838

MILLER, J. A. (1970) *Cancer Res. 30*, 559–576

MITCHELL, J. R., REID, W. D., CHRISTIE, B., MOSKOWITZ, J., KRISHNA, G. & BRODIE, B. B. (1971) *Res. Commun. Chem. Pathol. Pharmacol. 2*, 877–888

MITCHELL, J. R., JOLLOW, D. J., POTTER, W. Z., DAVIS, D. C., GILLETTE, J. R. & BRODIE, B. B. (1973*a*) *J. Pharmacol. Exp. Ther. 187*, 185–194

MITCHELL, J. R., JOLLOW, D. J., POTTER, W. Z., GILLETTE, J. R. & BRODIE, B. B. (1973*b*) *J. Pharmacol. Exp. Ther. 187*, 211–217

MITCHELL, J. R., JOLLOW, D. J., GILLETTE, J. R. & BRODIE, B. B. (1973*c*) *Drug Metab. Disposition 1*, 418–423

MITCHELL, J. R., POTTER, W. Z. & JOLLOW, D. J. (1973*d*) *Fed. Proc. 32*, 305

MITCHELL, J. R., THORGEIRSSON, S. S., POTTER, W. Z., JOLLOW, D. J. & KEISER, H. (1974) *Clin. Pharmacol. Ther.* in press

O'BRIEN, R. D. (1960) in *Toxic Phosphorus Esters*, pp. 73–113, Academic Press, New York

POTTER, W. Z., DAVIS, D. C., MITCHELL, J. R., JOLLOW, D. J., GILLETTE, J. R. & BRODIE, B. B. (1973) *J. Pharmacol. Exp. Ther. 187*, 203–210

PRESCOTT, L. F., WRIGHT, N., ROSCOE, P. & BROWN, S. S. (1971) *Lancet 1*, 519–522

RECKNAGEL, R. O. (1967) *Pharmacol. Rev. 19*, 145–207

REID, W. D. (1973) in *Toxicological Problems* (Loomis, T. A., ed.), (*Proc. V Int. Congr. Pharmacol.*, vol. 2), 62–74, Phiebig, White Plains, N.Y.

REID, W. D. & KRISHNA, G. (1973) *Exp. Mol. Pathol. 18*, 80–99

REID, W. D., CHRISTIE, B., KRISHNA, G., MITCHELL, J. R., MOSKOWITZ, J. & BRODIE, B. B. (1971*a*) *Pharmacology (Basel) 6*, 41–55

REID, W. D., CHRISTIE, B., EICHELBAUM, M. & KRISHNA, G. (1971*b*) *Exp. Mol. Pathol. 15*, 363–372

REYNOLDS, E. S. (1972) *Biochem. Pharmacol. 21*, 2555–2561
SINGER, S. J. (1970) in *Molecular Properties of Drug Receptors (Ciba Found Symp.)*, pp. 229–242, Churchill, London
SLATER, T. F. (1966) *Nature (Lond.) 209*, 36–40
SMUCKLER, E., ARRHENIUS, E. & HULTIN, T. (1967) *Biochem. J. 103*, 55–64
WEIHE, M., POTTER, W. Z., NELSON, W. L., JOLLOW, D. J. & MITCHELL, J. R. (1974) *Toxicol. Appl. Pharmacol.*, in press
WEISBURGER, J. H. & WEISBURGER, E. K. (1973) *Pharmacol. Rev. 25*, 1–66
ZAMPAGLIONE, N., JOLLOW, D. J., MITCHELL, J. R., STRIPP, B., HAMRICH, M. & GILLETTE, J. R. (1973) *J. Pharmacol. Exp. Ther. 187*, 218–227

Appendix

(1) *Further definitions for Fig.* 2

k_a = Rate constant for absorption of the foreign compound.
k_{13} = Rate constant for the formation of the reactive metabolite in compartment I.
k_{10} = Sum of the rate constants for the reactions by which the foreign compound is converted to inert metabolites in compartment I and for its excretion by lungs and kidneys.
k_{34} = Sum of the rate constants for the reactions by which the reactive metabolite covalently combines with the different kinds of macromolecules in compartment I.
k_{30} = Sum of the rate constants for the reactions by which the reactive metabolite is converted to inert metabolites in compartment I.
k_{12} = Rate constant for the passage of the foreign compound from compartment I to compartment II.
k_{21} = Rate constant for the passage of the foreign compound from compartment II to compartment I.
k_{25} = Rate constant for the formation of the reactive metabolite in compartment II.
k_{20} = Sum of the rate constants for the reactions by which the foreign compound is converted to inert metabolites in compartment II.
k_{56} = Sum of the rate constants for the reactions by which the reactive metabolite covalently combines with the different kinds of macromulecules in compartment II.
k_{50} = Sum of the rate constants for the reactions by which the reactive metabolite is converted to inert metabolites in compartment II.
$a = k_{10} + k_{13} + k_{12}$
$b = k_{20} + k_{25} + k_{21}$
$c = k_{30} + k_{34}$
$f = k_{50} + k_{56}$
$\alpha = 1/2\ [a + b + \sqrt{(a + b)^2 - 4\ [(k_{10} + k_{13})\ b + k_{12}\ (k_{20} + k_{25})]}]$
$\beta = 1/2\ [a + b - \sqrt{(a + b)^2 - 4\ [(k_{10} + k_{13})\ b + k_{12}\ (k_{20} + k_{25})]}]$
$\alpha\beta = (k_{10} + k_{13})\ b + k_{12}\ (k_{20} + k_{25})$
$R = \alpha\beta c\ (b - k_a)/b\ (\alpha - k_a)\ (\beta - k_a)\ (c - k_a)$
$S = k_a\beta c\ (b - \alpha)/b\ (\alpha - k_a)\ (\beta - \alpha)\ (c - \alpha)$
$T = k_a\ \alpha\ c\ (b - \beta)/b\ (\beta - k_a)\ (\beta - \alpha)\ (c - \beta)$
$U = k_a\ \alpha\beta\ (b - c)/b\ (c - k_a)\ (c - \alpha)\ (c - \beta)$
$W = \alpha\beta f/(\alpha - k_a)\ (\beta - k_a)\ (f - k_a)$
$X = k_a\beta f/(\alpha - k_a)\ (\beta - \alpha)\ (f - \alpha)$
$Y = k_a\alpha f/(\beta - k_a)\ (\beta - \alpha)\ (f - \beta)$
$Z = k_a\ \alpha\beta/(f - k_a)\ (f - \alpha)\ (f - \beta)$

(2) *Further definitions for Fig.* 3

k_{13} = Rate constant for the formation of the intermediate reactive metabolite.
k_{10} = Sum of the rate constants for the reactions by which the foreign compound is converted to other inert metabolites and for its excretion by the lung and kidneys.
k_{34} = Rate constant for the formation of the reactive metabolite.
k_{30} = Sum of the rate constants for the reactions by which the intermediate inert metabolites are converted to other inert metabolites and for the excretion of the intermediate metabolite by the lungs and kidneys.
k_{45} = Sum of the rate constants for the reactions by which the reactive metabolite covalently combines with the different kinds of macromolecules.
k_{40} = Sum of the rate constants for the reactions by which the reactive metabolite is converted to inert metabolites.
$a = k_{10} + k_{13}$
$b = k_{30} + k_{34}$
$c = k_{40} + k_{45}$
$E = bc/(b - a)(c - a)$
$F = ac/(b - a)(c - b)$
$G = ab/(c - a)(c - b)$

Discussion

Scott: If one pool takes a preferential absorption, obviously this pool will take it first.

Gillette: When we include the rate of absorption into a two-pool linear system, the rate constant for absorption doesn't even appear in the equation for ultimate amount of covalent binding.

Scott: But there is excretion at that early stage when the drug concentration is building up.

Gillette: Yes, the number of pools will affect the rate at which covalent binding occurs but not the ultimate amount of covalent binding.

Scott: I remain to be convinced of that.

Gillette: These points are discussed in the paper.

Riess: Do your kinetics refer to total radioactivity only or are you referring to concentrations measured by structure-specific analysis?

Gillette: Most of the covalent binding is to protein, but reactive metabolites may also react with other macromolecules. In our approach, we assume that changes in the covalent binding to one kind of macromolecule will result in proportional changes in binding to all the macromolecules after the various treatments. For example, the liver necrosis caused by carbon tetrachloride is thought to be caused by the reaction of the trichloromethyl free radical to phospholipid, but we have found that treatments which change the amount of covalent binding of the free radical to phospholipid also change the amount of covalent binding to protein to about the same extent.

Riess: But isn't it a little dangerous to take total radioactivity and use it for model considerations?

Gillette: No, not necessarily. We are not claiming that a given amount of covalently bound metabolite of a drug will necessarily result in toxicity. What we are suggesting is that when a toxic effect is mediated by a reactive metabolite, then treatments that change the magnitude of the covalent binding of the reactive metabolite to macromolecules will also cause parallel changes in the incidence and severity of the toxicity. In this view we have assumed that the proportion of the total covalent binding that is bound to target macromolecules remains relatively constant as the total binding is increased or decreased. The proportion may not be exactly the same, because we have not taken all the factors into account—for example the diffusion rates of reacting metabolites. Nevertheless, the equations provide reasonable approximations of the kinds of changes that would be expected from a system that approaches first-order kinetics. As I have pointed out, however, the formation of the mercapturic acid of bromobenzene is no longer first-order after glutathione is depleted and thus some of the other kinetic aspects of drug metabolism become important. But if we had not realized the importance of the ratios A and B in the linear kinetic model, we probably would not have discovered the importance of glutathione in limiting the toxicity of bromobenzene or paracetamol, or the reason for the dose thresholds.

Beckett: Are you sure that it is covalent bonding?

Gillette: Yes. We first extract the tissue macromolecules by Soxhlett extraction with organic solvents until we can no longer remove any radiolabel from the precipitate. Then we solubilize the precipitate with sodium hydroxide and extract it again, on the basis that some of the reversibly bound radiolabel may be trapped in the protein. Thirdly, we hydrolyse the protein with pronase, treat the amino acids with dinitrofluorobenzene, and show that we indeed have radioactivity associated with the amphoteric substances.

Beckett: What do you envisage as the actual covalent bond?

Gillette: We have not yet identified the amino acid conjugates, but since the reactive metabolites react with thiol groups we think they are conjugates of cysteine or perhaps methionine.

Beckett: Are you involving the epoxide of bromobenzene in the actual interaction?

Gillette: Yes.

Beckett: If you have N-OH, which is of an amide group, not of an amine, how would you envisage the mechanism?

Gillette: It is difficult to answer that. The current view is that metabolites such as the N-OH metabolite of fluoren-2-ylacetamide must be further activated through the formation of the N-O-sulphate conjugate which labilizes the bond. However, the reactive metabolite of paracetamol does not require the formation of the sulphate ester. Perhaps the hydroxyl group on the para position may labilize the N-OH bond in some way and permit the OH group to leave.

Beckett: You have what you term covalent bonding, but isn't the problem that you cannot define any active site? It is a random sort of bonding so how can you possibly relate this to toxicity?

Gillette: We have proved that the toxicity is mediated by a reactive metabolite and that really is all we can prove. We cannot prove what the target macromolecule is or how the covalent binding results in tissue necrosis with this kind of study.

Widdop: Assuming that extrapolation from mouse to man is feasible, what you tell us means that a patient in whom induced microsomal enzymes are already present, because of drug therapy, is in far greater danger after an overdose of paracetamol than the patient in whom enzymes are functioning at normal rates. Does this not mean, then, that the laboratory should not only measure the concentration of paracetamol in the blood of the poisoned patient, but also screen the urine for the presence of drugs capable of bringing about enzyme induction?

Gillette: If the patient is exactly like the mouse, the increase in the excretion of the mercapturic acid of paracetamol after the administration of an inducer may be so small as to appear negligible. Indeed the kinetics of the covalent binding predicts that two animal species may metabolize the drug in exactly the same way at exactly the same rate, yet in one species the drug will be toxic and in the other it will be non-toxic.

Prescott: I am not sure how useful Dr Widdop's suggestion about such screening might be but our experience with paracetamol has convinced us that patients who are chronic alcoholics do extremely badly. Whether this is because they already have underlying hepatic disease which makes them more susceptible to a limited lesion, or whether the effect is mediated through a change in metabolism, we don't know.

Gillette: Alcohol is an inducer of some drug-metabolizing enzymes. However, I am not sure that it induces the formation of the reactive metabolite of paracetamol.

Riess: Are the dose ranges used in the animal far greater than those used in man?

Gillette: The point is that this effect is not seen at ordinary doses but occurs only after high doses. I believe that the suicidal doses taken by patients in Edinburgh (see R. W. Newton, this volume, pp. 5–11) must have been roughly equivalent to the levels in our animals. A dose of 150 mg/kg in mice would be equivalent to a total dose of about 10 g in man.

Riess: But there won't be induction of any sort in a suicide attempt.

Gillette: The argument is that if an individual has been taking barbiturates for many months he will already be induced. If he then takes a suicidal dose of paracetamol a greater proportion of the dose may be converted to the reactive metabolite. In other words, there is an increase in ratio A. In man, the proportion of a non-toxic dose of paracetamol that is excreted as the mercapturic acid is about 2.5 to 5.0%, and this proportion is doubled after treatment with phenobarbitone. However, there is so much individual variability in drug metabolism in man that it would be difficult to determine from the urinary methods alone whether the patient was already induced.

Brown: Your demonstration of a threshold dose level of paracetamol in mice is very interesting. In our early studies in Edinburgh (Brown *et al.* 1970) we had a suspicion, which we could never prove, that there was a threshold dose for hepatic necrosis. Dr Prescott, has more explicit evidence been found recently?

Prescott: I think there must be a threshold, in general terms. In a group of individuals who have taken overdoses of paracetamol there is a very wide range of susceptibility. One patient may develop a severe lesion after, say, 12 g, whereas another patient who has taken 12 g (as proved by urinary recovery studies) may be virtually unaffected.

Gillette: This is what we would predict. There is a complex interrelationship among the many rate constants. The threshold even in the same patient will be highly variable, but whatever the level there should be a threshold.

Beckett: If we assume that, in paracetamol, the N-OH compound is the active species which leads to covalent bonding and therefore to toxicity, what do we know about that particular mechanism? Can we discover anything about this so that we can do something helpful?

Gillette: The cysteine moiety of mercapturic acid is in the meta position. We think that the positive charge migrates to the meta position, and then the reduced glutathione (GSH) reacts with it.

Beckett: Has anyone made the *N*-hydroxy compound to test whether it is a highly toxic material?

Gillette: Dr D. Jollow, in our laboratory, has tried to make it but can't. He has made the hydroxylamine of *p*-chloroacetanilide but every time he has tried to make the hydroxylamine of paracetamol it decomposes.

Prescott: That is suspicious in itself.

Bridges: These epoxides are often so active that one might expect them to damage the cytochrome *P*-450 involved in forming them!

Gillette: They don't. We know that carbon tetrachloride and dimethylnitrosamine destroy cytochrome *P*-450. But bromobenzene does not cause any selective decrease in cytochrome *P*-450. Of course after the cell dies, the endoplasmic reticulum is broken and both cytochrome *P*-450 and cytochrome b_5 decrease. But the ratio of cytochrome *P*-450 to cytochrome b_5 remains relatively constant after bromobenzene.

Prescott: Does paracetamol do the same as bromobenzene?

Gillette: I think so.

Bridges: Cytochrome *P*-450 itself may have some protective mechanism.

Gillette: It may, or else the epoxide of bromobenzene is not very reactive chemically. We have evidence, for example, that bromobenzene epoxide is stable enough to reach the lung. In other words, most of the reactive metabolite that is covalently bound in the lung after bromobenzene administration is formed in the liver.

Bridges: This must be a relatively stable metabolite to get through to the lung.

Gillette: It has to be there long enough for blood to flow between the liver and the lung, which takes about 10 seconds.

Bridges: It is surprising it gets off the *P*-450.

Gillette: But for most metabolites, the dissociation requires about a millisecond or less. The metabolite of bromobenzene is at least stable enough to get out of the liver. Whether the reactive metabolites destroy the cytochrome *P*-450 may depend on their chemical reactivity. It may well be that those metabolites that have sufficient chemical reactivity to destroy cytochrome *P*-450 are also so chemically reactive that they cannot escape from the liver. We have evidence, for example, that carbon tetrachloride does not leave the liver as a free radical. Those metabolites that do leave the liver may have little or no effect on cytochrome *P*-450.

Goulding: In animals, is there any time relationship in liver protection between the dose of paracetamol and the glutathione? And does this work in man?

Prescott: It does work in man.

Goulding: How do you predict that the one you have thus treated is saved?

Prescott: We can measure the plasma paracetamol concentration in a patient at a given time after ingestion and can predict the probability of liver damage and the severity of that damage. We can treat patients who have concentrations in a given range and compare the results in treated and untreated patients. In this way we can show without any doubt that cysteamine (mercaptamine) has a remarkable protective effect, provided that it is given within 10 hours (Prescott *et al.* 1974).

Goulding: So your one criterion for prognosis is the paracetamol concentration, or a series of paracetamol concentrations?

Prescott: Yes.

Goulding: If your prognosis on paracetamol concentrations should not be absolutely reliable then your measurement for the success of therapy loses its basis?

Prescott: I don't think so. We can make accurate predictions on the basis of the concentrations. We can tell you, for example, that a patient with a certain plasma paracetamol concentration at a certain time has, say, a 70% ± 20% chance of sustaining liver damage with peak serum transaminase activity above a certain level. We can apply statistical methods. Ten untreated patients may have transaminase levels of 5000 i.u./litre while ten treated patients will have transaminase levels that are either normal or less than 200 i.u./litre.

Goulding: Your practical way of assessing liver damage is then by a biochemical test of liver function.

Prescott: Yes.

Parker: You have discussed the microsomal oxidation system in liver, Dr Gillette, but there are low levels of enzyme activity in other tissues.

Gillette: Yes. That is why it is important to find out whether a reactive metabolite is stable enough to leave the liver. Suppose that the reactive metabolite cannot leave the liver. In this case, theoretically, if one blocks the metabolism in the liver and if the only other way of getting rid of the compound is by metabolism in the extrahepatic tissues, the toxicity would be decreased in the liver but increased in some other tissue. Cytochrome *P*-450 systems in the various tissues, however, have different affinities for different drugs. Some metabolize relatively few drugs. Moreover, they may be induced and inhibited by different substances. In fact, we have used these differences to study the problem of stability of reactive metabolites. For example, pretreatment of animals with phenobarbitone does not increase the covalent bonding of bromobenzene to lung macromolecules by lung preparations *in vitro*. But pretreatment with phenobarbitone markedly increases the covalent bonding of bromobenzene to lung macromolecules *in vivo* to about the same extent as it increases the covalent binding to liver macromolecules.

Parker: As a corollary to what you have said, then a drug-induced leucopenia might involve a selective capability of the cytochrome *P*-450 system in the leucocyte to produce a toxic derivative of the drug?

Gillette: That is the idea.

Parker: It was recently suggested that leucocytes can be used as a biopsy tissue to attempt to look at induction of the *P*-450 system. From studies in bronchial asthma and other diseases it would appear that peripheral blood leucocytes and other circulating cells can provide valuable information on pharmacological, hormonal or biochemical tissue response patterns to drugs in different individuals (see, for example, Parker & Smith 1973).

Gillette: Whitlock *et al.* (1972) have shown that 3,4-benzopyrene hydroxylase in human lymphocytes treated with either phytohaemagglutinin or pokeweed mitogen was induced by benzanthracene *in vitro*.

References

Brown, S. S., Proudfoot, A. T., Raeburn, J. A. & Wright, N. (1970) Elevation of serum enzyme levels in acute poisoning, in *Clinical Enzymology* (Frei, J. & Jemelin, M., eds.) (*Proc. VII Int. Congr. Clin. Chem., Geneva 1969*), vol. 2, 173–182, Karger, Basel

Parker, C. W. & Smith, J. W. (1973) Alterations in cyclic AMP metabolism in human bronchial asthma. I: Leucocyte responsiveness in β-adrenergic agents, *J. Clin. Invest. 52*, 48–59

Prescott, L. F., Newton, R. W., Swainson, C. P., Wright, N., Forrest, A. R. W. & Matthew, H. (1974) Successful treatment of severe paracetamol overdosage with cysteamine. *Lancet 1*, 588–592

Whitlock, J. P., Jr., Cooper, H. L. & Gelboin, H. V. (1972) Aryl hydrocarbon (benzopyrene) hydroxylase is stimulated in human lymphocytes by mitogens and benz[a]anthracene. *Science (Wash. D.C.) 177*, 618–619

Separation and detection of unstable metabolites of amphetamines, analgesics and phenothiazines

A. H. BECKETT

Department of Pharmacy, Chelsea College, University of London

Abstract Many drugs are metabolized substantially *in vivo* and the detection and analysis of metabolites in the poisoned patient may thus be important. Before analysis, treatment of the biological fluids to liberate the conjugates of a drug and its metabolites may change the latter compounds; for example, acid hydrolysis of the conjugates of pentazocine can decompose the parent drug. Before analysis, separation techniques usually have to be used and the conditions can effect transformation in the compounds under investigation; for example, for the extraction of organic bases into organic solvents, the aqueous biological fluid is usually rendered alkaline and this can result in extensive decomposition of some drugs and their metabolites. Also, the solvent used in extraction can interact with some drugs, e.g. chlorohydrocarbon solvents, and quaternize many basic drugs and basic metabolites.

Although thin-layer chromatography and gas–liquid chromatography, especially when used in conjunction with mass spectrometry, constitute powerful tools for the analysis of drugs and metabolites, care must be taken to ensure that the analytical technique used does not lead to decomposition of the compounds being examined. The problems are illustrated by examples from work with amphetamines, phenothiazines and narcotic drugs.

The importance of understanding the metabolism of drugs and the chemistry of these metabolites is stressed.

Many compounds are reported in the literature as drug metabolites. Are these compounds, identified after extraction, separation, concentration and analytical techniques, the actual products of enzymic reaction with the drug, or do many of them represent the final product of chemical changes resulting from the techniques used? The answer to this is important when drug action, structure–activity relations, toxicology, pharmacokinetics and so on, have to be considered.

The properties of the metabolites in the conditions met in all steps before the final point of measurement are relevant; some of the more important characteristics of metabolites in this context are listed in Table 1.

TABLE 1
Drug metabolic products: their characteristics

(1) They are produced in aqueous systems as components of a complex mixture
(2) Many are *labile* and have different susceptibilities to
heat pH
light oxygen
traces of heavy metals
characteristics of solid surfaces
(3) Many have high water solubility and low lipid solubility
(4) A drug may produce a complex mixture of metabolites consisting of neutral, acidic and basic molecules
(5) The different metabolites of a drug may have different lipid–water partition characteristics and stabilities at different pH values
(6) Many of the metabolites are present in the aqueous complex system in low concentrations
(7) In general, before analysis, *separation techniques* have to be employed.

CHARACTERISTICS OF METABOLITES

It is not always realized that most metabolites are labile in the conditions usually used in metabolic and pharmacokinetic studies. I will draw on studies in my own laboratories to illustrate this statement. My selection will include work on amphetamines, analgesics and phenothiazines, i.e. aralkylamines possessing one or more aromatic rings, and I will further restrict my examples by considering only oxidative metabolic attack on the basic centres and their α-carbon atoms. Primary attack on the α-carbon atom produces highly unstable aminoalcohols; attack on the nitrogen atom in tertiary amines produces *N*-oxides which are relatively stable in aqueous solutions, whereas attack on secondary aliphatic amines produces relatively unstable secondary hydroxylamines, and attack on primary aliphatic amines produces unstable primary hydroxylamines. Examples for amphetamines, analgesics (methadone) and phenothiazines are shown in Figs. 1, 2 and 3, respectively.

The metabolites arising from attack on α-carbon atoms in general (if the nitrogen atom is not part of a ring) are quickly converted chemically in solution into single products, i.e. dealkylated or deaminated compounds, depending on which α-carbon atom has been attacked. Attack on the nitrogen atom yields *N*-oxygenated products possessing a whole range of stabilities; they break down to a variety of products (e.g. the secondary hydroxylamine metabolites in Fig. 4 and the primary hydroxylamines in Fig. 5).

In our laboratories, we have established that formation of hydroxylamines (Fig. 6*a*) is an important *in vitro* and *in vivo* metabolic route in ranges of diverse primary and secondary aliphatic amines (see Fig. 6*b*); the route is important whether or not the nitrogen atom is part of a ring system containing other heteroatoms.

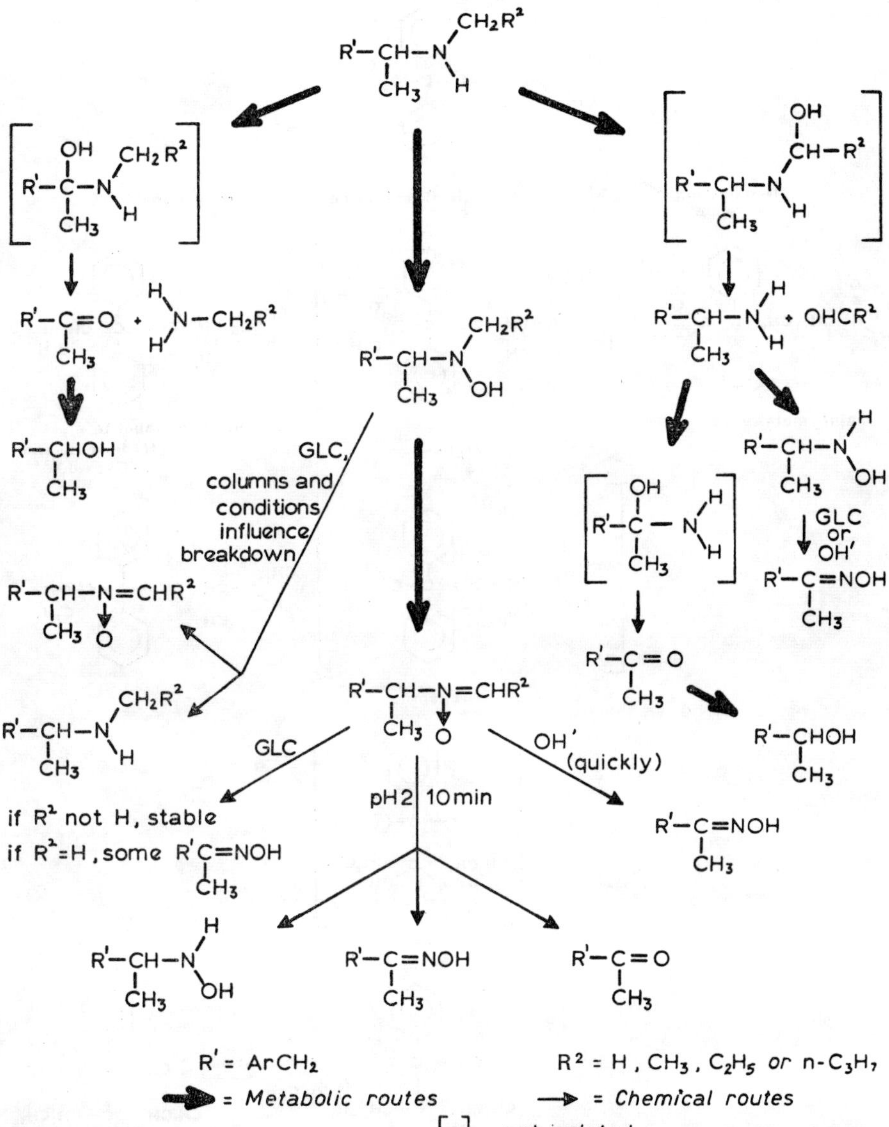

FIG. 1. The metabolism of aralkyl-secondary amines and the chemical changes of metabolites and metabonates during extraction.

PROBLEMS WITH SEPARATION TECHNIQUES

Many metabolites are changed chemically not only in the biological fluid in which they are produced, but also more drastically in the separation techniques

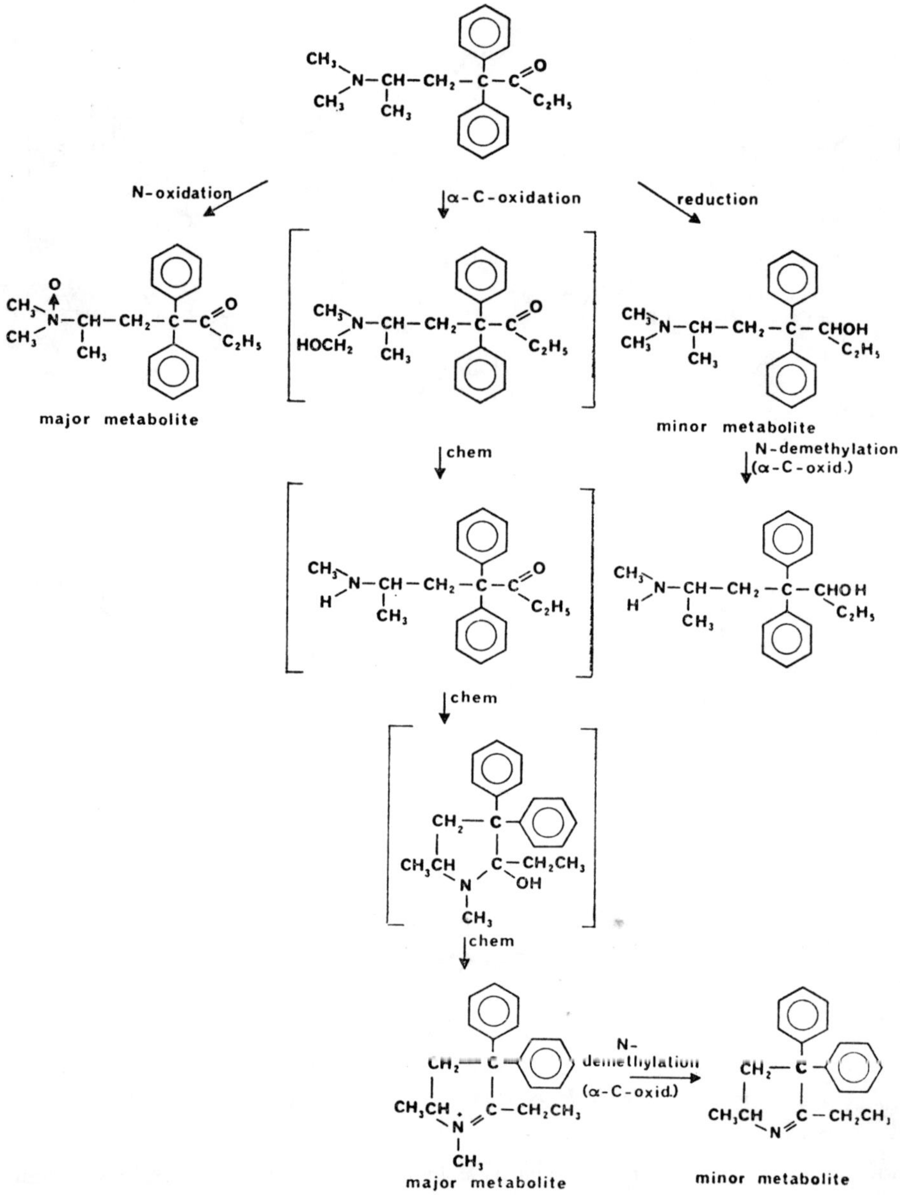

FIG. 2. The metabolism of methadone.

usually used before the final analytical technique. Table 2 records some of the problems which may be encountered in separation methods. A few examples will suffice to illustrate some of these problems.

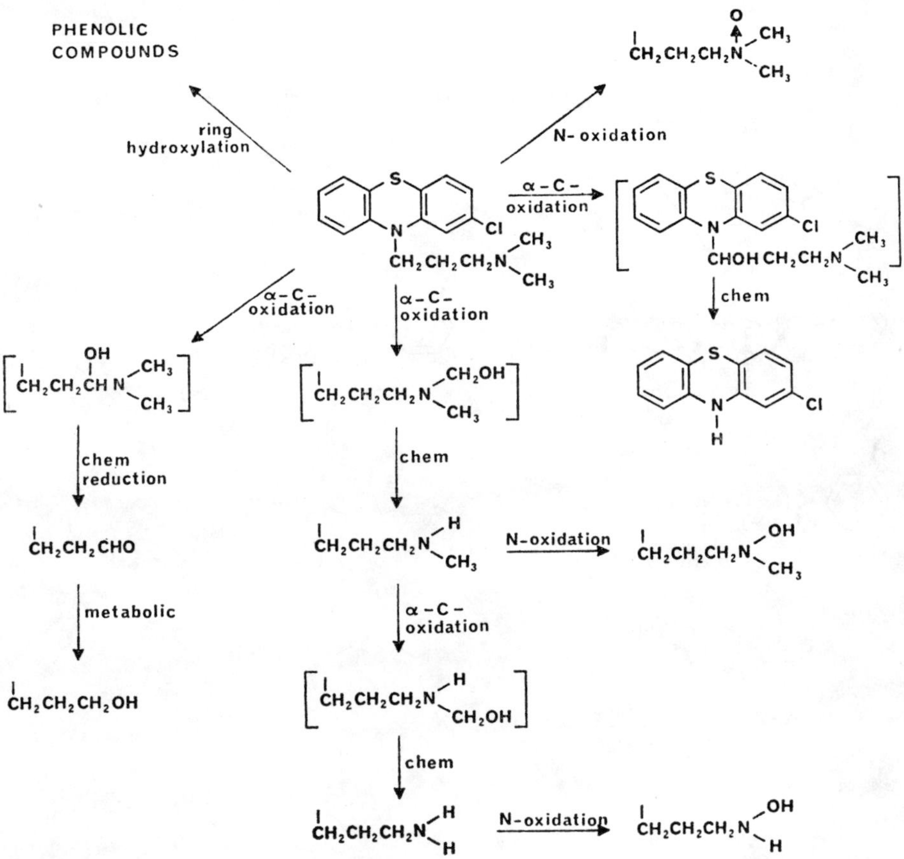

FIG. 3. Routes of metabolism of chlorpromazine.

Chemical changes when pH is changed

Phentermine (see Fig. 7; pK_a 10.1) (and chlorphentermine) is metabolized in animals and man to produce the hydroxylamine (pK_a 8.1), i.e. a much weaker base, and the *C*-nitroso compound, a neutral compound. If the aqueous solution is made alkaline before the drug is extracted, the hydroxylamine is converted into the nitroso and nitro compounds and the amount of change depends on how long the solution is kept at an alkaline pH (see Fig. 7); also, the nitroso compound is converted into the nitro compound at alkaline pH values.

Sometimes biological fluids are acidified before extraction. Fenfluramine gives a nitrone (Fig. 8) as a result of metabolic oxidation of the nitrogen and α-carbon atoms, as well as giving the hydroxylamine as a result of attack on only the nitrogen atom; the nitrone can be extracted from neutral aqueous solution, but

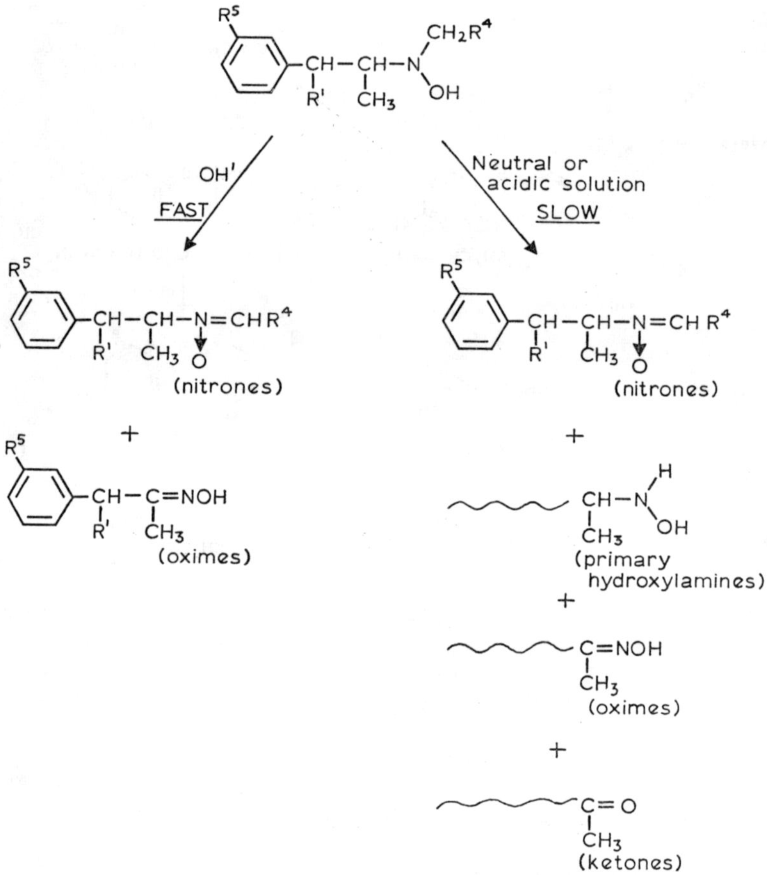

FIG. 4. Chemical changes of secondary hydroxylamines under aqueous conditions. If R^5=CF_3 or R^1=OH then hydroxylamines are more stable.

if the solution is acidified (e.g. pH 2.0) it is converted rapidly into a number of products, including the primary hydroxylamine, oxime and ketone (see Fig. 8).

Diethylpropion (amfepramone) (Fig. 9) is metabolized in animals and man by *N*-dealkylation and reduction of the carbonyl group; if the body fluid containing the amino-ketones is made alkaline to facilitate extraction of these compounds into an organic phase, they are changed chemically into the vinyl ketone, as shown in Fig. 9.

Amphetamine is metabolized *in vitro* and *in vivo* to the primary hydroxylamine (see Fig. 5), which in alkaline solution is rapidly converted into the oxime. The latter can be extracted into ether from alkaline solutions but if the pH is made more acidic (<4.0), it is rapidly converted into the ketone (see Fig. 10).

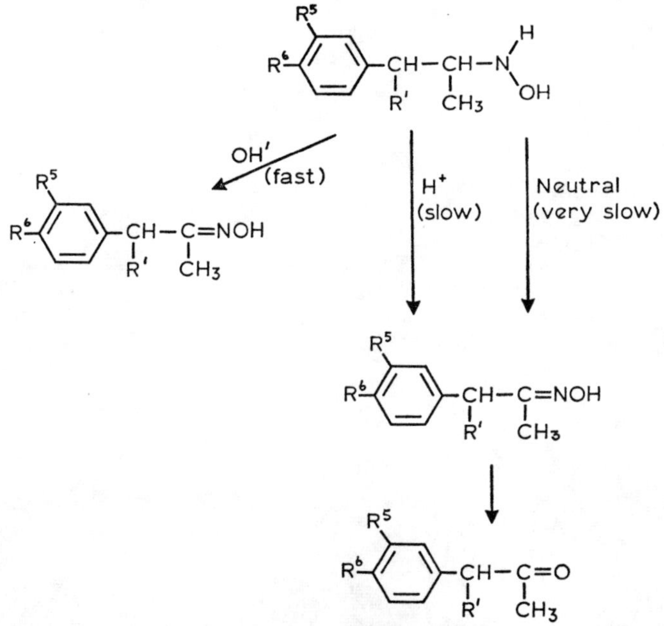

FIG. 5. Chemical changes of primary hydroxylamines under aqueous conditions.
Note: $R^5 = CF_3$ stabilizes the hydroxylamine;
$R^6 = OCH_3$ destabilizes the hydroxylamine;
$R^1 = OH$ stabilizes the hydroxylamine.

Chemical changes during conjugate hydrolysis

In man the analgesic pentazocine (Fig. 11) is excreted in urine both free and as a glucuronide conjugate. If the urine is heated with acid in conditions used for hydrolysis of conjugates, chemical change occurs in the parent molecule, in addition to glucuronide hydrolysis (Fig. 11); gas–liquid chromatography–mass spectrometry is complicated by the change.

Chemical changes involving interaction with solvents

The choice of organic solvent used in the extraction of metabolites may have an important influence on the observed result, because most organic solvents used for extraction in metabolic studies are not inert. For instance, the traces of peroxides present in ether attack primary and secondary amines. However, purified ether can be used to extract 'amphetamine hydroxylamine' without decomposition, whereas if ethyl acetate is the solvent it causes extensive decomposition of the metabolite. Purified ether can be used to extract the hydroxyl-

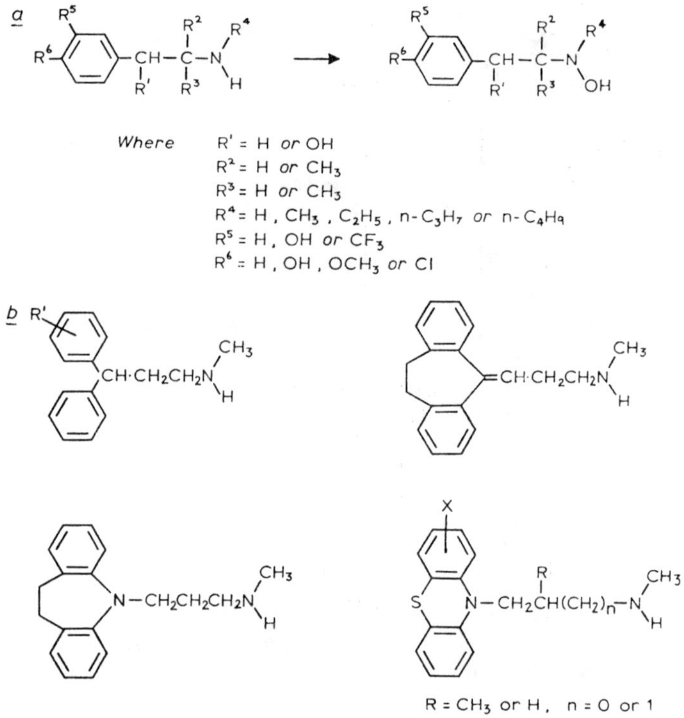

FIG. 6. Hydroxylamine formation from primary and secondary aliphatic amines—a general and important metabolic route.

amines from the mono- and di- demethylamines from promazine and chlorpromazine, whereas butanol can cause extensive decomposition (see Fig. 20 for some of the decomposition products).

Chlorohydrocarbon solvents and their impurities can interact with many basic compounds, e.g. dichloromethane reacts with the analgesics pethidine, dextromethorphan and methadone (see Fig. 12). If this solvent is used, and if the solution is concentrated before GLC analysis, more peaks may appear than with the parent drug (e.g. see methadone alone and evaporated with dichloromethane; Fig. 13); the mass spectrum may then suffer from interference from fragment ions. Sometimes *N*-oxides are extracted into chlorohydrocarbon solvents and the mass spectrum of the quaternary compound of solvent-drug interaction complicates that of the *N*-oxide.

PROBLEMS WITH ANALYTICAL TECHNIQUES

Many labile metabolites undergo chemical changes in the analytical techniques

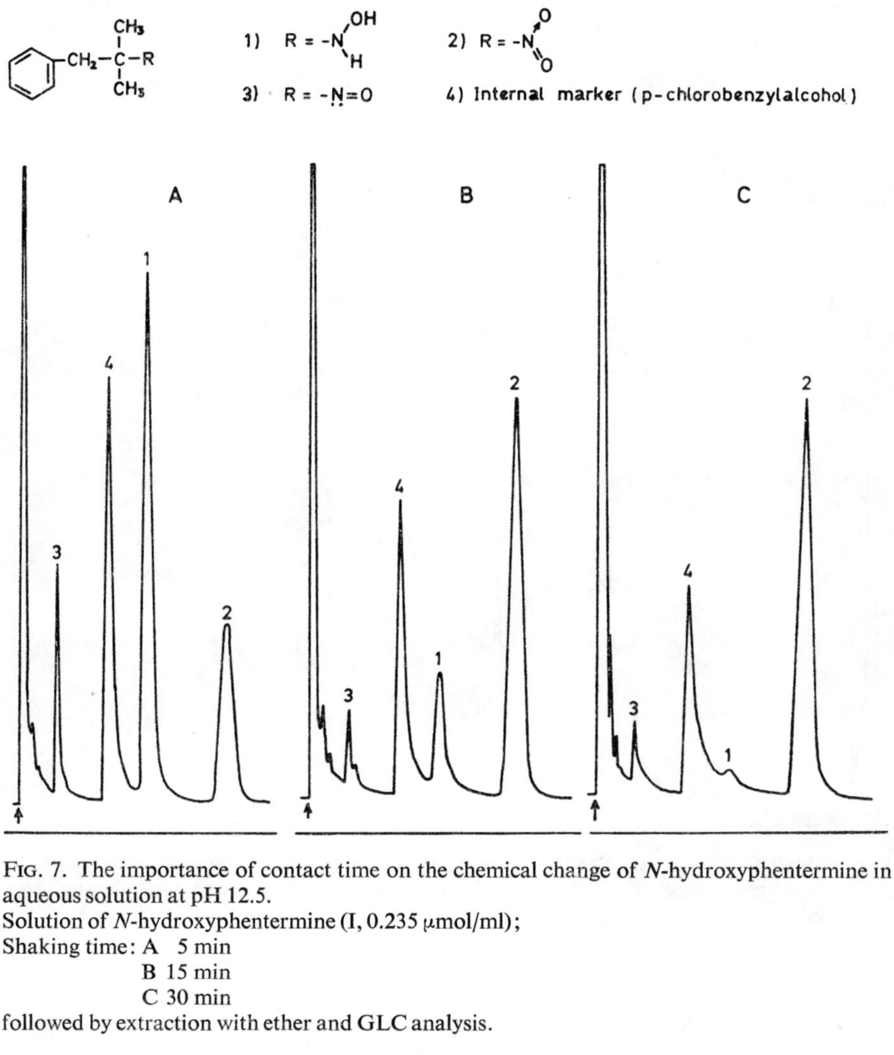

FIG. 7. The importance of contact time on the chemical change of *N*-hydroxyphentermine in aqueous solution at pH 12.5.
Solution of *N*-hydroxyphentermine (I, 0.235 μmol/ml);
Shaking time: A 5 min
B 15 min
C 30 min
followed by extraction with ether and GLC analysis.

used; some of the problems encountered are shown in Table 3. For instance, on GLC analysis secondary hydroxylamines break down by different routes and at different rates which are influenced by the columns, instruments and conditions used, as well as by the structures near the hydroxylamine group (see Fig. 14). Some of the decomposition products from the hydroxylamine metabolite of benzylamphetamine are shown in Fig. 15. The amount of breakdown may depend on the support and the stationary phase used (see Fig. 16 for 'amphetamine hydroxylamine'); the rate of injection may influence the amount of

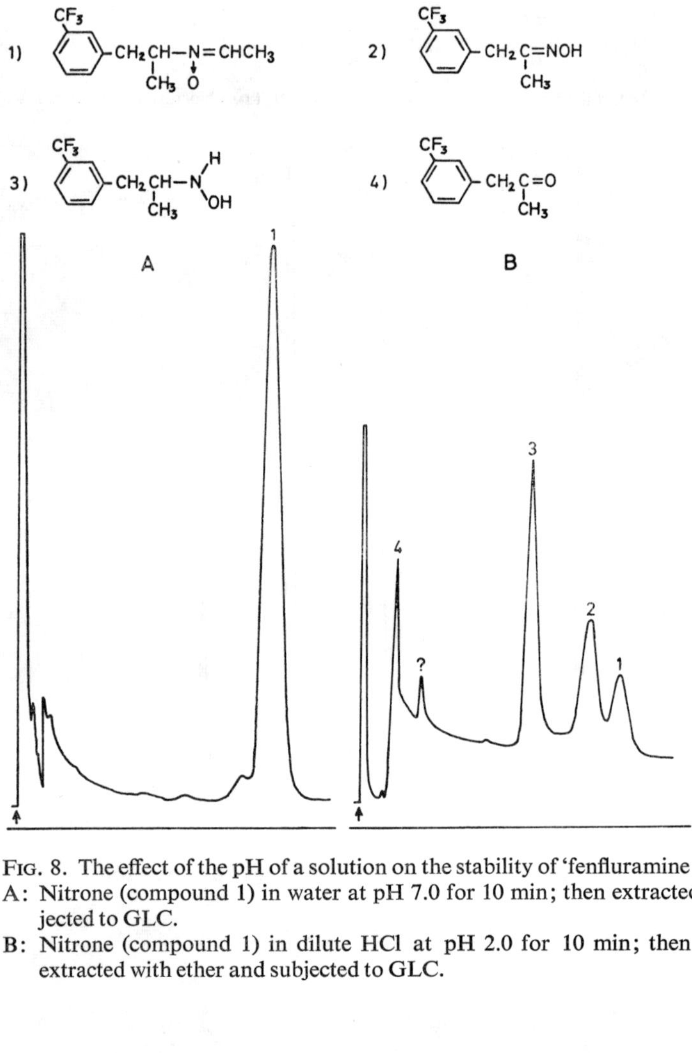

FIG. 8. The effect of the pH of a solution on the stability of 'fenfluramine nitrone'.
A: Nitrone (compound 1) in water at pH 7.0 for 10 min; then extracted with ether and subjected to GLC.
B: Nitrone (compound 1) in dilute HCl at pH 2.0 for 10 min; then adjusted to pH 7.0, extracted with ether and subjected to GLC.

breakdown (Fig. 17) and the instrument used may influence these chemical changes (e.g. see Fig. 18).

The *N*-oxidation products of promazine and chlorpromazine and of their demethylated products undergo chemical changes during GLC analysis (e.g. the *N*-oxides in Fig. 19 and the secondary hydroxylamines in Fig. 20).

The above examples indicate that attention to detail over the conditions of storage of biological fluids, and attention to detail and care in separation techniques are just as important as the final method of analysis if we are to detect most drug metabolites and determine them quantitatively. Increased

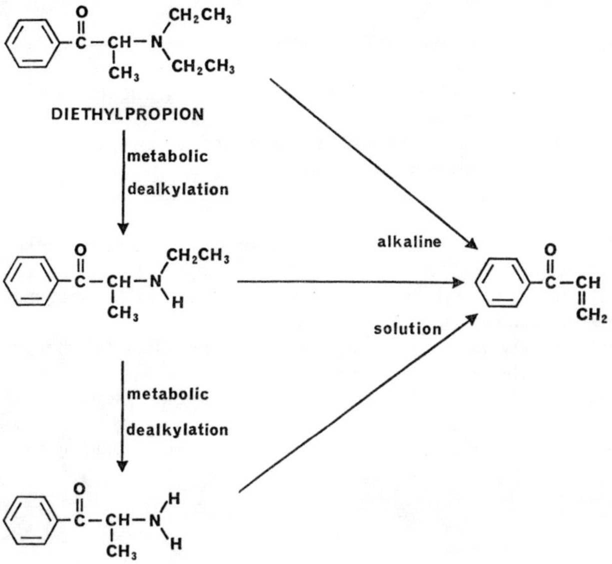

FIG. 9. Metabolic dealkylation of diethylpropion (amfepramone).

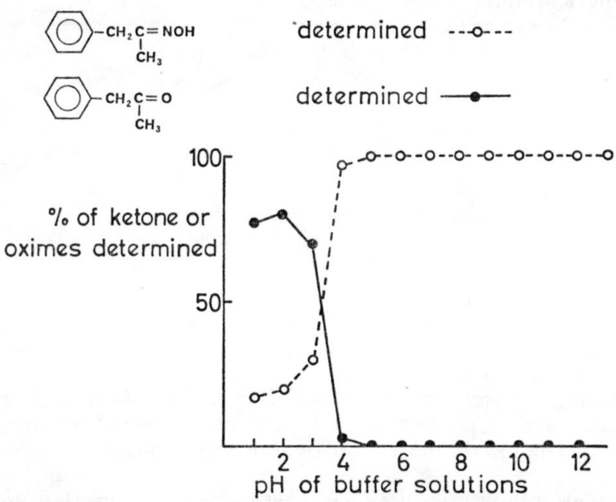

FIG. 10. Benzylmethyl ketoximes: conversion to benzylmethyl ketone during extraction into ether from buffer solutions of differing pH values. (Total time taken about 30 min.)

sophistication in analytical techniques alone will not guarantee success in these studies. Furthermore, continual emphasis must be laid on understanding the chemistry of the changes that occur in drugs and metabolites because of the

TABLE 2

Drug metabolic products: problems involved in separation techniques

(1) The metabolite has usually to be extracted from the aqueous to an organic liquid after conversion to a more lipid-soluble species by one of the following methods:
  (a) Change of pH to convert it into its more lipid-soluble un-ionized form—(metabolites may be decomposed by many routes and mechanisms).
  (b) Ion-pair formation by addition of compounds that form ion pairs.
  (c) Chemical changes of conjugates etc. by
    (i) acid hydrolysis at elevated temperatures—(many metabolites are changed other than by conjugate cleavage).
    (ii) enzymic hydrolysis—(the susceptibilities of many conjugates to the enzymes employed has not been established).
    (iii) reduction techniques, i.e. *N*-oxides to tertiary amines—(other chemical changes may occur during the reduction).

(2) The choice of organic solvent—(some solvents decompose labile metabolites, some extract unwanted compounds from complex mixtures).

(3) Concentration of the metabolites in organic solutions has usually to be effected by such techniques as—
    evaporation
    TLC
    GLC
  – (complex changes in metabolites can occur, depending on solvent and system employed; losses on vessel walls or by volatility can occur).

(4) Proteins are sometimes precipitated before extraction is carried out—(the reagents used decompose many metabolites and others are bound in the precipitate).

TABLE 3

Drug metabolic products: problems involved in analytical techniques

Many labile metabolites undergo chemical changes in the analytical techniques employed for their analysis, e.g. in the following techniques:

GLC	Different columns, supports, coating materials and batches of coating materials, injection blocks, temperatures, injection syringes, rate of injection, solvents containing the metabolites, etc. can cause different amounts and types of breakdown.
TLC	Different materials, solvents, temperatures, light intensity, etc. can lead to different amounts of decomposition of metabolites.
Polarography	Differences in solvents, pH of solution, presence of trace heavy metals, nature of antioxidants, etc. can produce differences in decomposition of metabolites.
Spectrophotometric and radiochemical techniques	Differences in solvents, pH, time taken for measurements, temperatures, exposure to light, traces of heavy metals, etc. can produce differences in the decomposition of metabolites.

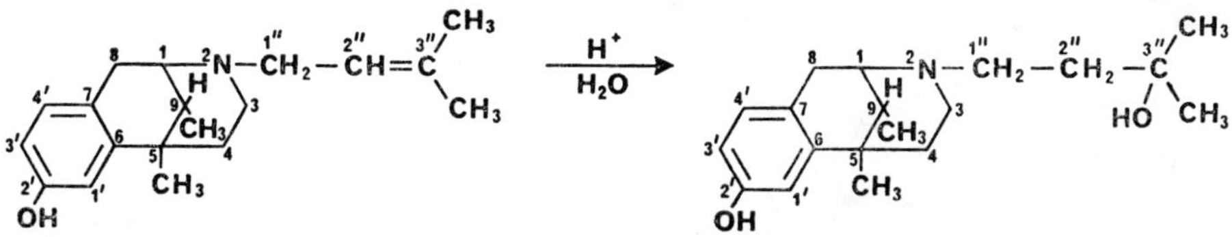

FIG. 11. Chemical change of pentazocine in the acid hydrolytic conditions used for the hydrolysis of glucuronides.

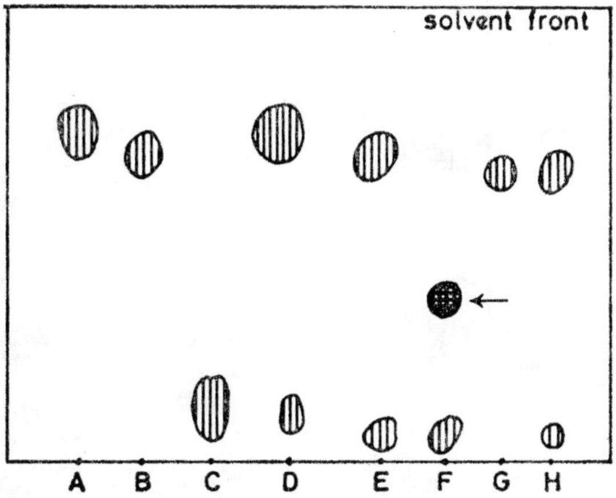

FIG. 12. The result of evaporation to low bulk at 42 °C of solutions of pethidine, dextromethorphan and methadone in methanol and in dichloromethane.
TLC analysis of concentrates and reference compounds on silica gel at 24 °C using solvent (benzene–methanol–triethylamine, 75:15:10); spot visualized with Dragendorff's reagent. ←yellow (picrate).
A: Dextromethorphan hydrobromide in methanol;
B: Pethidine hydrochloride in methanol;
C: Dextromethorphan chloromethochloride in methanol;
D: Dextromethorphan base concentrated in CH_2Cl_2;
E: Pethidine base concentrated in CH_2Cl_2;
F: Pethidine chloromethopicrate;
G: Methadone hydrochloride in methanol;
H: Methadone base concentrated in CH_2Cl_2.

techniques used. This is especially important if different metabolites are converted at different rates to a compound which is being measured as a so-called metabolite produced by a particular metabolic route; e.g. measurement of benzylmethyl ketone as a means of measuring deamination of dimethyl-

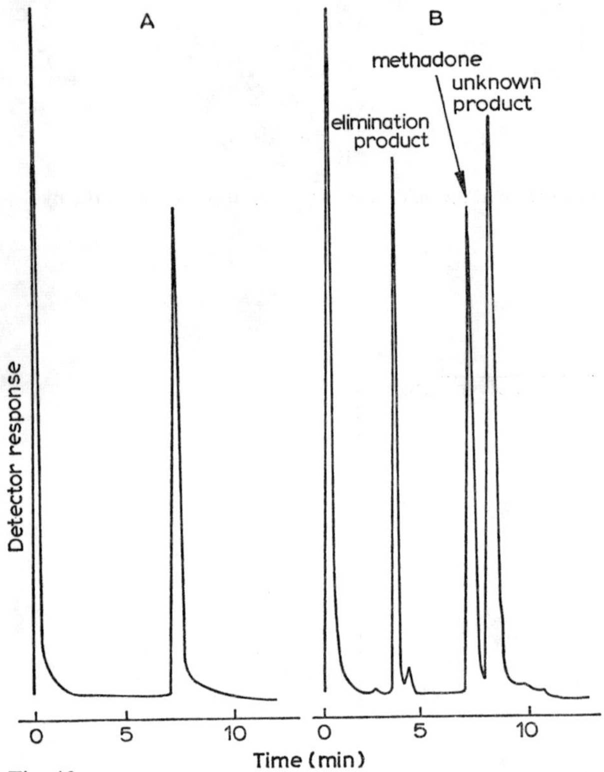
A
B
methadone
unknown product
elimination product
Detector response
0
5
10
0
5
10
Time (min)

Fig. 13

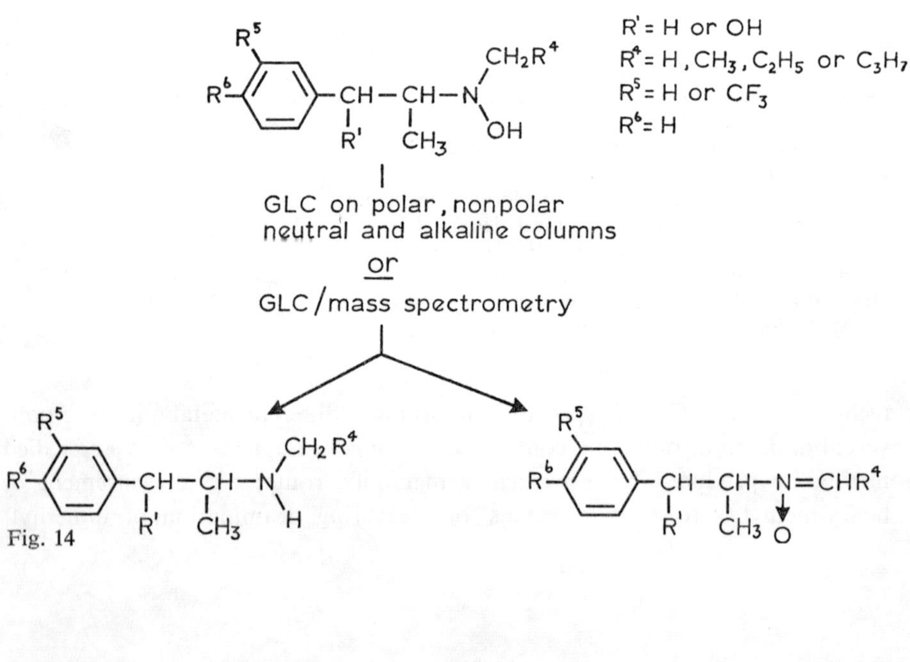
R' = H or OH
R⁴ = H, CH3, C2H5 or C3H7
R⁵ = H or CF3
R⁶ = H
GLC on polar, nonpolar neutral and alkaline columns
or
GLC/mass spectrometry

Fig. 14

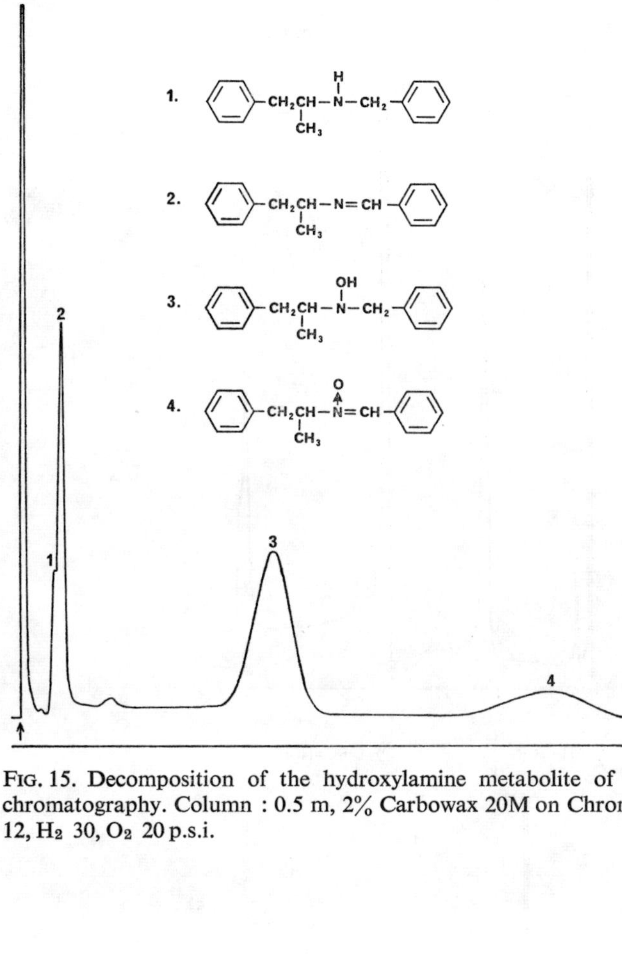

FIG. 15. Decomposition of the hydroxylamine metabolite of benzylamphetamine in gas chromatography. Column : 0.5 m, 2% Carbowax 20M on Chromosorb G Temp. 150°C; N_2 12, H_2 30, O_2 20 p.s.i.

FIG. 13. Gas chromatography (SE-30,200°C) of (A) methadone and (B) methadone solution in dichloromethane evaporated to small volume. (Elimination product has same retention time as 2-ethylidene-5-methyl-3,3-diphenyltetrahydrofuran.)

FIG. 14. Chemical changes of secondary hydroxylamines in GLC and GLC–mass spectrometry.
Note: 1. If R^5=CF_3, less breakdown in GLC;
2. Much more breakdown in GLC–mass spectrometry than in GLC;
3. When R^4=H, the oxime rather than the nitrone is produced.

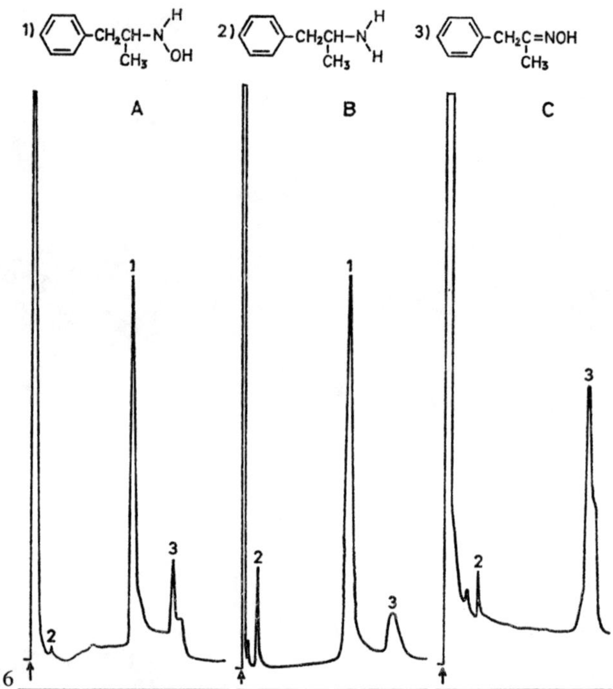
1) CH₂CH–N H OH CH₃
2) CH₂CH–N H H CH₃
3) CH₂C=NOH CH₃
A
B
C
1
2
3
1
2
3
2
3

Fig. 16

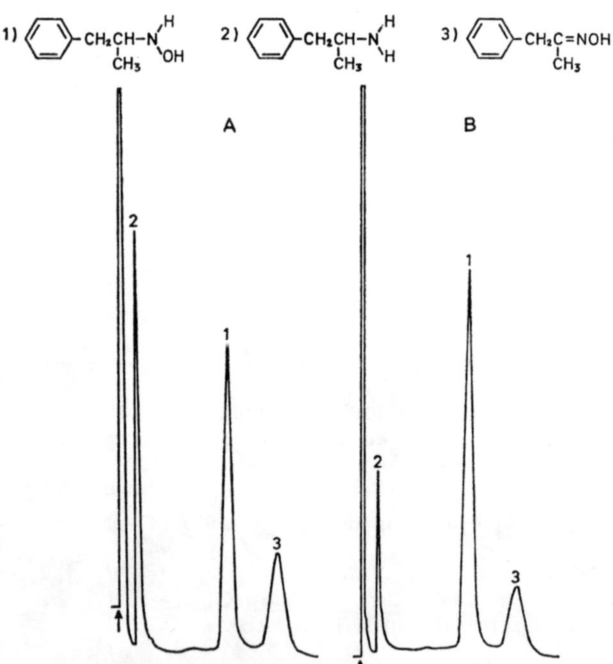
1) CH₂CH–N H OH CH₃
2) CH₂CH–N H H CH₃
3) CH₂C=NOH CH₃
A
B
2
1
3
1
2
3

Fig. 17

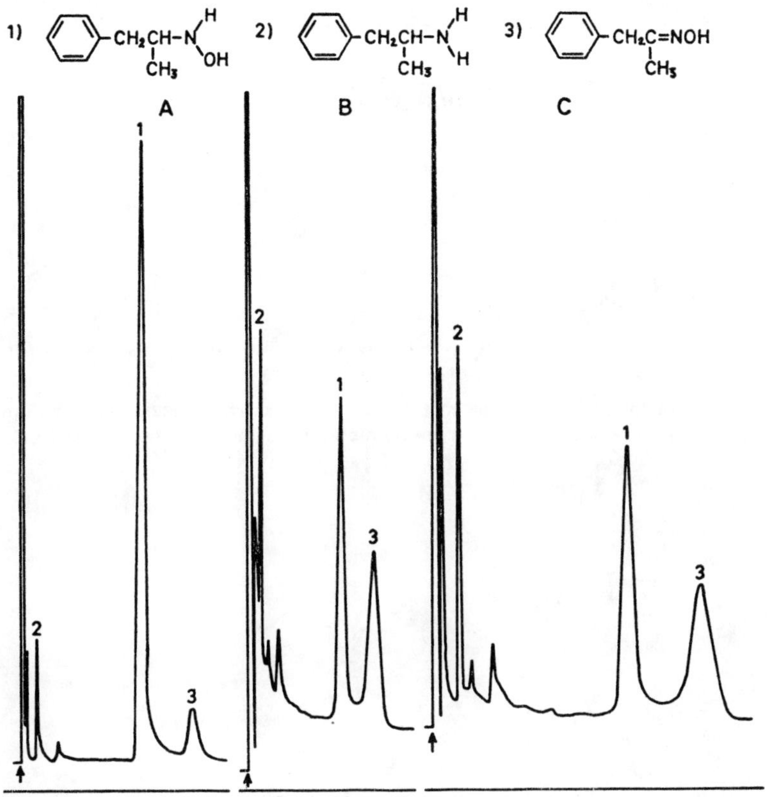

FIG. 18. The effect of change of GLC instrument on the breakdown of *N*-hydroxyamphetamine.
Column: 2 m glass, Carbowax 20M (sample *a*) 7.5% on Chromosorb W 80–100 mesh (sample *b*)
A: *F 11 instrument* N_2 30, air 20, H_2 20 p.s.i.
B: *F 30 instrument* N_2 99 ml/min, air 25, H_2 20 p.s.i.
C: *As B* but oven temp. lowered to 160°C

←

FIG. 16. The effect of different batches of support and of stationary phase on the breakdown of *N*-hydroxyamphetamine in gas chromatography. Instrument: Perkin–Elmer F11; 2 m glass column; N_2 30, air 20, H_2 20 p.s.i. Oven temp. 162°C for A, 167°C for B and C. Inj. temp. 215 °C, 7.5% Carbowax 20M on Chromosorb W AW DMCS
A: Carbowax (sample *a*), 100–120 mesh Chromosorb W (sample *a*)
B: Carbowax (sample *a*), 80–100 mesh Chromosorb W (sample *b*)
C: Carbowax (sample *b*), 80–100 mesh Chromosorb W (sample *c*) (Carbowax, sample *b* on 100–120 mesh Chromosorb W (sample *a*) gave similar results)

FIG. 17. The effect of rate of injection on the breakdown of *N*-hydroxyamphetamine in GLC.
Instrument: Hewlett Packard 5700 A;
Column: 0.9 m glass, 7.5% Carbowax 20M on Chromosorb W AW DMCS, 80–100 mesh, oven temp. 150°C, N_2 rate 60 ml/min.
Note: Injection point not heated; metal injection needle.
A: Normal injection rate. B: Very fast injection

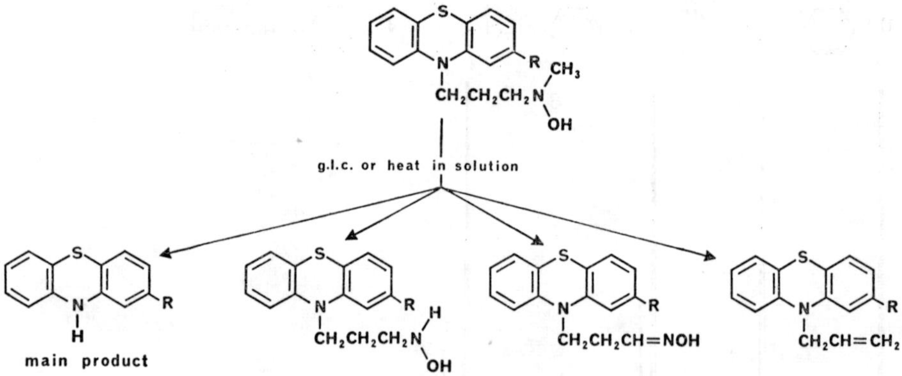

FIG. 19. Decomposition of hydroxylamine metabolites of demethylpromazine (R=H) and demethylchlorpromazine (R=Cl) in solution in organic solvents and in gas chromatography.

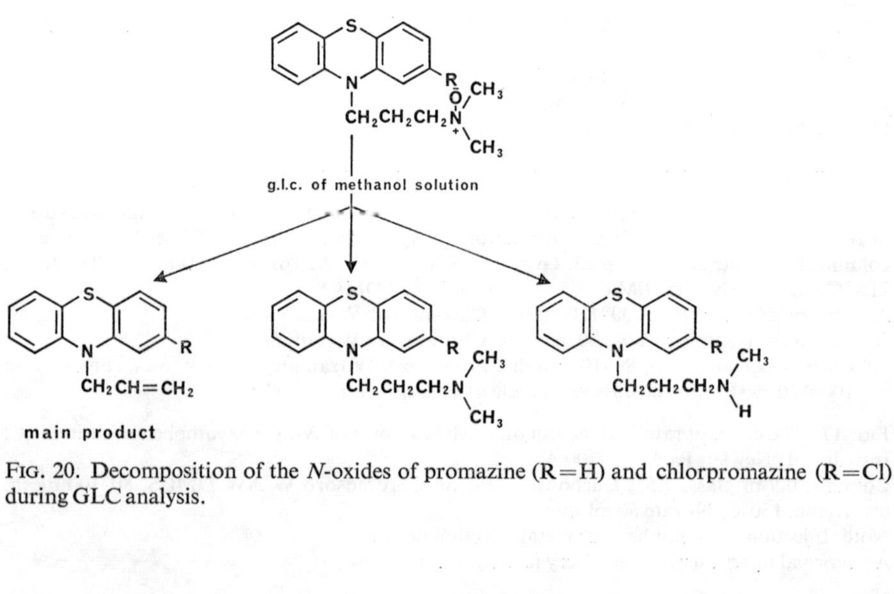

FIG. 20. Decomposition of the *N*-oxides of promazine (R=H) and chlorpromazine (R=Cl) during GLC analysis.

amphetamine is meaningless since this ketone is produced by a number of different routes and by different chemical reactions after metabolism.

Recently, because of the problems I have described here, we have given much attention to separating drugs and metabolites quickly from biological fluids and putting them into organic solvents rendered as inert as possible; the aqueous solution is kept neutral by the processes used for extraction. The use of techniques involving ion-pair formation has facilitated these studies. Transfer of solutions is, as far as possible, eliminated. Solutions should be concentrated in inert atmospheres in subdued light. Direct insertion mass spectrometry is used when the characteristic ions of the drugs, metabolites, and the subsequent metabonates have been identified.

ACKNOWLEDGEMENTS

The material in this paper is based primarily on the experimental work of my doctoral and post-doctoral students, some of which has already been published in the papers recorded in the bibliography below. I thank those students for their collaboration and enthusiasm. I also thank the Medical Research Council, the Home Office and the Research Council of Canada for financial support for various aspects of this research.

Bibliography

BECKETT, A. H., VAN DYK, J. M., CHISSICK, H. H. & GORROD, J. W. (1971*a*) Metabolic oxidation on aliphatic basic nitrogen atoms and their α-carbon atoms—some unifying principles. *J. Pharm. Pharmacol. 23*, 809–812

BECKETT, A. H. (1971*b*) Metabolic oxidation of aliphatic basic nitrogen atoms and their α-carbon atoms. *Xenobiotica 1*, 365–383

BECKETT, A. H. & AL-SARRAJ, S. (1972*a*) The mechanism of oxidation of amphetamine enantiomorphs by liver microsomal preparation from different species. *J. Pharm. Pharmacol. 24*, 174–176

BECKETT, A. H., VAUGHAN, D. P. & ESSIEN, E. E. (1972*b*) *N*-oxidation—an important route in the metabolism of methadone in man. *J. Pharm. Pharmacol. 24*, 244

BECKETT, A. H. & SALAMI, M. A. (1972*c*) A note on the identification of *N*-hydroxyphenmetrazine as a metabolic product of phendimetrazine and phenmetrazine. *J. Pharm. Pharmacol. 24*, 900–902

BECKETT, A. H. & AL-SARRAJ, S. (1972*d*) *N*-oxidation of primary and secondary amines to give hydroxylamines—A general metabolic route. *J. Pharm. Pharmacol. 24*, 916–917

BECKETT, A. H., COUTTS, R. T. & OGUNBONA, F. A. (1973*a*) *N*-ethyl-α-methyl-α-(*m*-trifluoromethylbenzyl) nitrone—the major *in vitro* metabolic product of fenfluramine in guinea pig liver microsomal fractions. *J. Pharm. Pharmacol. 25*, 190–192

BECKETT, A. H. & AL-SARRAJ, S. (1973*b*) The identification, properties and analysis of *N*-hydroxy-amphetamine—a metabolite of amphetamine. *J. Pharm. Pharmacol. 25*, 328–334

BECKETT, A. H. & ESSIEN, E. E. (1973*c*) Chlorpromazine 'hydroxylamines' in red blood cells as major metabolites of chlorpromazine in man. *J. Pharm. Pharmacol. 25*, 188–189

BECKETT, A. H. & AL-SARRAJ, S. (1973*d*) Metabolism of amitriptyline, nortriptyline, imipramine & desipramine to yield hydroxylamines. *J. Pharm. Pharmacol. 25*, 335–336

BECKETT, A. H., COUTTS, R. T. & OGUNBONA, F. A. (1973*e*) Metabolism of amphetamines. Identification of *N*-oxygenated products by gas chromatography and mass spectrometry. *J. Pharm. Pharmacol. 25*, 708–717

TESTA, B. & BECKETT, A. H. (1973) Metabolism and excretion of diethylpropion in man under acidic urine conditions. *J. Pharm. Pharmacol. 25*, 119–124

VAUGHAN, D. P. & BECKETT, A. H. (1973) A note on the chemical change of pentazocine in aqueous acidic media. *J. Pharm. Pharmacol. 25*, 993–995

Discussion

Riess: We have a problem similar to yours when we are developing new drugs and want to study their metabolism in detail, Professor Beckett. Our way out of the dilemma is to use an internal standard which is the same substance as the one we want to measure. One can either label the internal standard with a stable isotope and use mass spectrometric techniques or take a ^{14}C-labelled compound as the internal standard and use a radioisotope derivative method. Of course, when trying to measure metabolites we have to provide the metabolite in labelled form first. A practical way of doing this is to administer a labelled drug to animals, isolate the relevant metabolite in labelled form, and then use it as an internal standard for analysing biological fluids in man.

Beckett: Routinely we use either hepatic 10 000 g supernatants or microsomes and concentrate on the actual chemistry. Time invested in the problems of handling the materials and looking at them is well worth while but I don't think there is any short cut from studying the chemistry of the actual compounds. Of course, we don't know how to look for compounds if we don't know whether they exist, but the principles of metabolism have been established so we ought to know the possible compounds for which to look. I now look routinely for nitroxides, hydroperoxides etc., some of which are stable enough to handle. As we begin to understand more about *N*-oxidation mechanisms we realize the importance of investigations of this type of structure. In the future we will know more of the chemistry and avoid the mistakes of the past.

Holmstedt: If the ideal internal standard, labelled with a stable isotope, is added at the beginning of the procedure, then with GLC-MS one would end up with the same number of chemical artifacts for both the stable isotope compound and the other one. Those wouldn't be got rid of even though the internal standard is ideal for measuring the parent drug.

Curry: True, and you might have more gas phase reactions going on too. There are so many breakdown products now that you can get, not just four, but eight on one column.

Holmstedt: Yes, but if you have a sufficiently specific detector, you wouldn't notice that.

Prescott: Is the instability that you found in the metabolites of basic drugs present also in other major groups of compounds, Professor Beckett?

Beckett: Yes. The key is the oxidation of the α-carbon to the nitrogen atom in tertiary bases to give unstable aminoalcohols which dealkylate. We know about such unstable compounds only by inference. With slightly more stable compounds as hydroxylamines and nitrones, we can get our quantitative answers directly by analysis. We can build this information into our consideration of rate processes. In all our work we are trying to establish certain key compounds and rates and then use analogue and digital computer programs for whole processes. This will help us to understand metabolic processes inside man. This applies to any metabolic products. I doubt now whether there are any really true metabolites for basic compounds on the basic centre except *N*-oxides, hydroxylamines, nitroxides and nitrones.

Prescott: In clinical practice we are obliged to think about the concentration of a barbiturate rather than hydroxylated side-chain derivatives. Do problems of the same magnitude arise with the parent drugs?

Beckett: Not if we are careful. We ought to know the chemistry of the parent drug, how it interacts with solvents and how to analyse it without breakdown. That puts most parent drugs into a different category from the labile metabolites, which may not be readily synthesized. Recently we have been able to synthesize many hydroxylamines and nitrones from widely used drugs. Now we are beginning to investigate their toxicity, pharmacology, etc. To begin with, many investigators thought that because they couldn't find them these hydroxylamines we were reporting were figments of our imagination. This illustrates the difficulty of judging unstable metabolites when their chemistry is not yet established.

Gillette: Dihydrodiols and mercapturic acids are classic examples of what you are talking about. The biochemistry books used to show the mercapturic acid of bromobenzene with a phenyl group. The compound actually excreted in the urine, however, is a dihydro-3-hydroxy analogue of the mercapturic acid. The original workers acidified urine in order to extract the mercapturic acid into organic solvents. But under acidic conditions the metabolite is dehydrated to form the bromophenylmercapturic acid. The same thing happens with the dihydrodiol of bromobenzene. Acidification dehydrates it to bromophenol. For many years, other dihydrodiol metabolites of drugs, such as diphenylhydantoin (phenytoin), which is now known to be excreted as a dihydrodiol, couldn't be found because investigators first acidified the urine before they extracted the metabolites into organic solvents. Another classic example is thalidomide. On a gas chromatography column some of the metabolites can become dehydrated to form thalidomide again, so what appeared to be unchanged thalidomide was really a metabolite.

Beckett: Metabolic work and kinetic studies will get more complicated. Some drugs metabolize to hydroxylamines and to primary amines but then we have a reverse metabolic reaction going on all the time. Some primary amines are methylated fast *in vivo* whereas their parent dimethylamine compounds are demethylated. We are trying to work out the rate processes in the *in vivo* situation. *N*-oxides are primary metabolites of some drugs *in vitro* but frequently one doesn't find more than low concentrations in urine because *in vivo* *N*-oxide reductases are present. In the end we must place metabolic studies on a kinetic basis. This means that we must be sure that the structures we are measuring are not artifacts of the separation and analytical techniques being used.

Scott: Most of my time is spent on instrumental methods of analysis and I find it very refreshing—but depressing—that you should bring these points out. We have been trying to improve the situation. One of the gentlest methods of separation is high pressure liquid chromatography. This can be run at sub-ambient temperatures, if necessary, to slow down many reactions that may occur. I think we must modify our separation techniques, not just to get better resolution but to maintain stability in the separation system. Liquid chromatography at low temperatures shows great promise in this direction.

Jackson: Your warning about the extraction method is very useful, Professor Beckett. Do you think comparative extraction has a place in determining whether what is identified has been produced during extraction or is real? That is, could you do an extraction with ether and compare that with results you get by extraction with dichloromethane or hexane?

Beckett: Once I have obtained the metabolites as chemical entities the problems become soluble. Until one has obtained the compounds, one doesn't know where the problems lie. After that, we use different analytical methods and compare the results. For some of these hydroxylamines we routinely use four or five different analytical techniques to try to find accurately how much is present.

Jackson: What you say implies that the clinical and forensic toxicologists, who don't know what they are looking for to start with, should not rely on one particular extraction method.

Beckett: Yes, of course. We all know the problems but perhaps we don't pay enough attention to the losses. Once we know the chemistry of compounds in systems being used we can advise people what to do. Many chlorohydrocarbons are used to extract bases. Then the evaporating techniques cause problems: simple transfer of some drugs in solution from tube to tube leads to substantial losses of the drug on the glass surfaces.

Sunshine: I am shattered by these findings, Professor Beckett. When you compared the injection of the same material into different gas chromatographs, you obtained different materials. Did you mean that this was because the injection points were different, that is the physical parameters on each of those instruments were different and consequently the labile compound reacted differently?

Beckett: Yes. Some compounds are broken down by ionization of the gas. There are metal-catalysed reactions of some compounds and where a metal needle is being used the solution must be injected quickly, if heat is conducted to the needle in the instrument used. Even instruments of the same make and model number can differ slightly, in terms of injection block, metal surfaces, etc. For our work on hydroxylamines of aralkylamines, two instruments lead to little breakdown of compounds, but others of the same make and model lead to extensive breakdown even when the same columns are used.

Prescott: We have seen the same thing when just a simple mixture of barbiturates was injected into an injection port with a hot metal liner.

Scott: In this type of work, if you have a gas chromatograph with a high temperature injection system I would advise you to throw it away and use on-column injection.

Beckett: Some of the injection ports were not heated.

Scott: They were not on-column injections?

Beckett: No. The problem is that the gas is carrying the compounds through the column and if the gas is ionized direct on-column injection still leads to breakdown.

Scott: Invariably it will help, because the solution will rapidly get to the stationary phase and in doing so become diluted.

Beckett: You still have the same problem.

Holmstedt: How do these experiments come out if you use capillary columns?

Beckett: We have not used them for this work.

Leach: Many of these difficulties are due to injection port heaters—large lumps of reactive metal at high temperatures.

Curry: What is an inert solvent, Professor Beckett?

Beckett: If we had to use a heavier than water solvent we would normally use a chlorohydrocarbon. We make use of the very simple chemical principle that the attack of the nitrogen is a nucleophilic attack on the carbon of the chlorohydrocarbon and we alter the rate of the reaction by altering the polarity of the solvent. We therefore use mixed solvents and alter the rate of quaternization by increasing the hydrocarbon component in the mixture sufficiently to depress that rate process as far as possible but with retention of sufficient extracting power in the mixture. Carbon tetrachloride is a much more inert solvent than is chloroform or methylene dichloride.

Scott: We have a system similar to yours. It is a continuous procedure. We put a sequence of 12 solvents through a liquid chromatographic column, starting with a completely non-polar solvent, heptane, and ending with water. In our experience decomposition takes place when one uses a solvent that is more polar than is needed to obtain solubility. One of our standard procedures is to inject, say, a sample of a fermentation broth onto the front of a column and then progress stepwise through these series of solvents. We get perfectly good and reproducible chromatograms because we always extract each solute with the solvent of lowest possible polarity.

Beckett: That is a good point about polarity. I agree with you. However, for nitrogen compounds, solvents with the same polarity may have different reactivities with the basic group.

Leach: When you do the gas chromatography what solvent is injected? We are worrying about the reactivity of what are generally thought to be inert solvents, yet we dissolve a compound in a similar solvent and inject it into something heated to over 100 °C. Something is quite likely to happen at that stage, no matter what has happened earlier.

Beckett: It depends on the solvent. If ether is purified, it is not a bad solvent for most of this work. Obviously, a trace of ether peroxide will destroy many primary and secondary amines. Simple hydrocarbon solvents are useful but of course do not extract many of the main polar drugs and metabolites. I would not use chlorohydrocarbon solvents unless I wanted a heavier than water solvent for some reason.

Curry: The clinicians need to know what the figures mean.

Brown: It would be very helpful if clinicians knew the scope and the limitations of our analytical methods. One basic problem is the reproducibility of columns in gas–liquid chromatography. A GLC column may work wonderfully for a particular separation for several months, but after that time its performance deteriorates and we may never get another column like it. This obviously bears on the general problem of performance and usefulness of GLC assays.

Leach: If one or two columns are being used for a number of purposes, after a short time the columns contain a lot of totally unknown residues. It is not the stationary phase alone that is being chromatographed then but also bits of liver fat and all the other things that have been injected. Again, a column may not work at first but after a short time it does work, simply because enough impurities have been added.

Scott: That explains how it changes, but how do we get another column the same? This really needs stringent standardization of the apparatus, the support and the stationary phase. To run a standard and repeatable analysis by gas chromatography it is advisable to buy a stock of a particular stationary phase or a particular support and keep it only for the purpose.

Agurell: We were all much happier a few years ago when things were much more stable than they are today! We used to collect urine under what we thought were normal conditions, with preservative, etc. However in one study, after collecting the urine in a glass tube cooled with carbon dioxide, we found that the pattern of the metabolites was quite different. Now we have been trying to use less sophisticated techniques, such as TLC, to check that we have the same metabolite pattern all the way, including throughout the isolation procedure.

Beckett: The biological specimens themselves should certainly have the same attention as the analysis. When an internal standard compound is used as well as the compound being measured, many workers without much experience can produce a calibration curve, but almost invariably they draw through the origin. But the curve doesn't have to go through the origin at all when extraction from biological specimens is involved. Then inexperienced workers often use a calculation factor rather than the actual slope. Also, if the analysis involves precipitating protein, the difference between the loss of the internal standard compound and what we are trying to measure can be great. How accurate are figures obtained for lignocaine (lidocaine) in blood, for example if the added compound is bound to a different extent than is lignocaine?

Curry: What effect do trace elements have on samples in syringes or in plastic containers?

Prescott: And what happens to the sample between the time it leaves the patient and the time it arrives in the laboratory? It may be left on a shelf over a radiator, where bacteria can grow in it for a day.

Curry: Are we perhaps falling into our own trap by calling chloroform or ethylene dichloride pure when they are only 99% pure?

Beckett: The material in chloroform reacting fastest with bases is the impurity contained in that chloroform. This fact emerged many years ago in alkaloidal chemistry.

Sunshine: Some work has been done on the storage of samples of urine in glass and various types of plastic containers. This storage problem could be a Pandora's box.

Scott: The point about solvents ought to be amplified a little. In the system with 12 solvents that I mentioned, ordinary spectroscopically pure solvents are run in a series of increasing polarity through a liquid chromatographic column. Each time the solvent is changed, we get a peak of materials with high boiling points that were in the previously used 'pure' solvents. We found that to get anything like pure solvents we had to run them through a layer of molecular sieve, a layer of charcoal and then a layer of silica gel. The product is still not 100% pure but it is much improved. This sort of purification is essential for solvents used for either extraction or liquid chromatography, otherwise one obtains spurious results from the solvent impurities.

Prescott: Selective detectors can help with the solvent impurity problem, in certain circumstances.

Curry: With the simple test for salicylate that Dr Newton uses, he detects concentrations of 50 mg/100 ml blood. Later we will be talking about nanograms —a million times smaller. It is impossible to clear out impurities in the solvents at this level, and I wonder what the analytical complications will be there. These few parts per million assume massive proportions when one is dealing with such small quantities.

Beckett: At these levels most compounds simply decompose in the systems used.

Sunshine: If a person has taken amphetamine, for forensic or clinical purposes all I need to know is whether he has taken more than a therapeutic dose or even an enormous dose, not whether amphetamine metabolites are present or the concentration of each of these. For example, I may want to know whether, in the race that he just ran, he was jazzed up enough for the amphetamine to have contributed to his performance. Was it there at all and, if so, was it there in very large amounts? Where does what you discussed so well fit into that picture, Professor Beckett?

Beckett: What I discussed does not apply to compounds as stable as amphetamine unless one has used an incorrect solvent, for example ether containing peroxides. We can obtain the right figure for the drug in the urine collected at a particular time but this figure does not indicate how much the man took, unless it is known when he took it and the urinary pH, etc. From the pH of the urine and the time of dose and of urinary collection I can get a rough idea of the dose taken.

Curry: But can we still rely on these standard chemical methods?

Beckett: Providing we are dealing with reasonably stable compounds, as most of the parent drugs are—at least we can devise techniques which don't break them down—then we can rely on the figure we get.

Curry: I would like to draw attention to the increasing use of the internal standard technique over the last four years. Surely this is our best approach?

Jackson: There has also been an increasing use of non-polar solvents.

Evaluation of chromatographic and spectroscopic procedures*

A. C. MOFFAT

Home Office Central Research Establishment, Aldermaston, Reading, Berkshire

Abstract Chromatographic and spectroscopic techniques are widely used for identifying drugs extracted from biological fluids. The most important features of an analysis are (*a*) speed, (*b*) sensitivity, (*c*) distribution of the physicochemical constants among the substances tested, (*d*) reproducibility and (*e*) correlation of results when more than one system is used. The last three features may be considered together by measurements of the discriminating power, defined as the probability that two drugs selected at random from a large number will be discriminated.

Paper chromatographic (PC) and thin-layer chromatographic (TLC) systems can have discriminating powers of 0.78, whereas the best gas–liquid chromatographic (GLC) system has a much higher discriminating power (0.967); GLC is also a much more sensitive technique than either PC or TLC. Different stationary phases used in GLC have high correlation coefficients (0.71 to 0.99), which makes the use of more than one column of little value, but five PC and TLC systems have very low correlations and can therefore be used together.

The best technique is infrared spectroscopy (discriminating power 0.998 with six peaks). Ultraviolet spectroscopy in 0.05M-sulphuric acid has a discriminating power of 0.88, which rises to 0.908 when the spectrum is re-run in strongly alkaline solution.

Discriminating power can therefore be used to evaluate and compare the effectiveness of different techniques used for identifying drugs.

Before an unknown drug in a biological fluid can be identified it must be extracted and examined by appropriate physicochemical techniques. The characteristics observed can then be compared with data from reference collections until a unique identity is found for the drug being tested. The techniques most popular for this purpose are those of chromatography and spectroscopy, and I shall describe how they may be evaluated so that a drug may be identified with the minimum of work and in the shortest possible time. We may even get close to answering the question 'How much information is required before a drug can be said to be identified?'

METHOD OF EVALUATION

Before a technique can be evaluated, its important features must be recognized and a method of measuring its effectiveness must be devised so that comparisons can be made. Excluding the capital cost of equipment, the important features to be considered are:

(*a*) Sensitivity: in general, the more sensitive techniques are the most useful, especially when an extract is being screened for drugs;

(*b*) Time taken for the analysis: this should be as short as possible;

(*c*) Distribution of the measured values of all the possible drugs over the useful range of the technique: as many drugs as possible should have different values so that they may be discriminated;

(*d*) Reproducibility of the measurements: the interlaboratory reproducibility should be as good as possible;

(*e*) Correlation of results between systems or techniques: if two systems are closely correlated, as some chromatographic systems are, the use of the second system will give no further useful information.

A way of measuring the effectiveness of a procedure for identifying a drug has been devised which takes (*c*), (*d*) and (*e*) into account and expresses the result as a single figure (Moffat *et al.* 1974*a*). This measurement is 'discriminating power', defined as the probability that two drugs selected at random from a large number will be discriminated. It is calculated by comparing the measured physicochemical constants (e.g. R_f values) for each drug in turn with the constants for each of all the other drugs. If the constants are within a predetermined error (E), they are considered to be undiscriminated (or matched) and the total number of matches from all the drugs is designated M. The total number of possible matches is $N(N-1)/2$ (where N = total number of drugs) and therefore the probability of two drugs selected at random being matched is $2M/N(N-1)$. Hence,

$$\text{Discriminating power} = 1 - 2M/N(N-1)$$

Provided that the measured values are rectangularly distributed over the total population, the maximum discriminating power (DP) that can be obtained from a single system can be calculated from the expression

$$DP_{max} = 1 - 2E + E^2$$

Discriminating power will be used here to evaluate a number of chromatographic and spectroscopic techniques used for the identification of basic drugs (that is, drugs extracted from alkaline aqueous solutions by organic solvents).

CHROMATOGRAPHY

The techniques of paper chromatography (PC), thin-layer chromatography (TCL) and gas–liquid chromatography (GLC) are well established. With the newer high pressure liquid chromatography (HPLC), they are among the techniques most useful in drug analysis since they separate drugs as well as identify them. Only PC, TLC and GLC are considered here as too little information is available for a complete evaluation of HPLC.

Paper chromatography and thin-layer chromatography

PC is the least sensitive of the chromatographic techniques, requiring 10–20 μg of drug whereas TLC requires only 1–5 μg. The detection limits of both PC and TLC can be improved by an order of magnitude if an appropriate spray reagent is chosen, or in some cases by using ultraviolet (UV) light. Successive spraying of a drug spot with different reagents may be the best way of ensuring that a spot is detected.

One of the major disadvantages of PC is that it may take between 5 and 18 hours for analysis to be completed, depending on whether the run is made in descending or ascending conditions. In contrast, a reversed-phase paper system that uses aqueous buffer solution at a high temperature may only take 20 minutes for a 10 cm run (Street 1962*a*,*b*), while with TLC an 0.25 mm plate normally takes 1–1.5 hours to run 10 cm. Better spots may be obtained with smaller quantities of material and thinner TLC plates, e.g. of 0.10 mm thickness, but the slower running time (2–4 h) is a severe disadvantage.

Table 1 lists 14 PC and TLC systems which we have studied in detail. The R_f values of 100 drugs chemically and pharmacologically representative of the basic drugs in common use have been determined with these systems and their discriminating powers have been measured.

Fig. 1 shows two systems with vastly different distributions of R_f values across the plates. In System 8, 61 % of the R_f values were less than 0.10 and this explains why it has such a poor discriminating power ($DP_8 = 0.55$). On the other hand, System 3 has a very good distribution of R_f values and consequently a good discriminating power ($DP_3 = 0.75$).

In the past, PC has been more reproducible than TLC, but with modern precoated plates the errors of measurement of R_f values are about the same with either form of chromatography. The errors can be reduced enormously if standards are run at the same time as the test drugs and a linear regression is used to calculate corrected R_f values (Galanos & Kapoulas 1964; Dhont *et al.* 1970). In this way the error factors can be kept as low as 0.10, and an error factor of 0.10 in each system was therefore assumed when the discriminating

TABLE 1

Paper and thin-layer systems studied

System No.	*Adsorbent or paper*	*Solvent*	*DP**
1	Silica gel dipped or prepared with 0.1M–KOH	Cyclohexane–benzene–diethyl-amine (75:15:10)	0.73
2	Silica gel dipped or prepared with 0.1M–KOH	Methanol	0.69
3	Silica gel dipped or prepared with 0.1M–KOH	Acetone	0.75
4	Silica gel dipped or prepared with 0.1M–$KHSO_4$	Methanol	0.66
5	Silica gel dipped or prepared with 0.1M-$KHSO_4$	Ethanol–water (95:5)	0.67
6	Whatman No. 1 paper dipped in 5% sodium dihydrogen citrate	Butanol–water–citric acid (87:13:0.48)	0.74
7	Whatman No. 1 paper dipped in 10% tributyrin in acetone	Acetate buffer (pH 4.58) run at 95 °C	0.75
8	Whatman No. 1 paper dipped in 10% tributyrin in acetone	Phosphate buffer (pH 7.4) run at 86 °C	0.55
9	Silica gel 60	Ethyl acetate–heptane–methanol–ammonia (0.88) (60:30:7.5:2.5)	0.72
10	Aluminium oxide (Type E)	Chloroform	0.71
11	Silica gel 60	Dioxane–chloroform–ethyl acetate–ammonia (0.88) (60:25:10:5)	0.57
12	Silica gel 60	Methanol–ammonia (0.88) (100:1.5)	0.63
13	Silica gel 60 sprayed with 0.1M-NaOH	Cyclohexane–toluene–diethylamine (75:15:10)	0.76
14	Silica gel 60 sprayed with 0.1M-NaOH	Chloroform–methanol (90:10)	0.78

* Discriminating power (DP) calculated using an error factor of 0.10 in R_f for each system.

powers given in Table 1 were calculated. From these data the best systems are Systems 14, 13 and 3. Although System 6 is a paper system and therefore the sensitivity of detection is not as good as that of a TLC system, a cellulose TLC plate (0.25 mm or 0.10 mm thickness) with the same solvent system will give equivalent R_f values, with equivalent reproducibility (Haywood & Moss 1968; Smalldon 1971).

When systems are highly correlated the order of running in one system is very similar to that in the second. The result of using two such systems is that little further information is gained and a two-dimensional chromatogram (e.g. Fig. 2) shows this to be true. The combined discriminating power of the two systems ($DP_{4,5} = 0.76$) is therefore not much better than the individual discriminating powers ($DP_4 = 0.66$; $DP_5 = 0.67$).

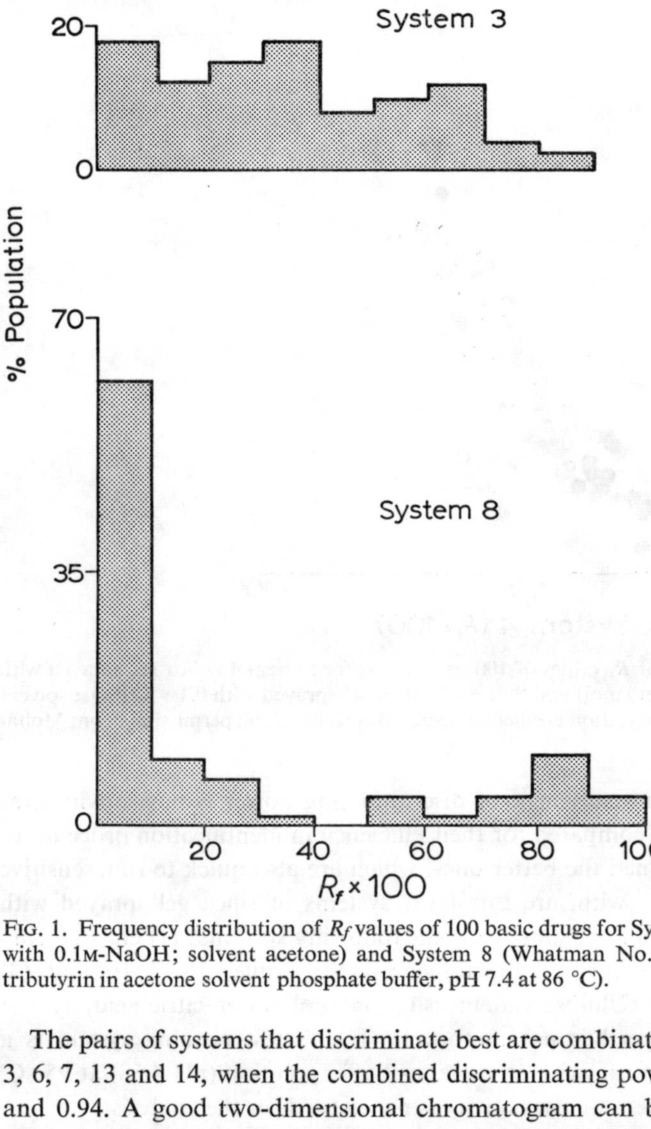

FIG. 1. Frequency distribution of R_f values of 100 basic drugs for System 3 (silica gel sprayed with 0.1M-NaOH; solvent acetone) and System 8 (Whatman No. 1 paper dipped in 10% tributyrin in acetone solvent phosphate buffer, pH 7.4 at 86 °C).

The pairs of systems that discriminate best are combinations between Systems 3, 6, 7, 13 and 14, when the combined discriminating powers are between 0.93 and 0.94. A good two-dimensional chromatogram can be obtained with two TLC systems, 13 and 14 (Fig. 3), and this is the best combination to choose when two systems are needed. Further combinations of systems enable even better discriminating powers to be obtained. The best combination of any three systems is 7, 13 and 14 ($DP_{7,\,13,\,14} = 0.982$), with any combination of three from Systems 3, 6, 7, 13 and 14 giving a combined discriminating power of 0.98. If four systems are to be used the discriminating power increases to 0.994 with Systems 6, 7, 13 and 14.

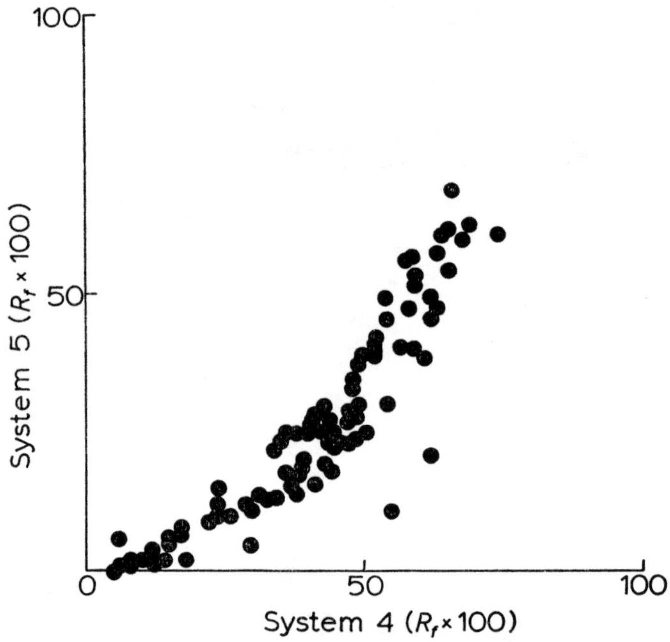

FIG. 2. The correlation of R_f values of 100 basic drugs for System 4 (silica gel sprayed with 0.1M-$KHSO_4$; solvent methanol) and System 5 (silica gel sprayed with 0.1M-$KHSO_4$; solvent ethanol–water, 95:5). Correlation coefficient 0.902. (Reproduced, by permission, from Moffat & Smalldon 1974.)

The value of the measurement of discriminating power is now obvious, as systems can easily be compared for their efficiency in identification procedures. Of the systems examined the better ones, which are also quick to run, sensitive and pleasant to work with, are thin-layer systems of silica gel sprayed with 0.1M-NaOH, dried and run using one of the following solvents: (1) chloroform–methanol, 90:10, (2) cyclohexane–toluene–diethylamine, 75:15:10 and (3) acetone. A thin-layer cellulose system using butanol–water–citric acid, 87:13: 0.48, is suitable if speed is not important. The fastest running system is a reversed-phase system run with an aqueous buffer solution (pH 4.58) at 95 °C, which can be used when high sensitivity is not needed for the analysis.

Gas–liquid chromatography

This is the most sensitive of the chromatographic procedures, the limits of sensitivity being about 10–100 ng with a flame-ionization detector. More specific detectors, e.g. halogen detectors, may not give an absolute increase in sensitivity, but because the background level is reduced a relative increase in

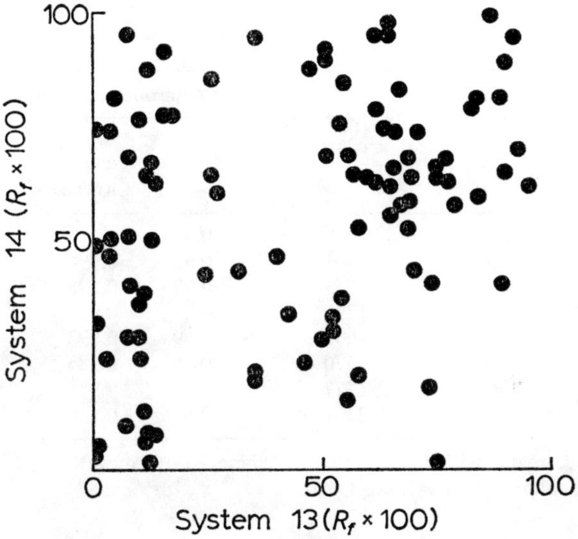

FIG. 3. The correlation of R_f values of 100 basic drugs for System 13 (silica gel sprayed with 0.1M-NaOH; solvent cyclohexane–toluene–diethylamine, 75:15:10) and System 14 (silica gel sprayed with 0.1M-NaOH; solvent chloroform–methanol, 90:10). Correlation coefficient 0.33.

both sensitivity and specificity may be obtained. The most sensitive detector, the electron capture detector, can detect picogram quantities of halogenated drugs or derivatives of drugs.

The time an analysis takes depends on the way the technique is used. A single gas chromatograph with a non-polar stationary phase can be programmed at 5 °C/min and cover a temperature range of 100–300 °C in 40 min, which should elute nearly all drugs with molecular weights of 100 to 400. If several gas chromatographs are available and are used isothermally, the analysis time can be reduced to 10–15 min/sample. Here the only disadvantage is the capital cost of the instruments compared to the negligible cost with PC and TLC.

Over 300 stationary phases have been used in GLC at one time or another, although only a handful have been extensively used for drug analysis. Columns with mixtures of phases have been prepared but single phases are more generally used, the choice usually being based on the polarity of the column. Table 2 lists eight GLC columns covering the complete range of polarities, as expressed by their McReynolds constants (McReynolds 1970), that can be used for the drug analysis.

The distributions of the retention indices of 62 drugs on the eight columns are practically the same (Fig. 4). However, only the SE-30 column elutes all the drugs, followed by the OV-17 column which elutes 58. The more polar columns

TABLE 2

Gas-liquid chromatographic data for eight GLC columns

*Stationary phase**	*Maximum operating temperature* (°C)	*McReynolds constant†*	*Discriminating power*	
			Alone	*In combination with SE-30*
SE-30	350	249	0.97	—
Apiezon L–KOH	300	301	0.90	0.990
OV-17	350	853	0.97	0.992
Carbowax 20M–KOH	230	1296	0.82	0.989
Carbowax 20M	230	1603	0.89	0.993
Cyclohexane–dimethanol succinate	230	1670	0.75	0.985
Diethylene glycol succinate–KOH	190	1777	0.76	0.984
Diethylene glycol succinate	190	2301	0.84	0.990

* On Chromosorb G (acid-washed, treated with dichlorodimethylsilane, 80–100 mesh)
† A measure of the polarity of the column (McReynolds 1970)

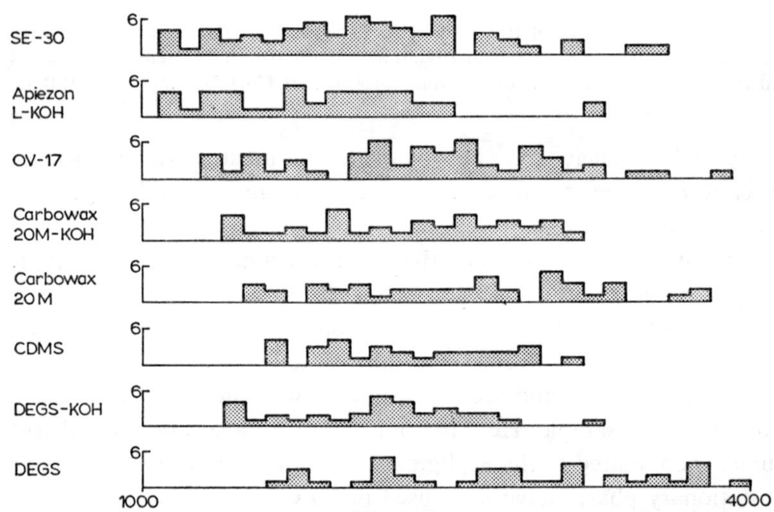

FIG. 4. Frequency distribution of retention indices of some basic drugs on GLC columns of different polarities. (Reproduced, by permission, from Moffat *et al.* 1974*b*). CDMS: cyclohexane–dimethanol succinate; DEGS: diethylene glycol succinate.

show varying degrees of success, with the cyclohexane–dimethanol succinate and diethylene glycol succinate–KOH columns eluting only about half the drugs (30 and 33 respectively). The lower operating temperature maxima explain why the more polar columns, compared with those of the low polarity phases, fail to elute substances of larger molecular weights. In addition, although KOH-

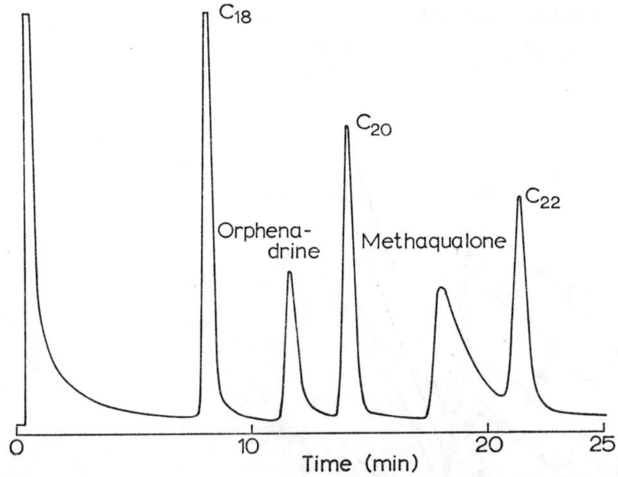

FIG. 5. Chromatogram of orphenadrine (retention index = 1927), methaqualone (retention index = 2095), and hydrocarbon standards on a 2% SE-30 column temperature programmed from 160 °C at 2 °C/min.

treated columns give better peaks because KOH reduces the adsorptive power of the support material, such treatment prevents the elution of phenolic bases and decomposes the more thermolabile alkaloids.

Whether retention indices are determined isothermally or methylene units × 100 are obtained by temperature programming, peaks that differ by more than 20 units can be distinguished easily (e.g. Fig. 5). However, the reproducibility of retention indices generally decreases as the polarity of the phase increases. On individual columns operated at one temperature, the indices are always within ± 10 on the non-polar and slightly polar phases and within ± 25 on the more polar columns. The interlaboratory variation in retention indices is probably about ± 30 and ± 50 respectively, and these values have been used as error factors in calculating the discriminating powers of the different stationary phases (Table 2).

As the polarity of the stationary phase increases the discriminating powers of the columns fall rapidly, due to fewer compounds being eluted and the greater reproducibility of retention indices of the low polarity phases. If only one column is to be chosen for drug analysis by GLC it should obviously be either the SE-30 or OV-17 column.

If more than one column is to be used, then the chosen columns should show different elution patterns for the drugs. Unfortunately, this cannot be achieved since the basic drugs on each chromatographic column behave similarly. In only two cases out of the eleven shown (Fig. 6) is the order of elution different on

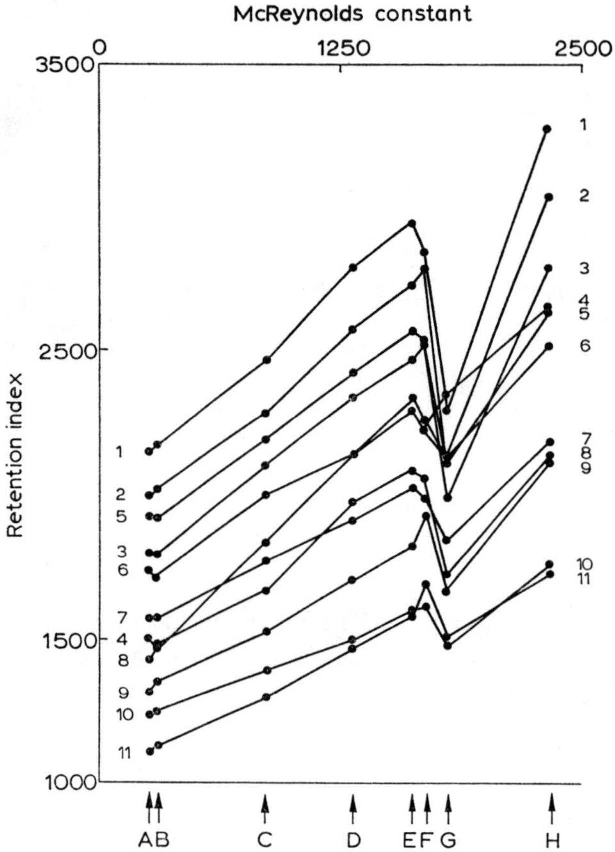

FIG. 6. Changes in retention indices of some basic drugs with the polarity of the GLC column. (A, SE-30; B, Apiezon L–KOH; C, OV-17; D, Carbowax 20M–KOH; E, Carbowax 20M; F, cyclohexane–dimethanol succinate; G, diethylene glycol succinate–KOH; H, diethylene glycol succinate; 1, bromodiphenhydramine; 2, chlorpheniramine; 3, pheniramine; 4, nikethamide; 5, orphenadrine; 6, pethidine; 7, amylocaine; 8, phenmetrazine; 9, chlorphentermine; 10, mephentermine; 11, amphetamine). (Reproduced, by permission, from Moffat *et al.* 1974*b*.)

the least polar phase from that on the most polar phase. Diethylene glycol succinate–KOH (G in Fig. 6) is a special case, and here the alkali is probably interfering with the polyester bonding to cause this change.

The correlation between columns makes the use of more than one GLC column of little value for the identification of basic drugs. If an SE-30 column is used first, then another with a low polarity phase, e.g. OV-17, will give almost the same elution pattern (correlation coefficient of retention indices = 0.991). If a more polar phase is used in conjunction with the SE-30 then the elution characteristics become slightly different (correlation coefficient of SE-30–diethylene glycol succinate–KOH = 0.71), but the more polar column elutes only half the drugs. Table 2 shows that the discriminating powers of the columns, in combination with an SE-30 column, are about the same, i.e. the lower correlations of the polar columns with the SE-30 column are completely offset by the smaller number of compounds they elute.

In conclusion, when large numbers of basic drugs of varying chemical and chromatographic properties have to be analysed, a non-polar column such as SE-30 is the best choice as a stationary phase. A second column is only of limited value and the use of another physicochemical technique is advocated unless sensitivity of detection is essential for the analysis.

SPECTROSCOPY

Spectroscopic techniques are amongst the oldest used for the identification of drugs and today ultraviolet (UV) and infrared (IR) spectroscopy play a large part in many laboratories. Nuclear magnetic resonance (NMR) spectroscopy is not so useful because of the large capital cost and lack of sensitivity (1–50 mg of drug are required), while fluorescence methods have only recently been used for more than a handful of drugs and few collections of data are yet available.

The information gained with spectroscopy is often of an absolute nature, i.e. particular molecular structures can be assigned to specific types of absorption, but searching techniques generally identify drugs by comparisons of absorption data with files of previously obtained data.

Ultraviolet spectroscopy

UV spectroscopy covers the range 230–400 nm in the electromagnetic spectrum. Below 230 nm problems from scattered light, bacterial metabolites in distilled water and solvent absorption effects are evident even when double-beam instruments are used.

Organic extracts from biological materials suspected of containing drugs are usually re-extracted into 0.05M-sulphuric acid and the spectrum is then run. A few drops of concentrated alkali are added to raise the pH to > 13 and any shift in absorbance is noted. These two steps complete the analysis and the data obtained are used for the search. The whole procedure takes about 10 min and is much quicker than chromatographic methods of analysis.

Experiments carried out in nine laboratories with 11 different spectrophotometers (all Perkin-Elmer or Pye Unicam instruments) indicated that an error of 2 nm is suitable for spectra obtained from both acid and alkaline solutions

(A. C. Moffat & G. W. Owen, unpublished). Better results are claimed by the instrument specifications (less than ± 1 nm from 200–500 nm) but other factors, such as the difficulty of assigning the position of maximum absorbance of a fairly flat peak, must be considered. Shifts of maxima after the 0.05M-sulphuric acid solution has been made alkaline can only be recognized if they are larger than about 2 nm, since small changes may be due to the different absorption characteristics of the new solvent.

Spectra of 100 drugs were obtained in 0.05M-sulphuric acid and in strongly alkaline solutions. The drugs could be divided into five main groups, according to the intensity of absorption:

(1) Virtually no spectrum at all: these are drugs which are fully saturated, or contain a single bond, and therefore do not absorb, e.g. cyclopentamine.

(2) Sufficient absorptions to be detected, but with no absorption maximum between 230 and 400 nm: the high background absorbance of co-extracted material means that peaks below 230 nm cannot be used, e.g. that for pyrrobutamine.

(3) Spectra with peaks between 230 and 400 nm but with extinction coefficients ($E^{1\%}_{1\,cm}$) of less than 20: drugs extracted from biological material will generally not be seen, due to the low absorbance of the molecule, e.g. benzenoid drugs such as amphetamine, lignocaine (lidocaine), etc.

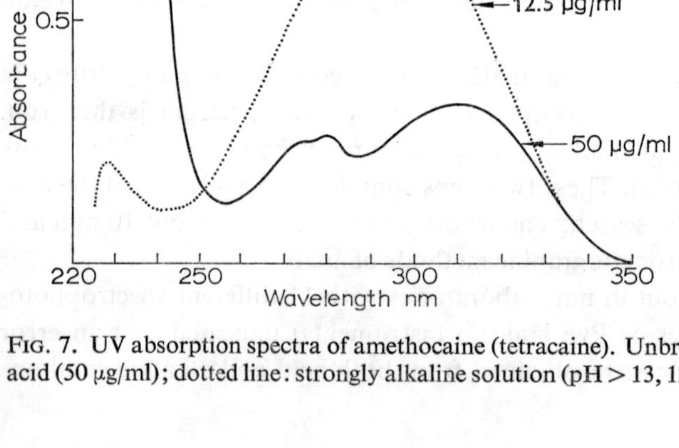

FIG. 7. UV absorption spectra of amethocaine (tetracaine). Unbroken line: 0.05 M-sulphuric acid (50 µg/ml); dotted line: strongly alkaline solution (pH > 13, 12.5 µg/ml).

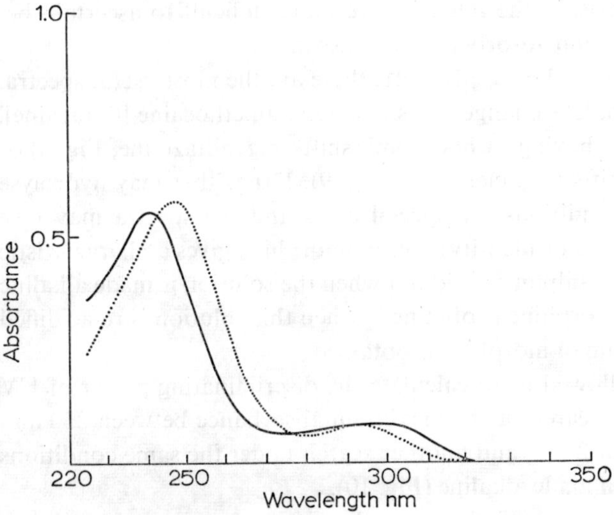

FIG. 8. UV absorption spectra of antazoline (10 μg/ml). Unbroken line: 0.05M-sulphuric acid; dotted line: strongly alkaline solution (pH > 13).

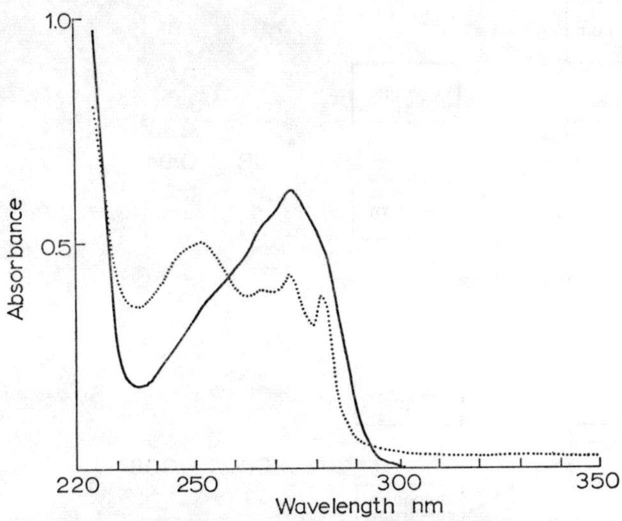

FIG. 9. UV absorption spectra of clemizole (20 μg/ml). Unbroken line: 0.05M-sulphuric acid; dotted line: strongly alkaline solution (pH > 13).

(4) Good spectra but with no detectable changes in the position of maximum absorbance when the solution is made alkaline: this would include all those drugs which precipitate under alkaline conditions (e.g. benzphetamine) as well as those which have no pH shift, e.g. caffeine and

meclozine. Changes in the intensity are more difficult to ascertain because the background absorbance may also alter.

(5) Good spectra which show a pH shift: these are the most useful spectra, some being complete changes in shape (e.g. amethocaine [tetracaine], Fig. 7) and others having bathochromic shifts (e.g. antazoline, Fig. 8) or hypsochromic shifts (e.g. clemizole, Fig. 9). Drugs that may hydrolyse under alkaline conditions are special cases and the spectra may give conclusive evidence of identity: e.g. diamorphine gives a characteristic spectrum in 0.05M-sulphuric acid but when the solution is made alkaline the spectrum of morphine is obtained; when this solution is re-acidified the acidic spectrum of morphine is obtained.

These classifications allowed us to calculate the discriminating power of UV spectroscopy, based on a search of the maximum absorbance between 230 and 400 nm, an error factor of 2 nm, and another search under the same conditions after the solution has been made alkaline (Fig. 10).

With fairly strong solutions of the pure drug, e.g. from a tablet, injection or syringe washing, only five drugs (in groups A and B above) out of

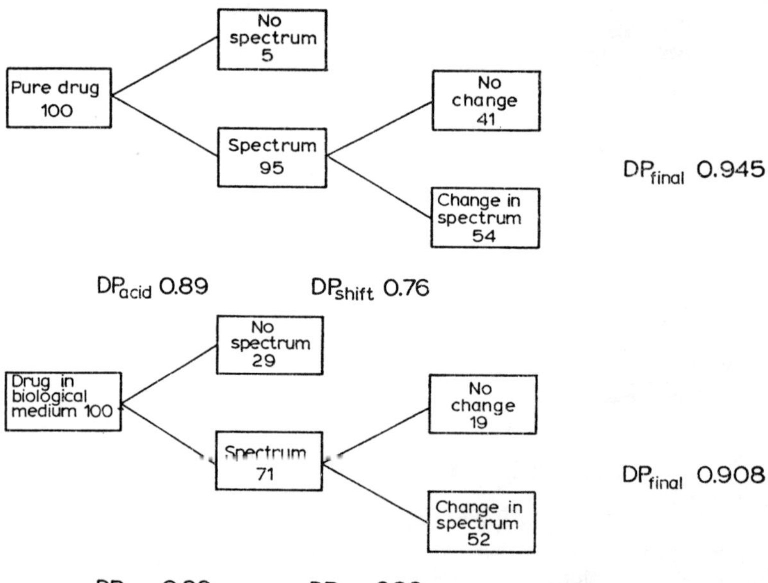

FIG. 10. Flow chart for the identification of 100 basic drugs by UV spectrophotometry. The first stage is the measurement of the absorption maximum in the spectrum between 230 and 400 nm. The second stage is the measurement of the shift of the maximum after the pH of the solution has been made strongly alkaline (pH > 13). The discriminating powers of each stage and of the procedure as a whole are calculated using error factors of 2 nm.

the 100 gave no spectrum and 54 of the other 95 produced pH shifts of spectral properties, giving a final discriminating power of 0.945. Drugs extracted from biological fluids were in much lower concentrations than the pure forms, and because of the interfering substances extracted at the same time 29 drugs had no spectrum. Of the remaining 71 drugs, 52 showed a change in spectrum and the final discriminating power was 0.908.

Infrared spectroscopy

IR spectroscopy is probably of more value in identifying an unknown drug than any of the other techniques I have referred to so far. The drug must be purified before analysis but this can often be done easily by elution from a paper or thin-layer chromatogram or by condensation of the effluent from a gas chromatograph. The main disadvantage is that hundreds of micrograms of material must usually be used unless an expensive instrument is available, such as the Perkin-Elmer 225 infrared spectrophotometer, or unless micro-discs are used in conventional instruments, when as little as 10 μg of material can give a spectrum of practical use. Analysis takes about half an hour, provided that a purified sample is available.

With a few exceptions every drug will give a different IR spectrum. Once a spectrum has been obtained for an unknown drug it is only necessary to reduce the number of possible identities to a reasonable level and then match the spectra. Our system (Curry *et al.* 1969) makes use of the major peaks in the 5.0–15.0 μm range of the spectrum. Peaks in the 6.7–7.6 μm range are excluded so that complications in examining the spectra obtained from Nujol mulls can be avoided. In the IR spectrum of zoxazolamine base (Fig. 11) the six major

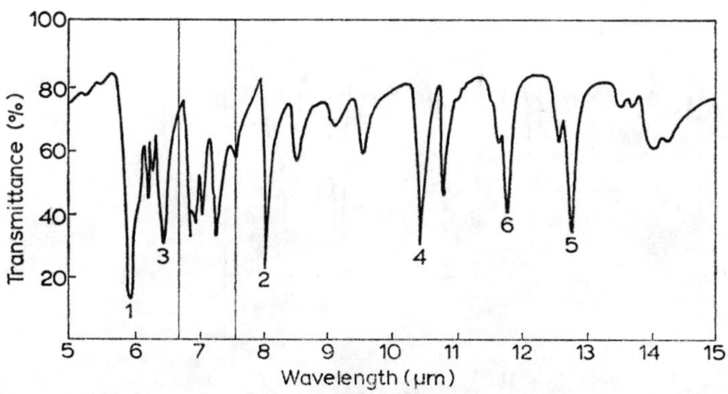

FIG. 11. IR spectrum of zoxazolamine (KBr disc). The six major peaks between 5 and 15 μm, but excluding the region 6.7–7.6 μm, are numbered in descending order of intensity.

TABLE 3

Discriminating power (DP) of infrared spectroscopy when several peaks are used in the search procedure

No. of peaks used	*DP, ignoring peak intensity*	*DP, using descending order of peak intensity*
1	0.69	0.900
2	0.89	0.985
3	0.958	0.997
4	0.984	0.9992
5	0.993	0.9998
6	0.998	1.0000

peaks are easily seen and are recorded correct to the nearest 0.1 μm. In an interlaboratory trial—10 laboratories with 12 different IR spectrophotometers—we showed that an error factor of 0.1 μm could be achieved (A.C. Moffat & G. W. Owen, unpublished).

Table 3 gives the discriminating powers of different searches with the method just described. The discriminating power rises as more and more peaks are used in the search, but three peaks in descending order of intensity are about as useful as six peaks when the intensities are ignored. Six peaks obtained in order of intensity should identify the compound every time. Unfortunately, obtaining peaks in ascending order is far more difficult than just choosing the six largest peaks and in our interlaboratory trial there was disagreement on the order of intensity of the peaks, although there was good agreement on the choice of the six peaks.

The more peaks that are used the higher the discriminating power, but often it becomes more difficult to choose the fifth or sixth peaks. Fig. 12 shows the

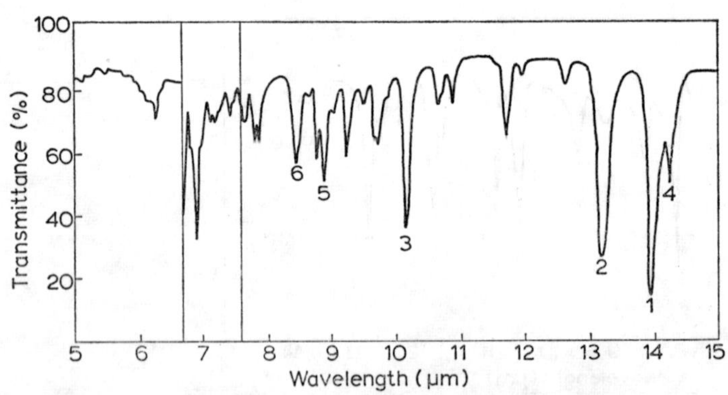

FIG. 12. IR spectrum of cyclizine hydrochloride (KBr disc). The six major peaks between 5 and 15 μm, but excluding the region 6.7–7.6 μm, are numbered in descending order of intensity.

IR spectrum of cyclizine hydrochloride and here the choice of the sixth peak was 8.5, although those at 8.8 and 9.3 have very similar transmittances.

These data indicate that using only four or five peaks to make sure that the unknown drug is included in those retrieved by the search may be better than trying to obtain a large discriminating power with six peaks and risk not finding the appropriate identity.

DISCUSSION

Once the chromatographic and spectroscopic techniques have been evaluated by measurements of their discriminating powers, a 'league table' of effectiveness can be constructed (Table 4). However, the figures in Table 4 are minimum values, since the identification procedures for each technique can be significantly increased. For example, the reaction with different spray reagents is useful in PC and TLC, derivatives may be used in GLC, and more peaks may be used for searches by UV and IR spectroscopy. Nevertheless, the values in Table 4 are a sound basis for any comparison of the techniques. Only speed of analysis, sensitivity, capital and running costs then need to be taken into account in deciding the best procedure to use for identification of an unknown drug.

One advantage of the discriminating power is that, since it is a probability, it can be used to give the average number of possible identities retrieved during a search programme. For example, one PC system has a discriminating power of 0.78, that is 78 out of every 100 drugs can be excluded and 22 are possible identities. The discriminating powers can also be multiplied together, provided that there is no correlation between them; that is, the combined discriminating power ($DP_{1,2}$) of two non-correlated systems of discriminating powers DP_1 and DP_2 is given by

$$DP_{1,2} = 1 - (1 - DP_1)(1 - DP_2)$$

TABLE 4

Summary of discriminating powers of chromatographic and spectroscopic techniques

Technique	*No. of systems used*	*Discriminating power*
PC	1	0.78
and	2	0.940
TLC	3	0.982
GLC	1	0.967
	2	0.993
UV	Acid spectrum	0.88
	+ alkaline spectrum	0.908
IR	4 peaks	0.984
	6 peaks	0.998

If the two systems are correlated, with a correlation coefficient of r, then the appropriate formula is

$$DP_{1,2} = 1 - (1 - DP_1)\,(1 - DP_2)\,/\sqrt{\,(1 - r^2)}$$

Discriminating powers allow a minimum probability of identification to be assigned to an analysis, and the question of how much information is needed before a drug can be identified is almost completely answered. The only thing left for the analyst to do is to decide how many possible drugs there are.

References

CURRY, A. S., READ, J. F. & BROWN, C. (1969) A simple infra-red spectrum retrieval system. *J. Pharm. Pharmacol. 21*, 224–231

DHONT, J. H., VINKENBORG, C., COMPAAN, H., RITTER, F. J., LABADIE, R. P., VERWEIJ, A. & DE ZEEUW, R. A. (1970) Application of R_f correction in thin-layer chromatography by means of two reference R_f values. *J. Chromatogr. 47*, 376–381

GALANOS, D. S. & KAPOULAS, V. M. (1964) The paper chromatographic identification of compounds using two reference compounds. *J. Chromatogr. 13*, 128–138

HAYWOOD, P. E. & MOSS, M. S. (1968) Screening for alkaloids in toxicology by using thin-layer chromatography: A rapid system simulating paper chromatography. *Analyst (Lond.) 93*, 737–739

MCREYNOLDS, W. O. (1970) Characterization of some liquid phases. *J. Chromatogr. Sci. 8*, 685–691

MOFFAT, A. C. & SMALLDON, K. W. (1974) The optimum use of paper, thin-layer and gas-liquid chromatography for the identification of basic drugs. 2. Paper and thin-layer chromatography. *J. Chromatogr. 90*, 9–17

MOFFAT, A. C., SMALLDON, K. W. & BROWN, C. (1974*a*) The optimum use of paper, thin-layer and gas-liquid chromatography for the identification of basic drugs. 1. The determination of effectiveness for a series of chromatographic systems. *J. Chromatogr. 90*, 1–7

MOFFAT, A. C., STEAD, A. H. & SMALLDON, K. W. (1974*b*) The optimum use of paper, thin-layer and gas-liquid chromatography for the identification of drugs. 3. Gas-liquid chromatography. *J. Chromatogr. 90*, 19–33

SMALLDON, K. W. (1971) A search for uncorrelated thin-layer chromatographic systems for the identification of basic drugs. *J. Forensic Sci. Soc. 11*, 171–176

STREET, H. V. (1962*a*) Rapid separation of drugs and poisons by high-temperature reversed-phase paper chromatography. II: Phenothiazine tranquillizers and imipramine. *Acta Pharmacol. Toxicol. 19*, 312–324

STREET, H. V. (1962*b*) Rapid separation of drugs and poisons by high-temperature reversed-phase paper chromatography. III. Alkaloids. *Acta Pharmacol. Toxicol. 19*, 325–329

Discussion

Dole: In the early days of screening for narcotics, when we needed simple methods for identifying them in the urine we were of course much concerned with the possibility of false positives. At the same time we were limited because we had to examine large numbers of people. Gas chromatography was quite out of the question for routine monitoring of 5000 people. But a series of sprays on the same thin-layer plate means that, in effect, several tests have been done. We reported as positive only those that were clearly positive on primary identification and which had positive confirmatory identification on the same plate.

Moffat: The laboratory adjacent to ours routinely sprays plates first with FPN reagent (ferric chloride, perchloric acid and nitric acid), which shows up all the phenothiazines, then with Dragendorff spray, which shows up most of the amines and alkaloid-type drugs, and finally with potassium iodoplatinate. So on the same spot they have three extra bits of information. However, I think it is sometimes quite dangerous to base any identities on the colours given by, say, an iodoplatinate spray. Dr Sunshine (1969) quotes all these sprays as functional group sprays. One should include information like this but I wouldn't like to use it in a searching system. The fact that the FPN spray didn't work wouldn't eliminate phenothiazines. If you put all the information available into the computer, then not only will it kick back the possible identities, but it will show the other systems in which the drugs could be discriminated and tell you how the spray reagent should have worked with that drug.

Dole: I certainly see that as a clinician. Of course, for security one has to include standards for morphine and other drugs. The standards should be spotted on every plate to verify performance of the system.

Moffat: The way we see it, we would probably have three or four standards. These would not only be picked out for their chromatographic properties, so they would be spread out over the plate; they would also be picked so that each spray reagent would be tested as well. Then one would know that if something was on that plate, the spray should have picked it up.

Holmstedt: To me, paper chromatography and thin-layer chromatography are separation methods. When you say that paper chromatography has a sensitivity of 10–20 μg, and thin-layer chromatography a sensitivity of 1–5 μg, what exactly do you mean?

Moffat: If 10 or 20 μg of any one of those 100 drugs is put on a paper chromatogram, it will be seen as a spot. With a highly fluorescent compound I could see, say, 0.1 μg. Amphetamine is a bad example: 40 or 50 μg for TLC and, say, 0.1 μg for GLC represents the comparative sensitivities of these chromatographic methods.

Sunshine: You have tried to make physical constants out of chromatographic data. I don't think they are constants. They will vary from day to day, place to place, and system to system. It is very difficult to get reproducible data that you can put into a data bank and get back. Infrared or ultraviolet spectra, on the other hand, provide true physical constants. If you put internal standards in the chromatographic system and compare the results visually, that is one thing. But to calculate these retention times or distances and then assume these numbers are reproducible is not valid. You have retention data for standards that have been chromatographed at the same time. What is the reproducibility of these values in your laboratory and how do they compare with those from other laboratories?

Moffat: We asked ten regional forensic laboratories to use TLC for testing six solutions that we sent them. If we use two standards and interpolate a spot, we get a standard deviation of just over 1%. If we extrapolate, it goes up to maybe 15%. If we use standards that are widely apart, we won't get that order of standard deviation. In system No. 3 (Table 1) we have one reference at about 0.2, and another at about 0.6 and we get a standard deviation of reproducibility of about 1–2%. If we have drugs at 0.6 and 0.8 the result is not so good. That is why I say we need at least three or four standards and we are hunting them down now. We want to pick out five systems that can be used in combination. Now we need to find out how reproducible these five systems are, and then how many standards we need so that we can cut down and use a very narrow band.

Beckett: Even infrared and ultraviolet spectra are not absolute figures but relative to some other standard. I see nothing wrong with your system in physical terms, Dr Moffat. Would it help if you also used UV spectra of compounds in two different organic solvents? Sometimes the solvent has a big effect on the observed spectra.

Moffat: Yes. The great joy with UV spectra is that once the substance is in the cell, it takes only two minutes for a scan. You can drop in concentrated alkali and run it again for just two extra minutes' work. If you extract it into an organic solvent and then put it into something else, you are making more work for yourself. But you have to balance that against how long it takes to do the chromatography, and whether you could be doing other things at the same time. If you split the sample, start off with GLC, then run TLC at the same time as you are doing a UV scan, you will have an awful lot of data at the end.

Beckett: You are going to extract the drug anyway; therefore you have to extract it into one organic solvent so it would be easy to use an additional solvent so that another curve could be obtained rapidly.

Moffat: It is really a non-destructive technique.

Curry: Until the experiment with 100 drugs ends, we shan't know how much more useful this method is. The problem is manpower. The object is cost–benefit analysis. Are scientists who are using these techniques day after day doing more work than they need do?

Scott: You have cooked the books a little by eliminating mass spectroscopy, the most discriminative spectroscopic technique available. With mass spectroscopy, your discriminating powers might be up to 0.9999.

Moffat: In fact, we had the mass spectra for our 100 drugs, some of which were taken from the collection at the Massachusetts Institute of Technology and some of which we ran ourselves, but we were only considering chromatography. An additional problem was how to code mass spectra. Should we pick out one peak in every 14 mass units? Or should we pick out three peaks in every 21 mass units? The difficulty lies not in deciding what the spectrum is but in coding the information. With the set-up at the moment, we could probably get a unique identity for each of our 100 drugs.

Scott: You have to have a reference spectrum. If you do a subtraction on a computer and get zero then your spectrum matches the unknown.

References

SUNSHINE, I. (ed.) (1969) *CRC Handbook of Analytical Toxicology*, CRC Press, Cleveland, Ohio

Use of gas chromatography–mass spectrometry in toxicological analysis

BO HOLMSTEDT and JAN-ERIK LINDGREN

Department of Toxicology, Swedish Medical Research Council, Karolinska Institutet, Stockholm

Abstract Since the introduction of the molecule separator about 10 years ago the combination of gas chromatography and mass spectrometry has come to play an increasing role in biomedical sciences. This combined instrument is of particular importance in toxicological analysis because of its ability to deliver positive evidence of the structure of compounds. If a computer is used, spectra of substances in a gas chromatogram can be more easily compared to experimental spectra from a large file of reference spectra of drugs and toxic compounds.

In mass fragmentography (also called multiple ion detection) the spectrometer is exclusively used for the mass specific recording of preselected ions. With this ion-specific detection, the intensity and abundance of the ions produced when the effluent from the gas chromatograph is ionized in the ion source may be recorded as continuous curves. The retention time is characteristic of the compound being examined and the peak area or peak height of every peak is proportional to the amount. In addition, the relative intensities of the ionic fragments should match those in the mass spectrum of the compound.

Mass fragmentography is not only a highly selective technique; amounts down to the picogram level can be determined; it also allows compounds labelled with stable isotopes to be used as internal standards. It is an ideal way of calibrating other methods, such as the various immunoassay techniques.

Mass spectrometry has existed for about fifty years but only within the last ten years has it been extensively used as a tool for detecting organic compounds in biological tissues and fluids and for elucidating their structure. During those ten years the technique has undergone a renaissance, as witnessed by its present widespread use for determining the structures of drugs and natural products. With the advent of various devices for coupling a gas chromatograph with a mass spectrometer, a vast new territory of particular use to the toxicologist and pharmacologist has been opened up. The combination of the separating ability of the gas chromatograph with the extremely high sensitivity of the mass spectrometer has led to these instruments being used to analyse complex mixtures of many sorts, including those obtained from body fluids of poisoned people.

The principles and uses of the combination of gas chromatography and mass spectrometry (GC–MS) in biomedical sciences have been repeatedly reviewed (see Hammar *et al.* 1969; Hammar 1971; Holmstedt & Linnarson 1972; Waller 1972; Jenden & Cho 1972; Costa & Holmstedt 1973).

If a computer of moderate size is available in addition to GC–MS, this on-line combination gives the analyst an even more powerful method. When the three are properly interfaced, all spectra of substances in a gas chromatogram can be automatically recorded and the experimental spectra can be compared with a file of authentic mass spectra of drugs and toxic compounds. With ancillary techniques using a computer, tasks such as monitoring selected masses to determine the presence and abundance of ions characteristic of certain structures, including metabolites of drugs (mass fragmentography, MF), can be performed.

PRINCIPLES AND EQUIPMENT AVAILABLE

The introduction of the molecule separator in 1964 allowed the gas chromatograph to be interfaced with the mass spectrometer (Ryhage 1964; Watson & Biemann 1964).

In Ryhage's design a two-step jet-diffusing system made it possible for the effluent from the gas chromatograph column to be introduced directly into the mass spectrometer. Mass spectra can thus be obtained without the compounds having to be isolated first. To maintain the necessary vacuum in the mass spectrometer the separator removes about 99% of the carrier gas. Separators built on other principles have been reported (see Waller 1972).

When the sample leaves the molecule separator it enters the mass spectrometer, which performs three different physical processes: the sample under investigation is *ionized* in a special ion chamber of the instrument; the ions produced are *separated* according to their mass, in either a magnetic or an electric field; and the ions are then directly or indirectly *recorded* by a detector placed after the ion separator. For all this to be technically possible an adequate vacuum has to be provided by two or more different pumping systems.

A suitable parameter of the ion-sorting system, or the magnetic or electric field, is gradually changed so that the ions are focused at the detector in order of mass. The signal from the detector can be seen on a fast recorder as a complex curve similar to a bar diagram.

The mass spectrometer most commonly used so far has been the *single-focusing magnetic instrument*. The standard ion source is of the electron bombardment or *electron impact* (EI) type. It consists of a filament which is heated to glowing by an electric current. Electrons are emitted from the filament and are then accelerated into a chamber where ionization takes place. Finally, they are collected on an anode. The accelerating potential is adjusted so that the electrons are loaded with a certain kinetic energy which is then transferred to the sample molecules to be ionized. The normal ionization energy is 70 eV. Most of the organic molecules are ionized in the range of 8 to 15 eV. The reason for using a higher energy is to create a *fragmentation of the molecule* in order to get information on its structure.

The degree of ionization and fragmentation depends on the electron energy and the constitution of the molecules, and also on the temperature of the ion source. The ion-accelerating voltage is usually kept at 3.5 kV. The accelerated ions leave the ion source through the electrical focusing lenses and the exit slit and enter the analyser tube which has a magnet around the central section. In the scanning process, the ions have to pass through a continuously varying magnetic field which deflects them according to their individual masses (m/e values). The scans can either be single ones or elicited repetitively.

The relationship between the mass (m), the strength of the magnet field (H) and the accelerating voltage (V) is expressed in the formula

$$m/e = H^2 r^2/2V$$

where e = the charge of the ion, r = radius, which is constant, and V which is usually also constant (the exception being mass fragmentography, see below). Most often one electron is lost. Because of this relationship only ions with a certain m/e value are able to pass through the collector slit near the end of the tube at a certain strength of the magnetic field. By the continuous variation of the magnetic field, ions of increasing masses are successively brought into focus and hit the multiplier. This type of detector can amplify the small ion signal by about a million times. A simplified picture of a magnetic mass spectrometer is shown in Fig. 1.

In the *electric field instruments* (quadrupoles, dodecapoles, etc.), the ions are generated and recorded in the same way as with the magnetic sector instruments. Mass analysis or mass separation of ions is, however, performed differently. The quadrupole mass filter consists of four metal electrodes or rods located in a square array. A combined radio frequency (RF) and DC voltage of increasing amplitude is applied to each diagonally paired set of rods. One pair (Y rods) receives an RF voltage and a positive DC voltage and the other pair (X rods) receives an RF voltage with 180° phase shift and a negative DC voltage.

By applying suitable RF/DC voltage ratios, it becomes possible to transmit through the mass filter only ions of a specific m/e value. These ions are in phase with the oscillating electric field. Ions which are not transmitted strike one of the rods, where they are neutralized and pumped away by the vacuum system.

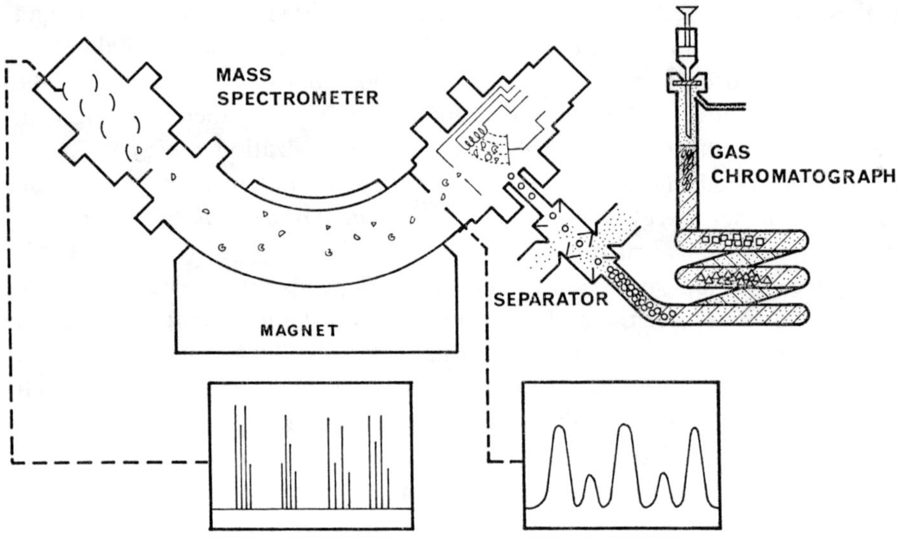

FIG. 1. Diagram of gas chromatograph–mass spectrometer.

During scanning, the RF and DC voltages are increased from zero to their maximum values; ions will then be transmitted sequentially in order of their *m/e* values, beginning at low mass and proceeding to higher masses. With the electric field instruments the final mass presentation is inherently linear, which makes identification of mass peaks easier. Because the mass scan is accomplished electrically, extremely fast scanning speeds are achieved which provide certain advantages.

Electric field instruments have been accused of producing mass discrimination, i.e. of having a lower sensitivity for ions of higher mass, but newer designs of quadrupole and dodecapole mass spectrometers have largely disposed of this disadvantage. The linear mass display, fast scanning and electrically adjustable resolution make for ease of computerization and computer-controlled operation.

Chemical ionization (CI) had its beginnings in 1966 when Munson & Field (1966) published their introductory paper on this subject. It is a comparatively recent addition to the available means of ion production, such as electron impact, described above. In ion production by chemical ionization the substance under investigation is made to react with a known and preselected set of ionizing reactant ions. Thus the reactant ions are to chemical ionization what the electrons are to electron-impact ionization. It is necessary, of course, to establish a condition which results in a primary ionization step. A complex series of reactions may occur (depending on the conditions in the ion source), yielding one

$$CH_4^{+} + CH_4 \longrightarrow \left.\begin{matrix} CH_5^{+} \\ C_2H_5^{+} \end{matrix}\right] \; 90\ \%$$

$$\text{Other} \quad 10\ \%$$

$M + CH_5^{+}$	$\longrightarrow MH^{+} + CH_4$	M + 1
$M + CH_5^{+}$	$\longrightarrow [M - H]^{+} + H_2 + CH_4$	M - 1
$M + CH_5^{+}$	$\longrightarrow MCH_3^{+} + H_2$	M + 15
$M + C_2H_5^{+}$	$\longrightarrow MC_2H_5^{+}$	M + 29

FIG. 2. Reactions between hypothetical sample molecules, *M*, and methane reactant ions.

or a few ions from the neutral molecules under study. A simplified scheme of what happens in chemical ionization is given in Fig. 2, where the reactant gas was methane.

Most mass spectrometers can be modified for chemical ionization with gases under pressures of 1 to 2 torr (~133 to 266 Pa) without the location of the source or inlet arrangements for the sample being changed, although the vacuum system may need modification. The CI source is usually operated with methane, isobutane, or nitrogen–ammonia but other reagents have been used.

The complex but structure-related character of electron impact spectra is much to be preferred to the one-peak approach of chemical ionization if one wishes to identify previously unknown or unexpected substances from drugs or metabolites (Costello *et al.* 1972). Fig. 3 demonstrates this.

In structure determination CI is at best a complement to EI. CI mass spectrometry may, however, offer certain advantages over EI mass spectrometry, particularly when one is trying to measure organic compounds and their metabolites present in low concentrations in body fluids. No separator between the gas chromatograph and the ion source is needed even when packed columns are used. This eliminates the possibility that samples present in low concentrations will be absorbed on the separator.

The quasimolecular ion or ions created by CI are of fairly high intensity and occur in the upper mass range, where less interference from biological compounds might be expected, although the possibility that interfering compounds are also chemically ionized and moved up the scale cannot be excluded. The quasimolecular ions may be used for mass fragmentography (see p. 114).

DATA PROCESSING AND SEARCH

A logical extension of the integrated GC–MS systems is the inclusion of

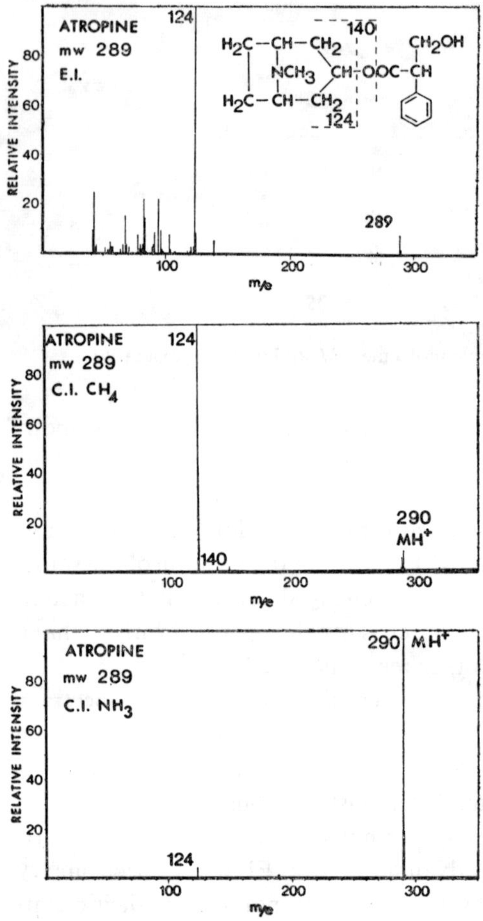

FIG. 3. Top: Electron impact mass spectrum of atropine.
Middle: Chemical ionization mass spectrum of atropine. Reactant gas, methane.
Bottom: Chemical ionization mass spectrum of atropine. Reactant gas, ammonia.

computer analysis. Evaluation of a mass spectrum from the recording on the ultraviolet-sensitive paper and construction of a bar diagram take a long time, sometimes several hours. It therefore comes as no surprise that several solutions to the computerization and digitalization of mass spectra have been achieved. Hites & Biemann (1968) were the first to publish a system. Waller (1972) has described all existing non-commercial systems. Commercially available units are listed in Table 1.

The generation of the data directly in digital form may not only permit a wide variety of presentation methods but also open the way for efficient, automatic evaluation of the spectra. The data can be presented in tabular form

TABLE 1

Companies producing GC–MS–computer systems

AEI Scientific Apparatus, Inc., Elmsford, NY 10523, USA
Bendix Corporation, Rochester, NY 14603, USA
Du Pont Instruments, Monrovia, Ca., 91016, USA
Finnigan Corporation, Sunnyvale, Ca., 94086, USA
Hewlett Packard Co., Palo Alto, Ca., 94304, USA
Hitachi, Tokyo, Japan
Jeol U.S.A. Inc., Cranford, NJ, USA
LKB Produkter AB, Fack, 16125 Bromma 1, Sweden
Varian-Mat, Bremen, West Germany

(using the line printer of the computer) or as 'bar-graphs', produced by an incremental plotter driven by the computer.

Because of the large number of spectra that can be recorded it is practically impossible for each one to be interpreted individually; it is therefore logical to use a computer for this task. 'Automatic' identification is obtained by searching the authentic mass spectra stored in the memory of the computer for identical or similar spectra (e.g. Finkle *et al.* 1972). A system of this kind is obviously more useful for problems involving a number of gas chromatograms of very complex mixtures rather than an occasional one involving only one or a few components. The former situation may often be encountered in toxicological problems. Several data acquisition systems which continuously sample the output of a mass spectrometer are now in use both for magnetic sector and electric field instruments.

Mass chromatography is an extension of the technique described above. It consists of the analysis of data from repetitively scanned mass spectra, stored for the most part on magnetic tape or disc, and from which a graph of specific ion abundance can be plotted against time. No previous knowledge of the masses being studied is needed, and any masses can be recalled (Hites & Biemann 1970). The sensitivity of mass chromatography is about the same as that of a single scan (10^{-7} g). Mass chromatography should not be mixed up with mass fragmentography, a much more sensitive technique, described below (pp. 114–120). Large files of mass spectra are now available from the computer (Heller 1972).

APPLICATIONS

Scanning of spectra

If conventional recording systems (i.e. oscillographs) are used, individual spectra can in practice be recorded only when a fraction of interest emerges from the gas chromatograph. This procedure calls for continuous decision-making during the experiment. Although it may lead to the loss of valuable, often unexpected, information represented by small peaks and shoulders on the gas chromatogram, for many practical reasons it may be regarded as sufficient. This is demonstrated by the following example.

> An 18-year-old girl (J.G.) had been taking phenmetrazine (Preludin) intravenously for about a month. One evening, with a girl friend, she visited two known addicts and received an intravenous injection of a drug from their supply. She reacted immediately by sitting limply in a chair and replied with difficulty when spoken to. The volume administered was reported to be between 2.5 and 4 ml but was presumably the latter.
>
> According to the statements of the addicts, her girl friend and a visiting medical student, the girl had reacted to the injection, within seconds, with paraesthesia and she complained about difficulties in seeing and keeping her eyes open, she had pin-point pupils, a reduced pulse rate and slow and irregular respiration, followed by unconsciousness, cyanosis and coma.
>
> The only compounds she could have taken were a 2% solution of morphine and a 3% solution of amphetamine. Injections of amphetamine were given by the addicts, as well as some kind of artificial respiration. However the girl died about six hours after the first intravenous injection.
>
> On autopsy and analysis by paper chromatography, amphetamine and phenmetrazine were recognized in the urine, kidney and liver. Strangely enough, no morphine was found in spite of the classical signs of morphine poisoning. The legal issue centred around what compound had caused death and who had given the first injection.

It was evident that the patient might have received 60–80 mg of morphine, a dose within the range considered to be toxic. Administered morphine leaves the blood rapidly but can be found in the urine, bile, kidney and liver more than 24 hours afterwards (Way & Adler 1960).

In view of the negative result for morphine the analysis was repeated, this time with GC–MS. A peak was found in the gas chromatogram with the same retention time as that of morphine base. When mass spectra were recorded from both the urine extract and the compound, *m*/*e* values of similar intensities were found in both spectra (Fig. 4). It was thus unequivocally established that morphine had been given to the girl instead of amphetamine, as had been stated. To the experienced toxicologist, the symptoms alone are enough for the diagnosis of morphine intoxication. GC–MS provides positive evidence for this, which in the case described was all-important to the legal issue.

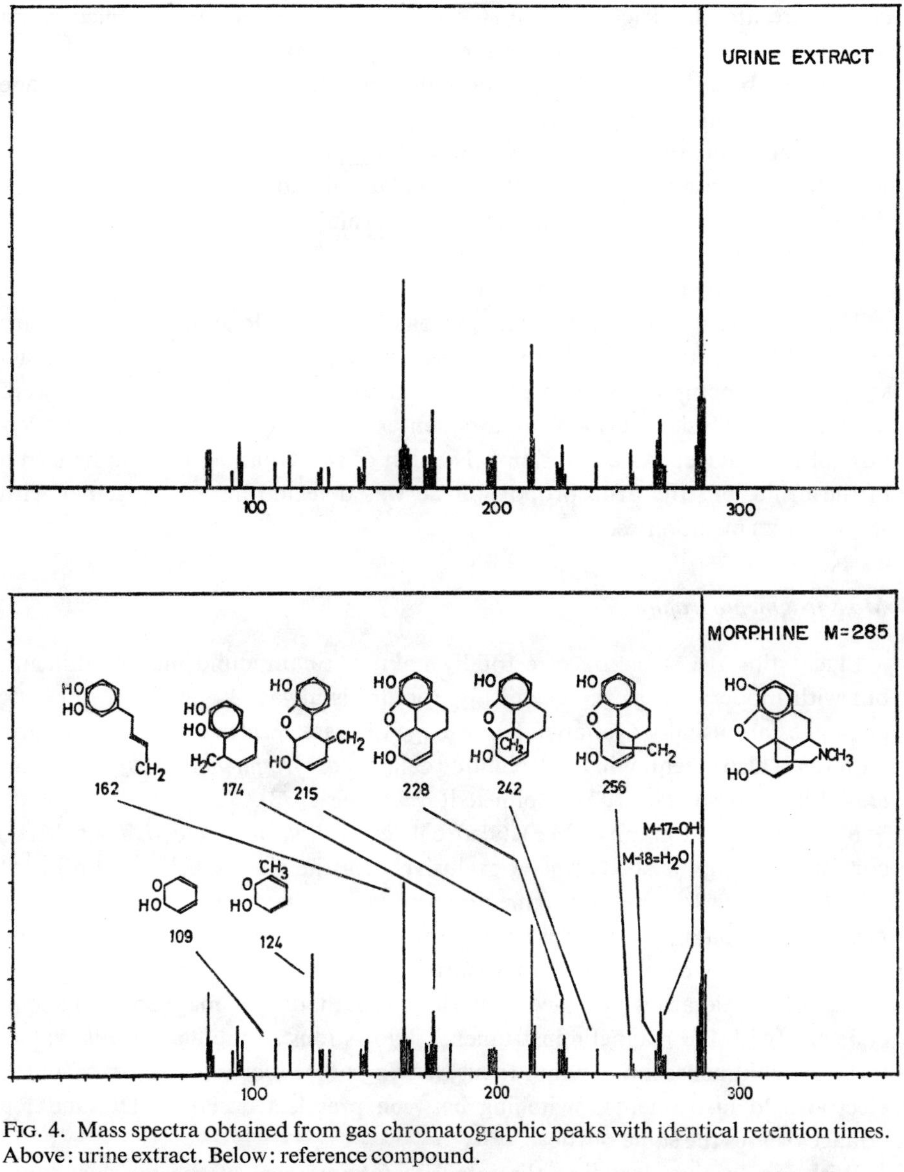

FIG. 4. Mass spectra obtained from gas chromatographic peaks with identical retention times. Above: urine extract. Below: reference compound.

In this case little effort was needed to obtain positive evidence by single-scan GC–MS. Naturally a computerized system would have picked out morphine as well.

Things may be more complicated when single-scan GC–MS is used to detect phencyclidine (Hog), as in a case described by Lindgren *et al.* (1969). Lindgren *et al.* were able to determine the structure of this compound, supplied as an unknown in a quantity of a few milligrams, by the following procedures:

(1) establishing through extraction and gas chromatography that only one amine-like component was present,
(2) recording the mass spectrum of that compound,
(3) measuring the masses of the molecular ion and certain fragments;
(4) selecting the most likely empirical formulas for these fragments; and finally
(5) searching the relevant literature.

The usefulness of repetitive scanning has been well documented by Althaus *et al.* (1970). Data obtained from a gas chromatograph–low-resolution mass spectrometer–computer system and other methods of gas-phase analysis were used in the analysis of urine from a patient suspected of having taken an overdose of chlordiazepoxide (Librium). No sign of this compound could be found in the urine, but the drug propoxyphene was detected instead, together with several of its metabolites.

Mass fragmentography

Elucidating the structure of a totally unknown compound may be difficult, but with modern drugs the chemical structure is always known and synthetic analogues are usually available. Knowledge of mass spectra and fragmentation patterns is also essential in the technique called *mass fragmentography* (Hammar *et al.* 1968; Borgå *et al.* 1973; Holmstedt & Palmér 1973).

Mass fragmentography (MF) (also called *multiple ion detection*, or MID) consists of using the spectrometer exclusively for the mass specific recording of *preselected ions*. A mass fragmentogram is obtained by on-line analogue processing of data and the mass spectrometer has to be focused beforehand on the ion masses which are to be measured. Rapid switching between selectable values of accelerating voltage, with the strength of the magnetic field kept constant (with the magnetic instrument), allows ions of the desired m/e values to be brought consecutively into focus, leaving other ions undetected. With the electric field instruments, switching between preselected sets of DC and RF voltages serves the same purpose.

With ion-specific detection the intensity (abundance) of the ions produced when the effluent from the gas chromatograph is ionized in the ion source may be recorded as continuous curves. Depending on the equipment used, different numbers of fragments typical of the compound to be analysed may be detected simultaneously. A mass fragmentogram is similar in appearance to a gas chromatogram and to a mass chromatogram. Like the latter it gives information about the retention time characteristic of the compound and the peak area or peak height (of any of the peaks) proportional to the amount. In addition, the relative intensities of the peaks should be the same as the relative intensities of the ion fragments in the mass spectrum of the compound. This is another criterion of identity. Several hardware systems for MF have been described by Holmstedt & Palmér (1973).

Recently, systems for multiple ion detection have been developed in which control of the GC–MS and signal processing are both done by a computer (Elkin *et al.* 1973; Holmes *et al.* 1973; Watson *et al.* 1973). The computer focuses on a certain mass by adding a voltage from a digital-to-analogue converter and booster amplifier to the accelerating voltage of the GC–MS. The digital treatment of the signals offers more satisfactory control of the baseline and gain; at the same time it allows the number of channels to be increased without modification of the hardware. The sampled data can be continually displayed on the oscilloscope of the computer and all questions and answers observed on the oscilloscope. The operator can set a baseline level, sample rate and gain for each channel. The data and calculated results displayed on the oscilloscope can be presented as hard copy on the teletype or plotter. A mass fragmentogram of this kind is demonstrated in Fig. 5.

MF has several advantages in toxicological analysis. It is one of the most sensitive of all the gas chromatographic detection systems known and can only be matched by an electron capture system for certain compounds. In general, MF is from 100 to 1000 times more sensitive than flame ionization detection (FID) and GC–MS. The sensitivity is obtained by selecting intense ions, wide optical slits and a favourable signal-to-noise ratio which cannot be obtained in repetitive scanning.

The ability of MF to utilize certain fragments or ions for detection provides a unique means of selectivity, which can easily be changed in such a way that either a single compound or a family of related compounds (e.g. metabolites) can be recorded. 'Partial mass spectra' characteristic of the compounds may be obtained by refocusing, even if the amounts available are too small for the scanning of a complete mass spectrum.

The technique of MF may, in contrast to electron capture detection, be applied to virtually any compound suitable for gas chromatography and which has a suitable fragmentation pattern. MF has already been used for quantitative analysis of drugs and endogenous compounds in biological samples such as blood or cerebrospinal fluid. It allows the ideal internal standards (i.e. compounds labelled with stable isotopes) to be used for quantitative determinations. It may also be used to check simpler and less expensive methods. Examples of this have already been given by Borgå *et al.* (1971) for nortriptyline and

Sample No. : 5
Waiting period 1 Sample period 3
Methaqualone and internal standard

Channel	Mass	Height	Ret. time	Ratio
1	235	480	1.52799	1
2	233	319	1.52799	.664583
3	250	176	1.52209	.366666
4	264	148	1.79800	.308333

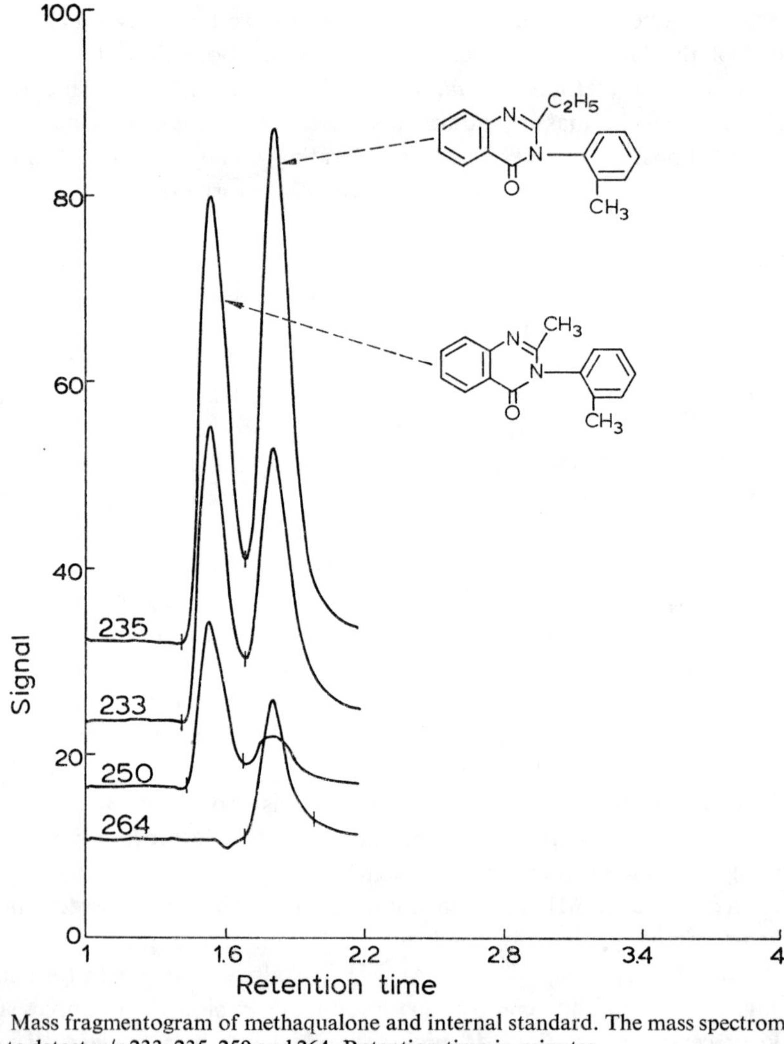

FIG. 5. Mass fragmentogram of methaqualone and internal standard. The mass spectrometer was set to detect m/e 233, 235, 250 and 264. Retention time in minutes.

by Palmér & Kolmodin-Hedman (1972) for 2,2-bis-(p-chlorophenyl)-1,1-dichloroethylene (DDE).

The usefulness of MF *per se* and for calibrating other methods will be further exemplified in the following case history:

> A 45-year-old man (J.H.) who was a known abuser of alcohol was operated on for a stomach ulcer. When he was discharged from hospital, methaqualone was prescribed (1–2 tablets nightly). J. H. took these tablets for about three months, sometimes with alcohol, but he strongly emphasized that he only took the tablets before going to sleep. One morning, after he had taken one tablet of methaqualone at about midnight, J. H. set out by car for a neighbouring city. After he had driven about 70 kilometres other drivers noticed that he was zigzagging along the road. Finally he hit a fence, wrecking the car but not hurting himself, and he was then taken to the nearest police station, where blood samples were taken. No smell of alcohol was noticeable but J. H. appeared to be drunk and was charged with drunken driving. His blood was sent for forensic analysis. No alcohol was found and the laboratory therefore proceeded to analyse for drugs, using UV-spectrophotometry after extraction with acid chloroform. With this method, 0.8 mg methaqualone/100 ml blood was found.

The method does not exclude the presence of metabolites and the figure is so high as to be incompatible with life, according to some authors. The legal issue was whether J. H. had taken one or several tablets the previous evening.

This case prompted a reinvestigation of the analytical methods for methaqualone and an exploration of its pharmacokinetics. First of all a sensitive mass fragmentographic method, using an analogous compound as an internal standard, was worked out for the drug (Alván *et al.* 1973) (Fig. 5). Plasma concentrations of methaqualone were then followed for several days after single oral doses in five healthy subjects. The plasma levels were interpreted according to a two-compartment model. The elimination rate of methaqualone was found to be much slower than previously reported, with half-lives in the β-phase ranging from 19.6 to 41.5 h (Fig. 6).

Methaqualone is generally considered to be a safe hypnotic drug which is rapidly absorbed and eliminated (FASS [Farmacevtiska specialiteter i Sverige] 1973; Physician's Desk Reference 1970), and this has been supported by a report (Morris *et al.* 1972) on plasma concentrations of methaqualone in man after single oral doses. By extending the period during which blood samples were taken, and by using MF, Alván *et al.* (1973) obtained results suggesting that after single oral doses the pharmacokinetics of methaqualone differs from the rates previously reported. The slope of the β-curve suggests that a steady-state plasma level could build up, for example in the individual described in the

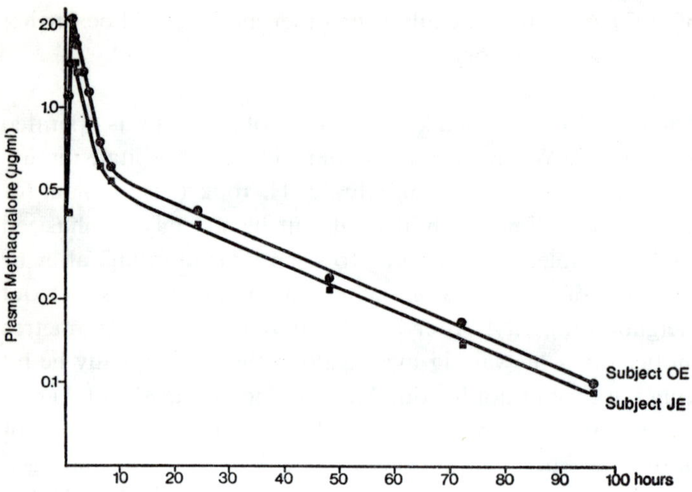

FIG. 6. Plasma concentrations of methaqualone in two subjects after a single dose of 4.0 mg/kg.

case history. Indeed steady-state plasma levels have been achieved experimentally (Alván *et al.* 1974) (Fig. 7).

These experiments with methaqualone were all carried out by MF. For the routine measurement of the drug in plasma it was desirable to use a simpler and less expensive method. For general use the following methods have been de-

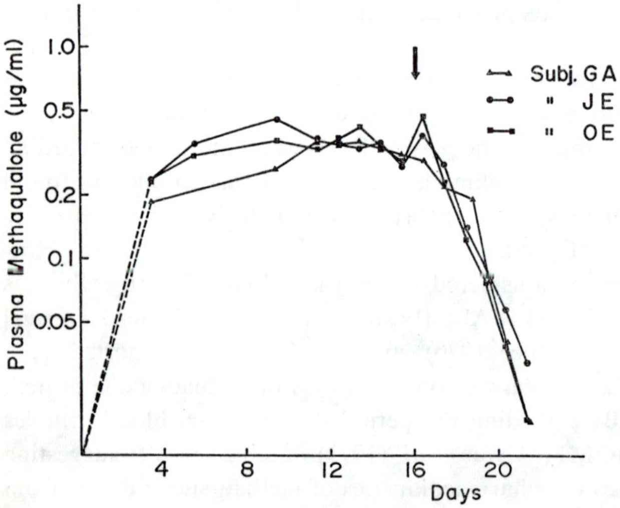

FIG. 7. Plasma concentrations of methaqualone in three subjects when the dose was 1.0 mg/kg once daily for 16 days. Arrow indicates the last dose taken.

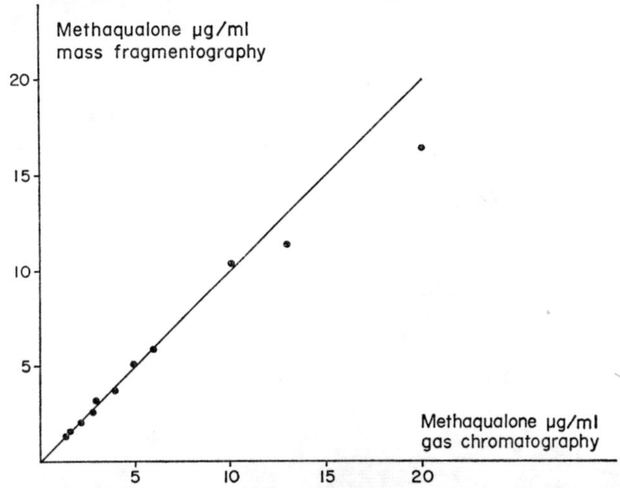

FIG. 8. Relationship between the concentration of methaqualone in plasma samples analysed with gas chromatography and mass fragmentography.

scribed: colorimetry, UV, fluorescence, NMR and gas chromatography (Höhlein 1966; Akagi *et al.* 1963; Brown & Smart 1969; Rücker *et al.* 1971; Goenechea *et al.* 1973; Mitchard & Williams 1972; Berry 1969). A gas chromatographic method in which a methaqualone analogue is used as an internal standard has recently been developed by A. Hanson working in the General Hospital, Malmö (unpublished). It was decided to test this method against MF by using identical plasma samples taken at various time intervals from an intoxication case. The result of this comparison can be seen in Fig. 8.

As is evident, there is a good correlation between MF and GC below a value of 15 µg/ml blood plasma. The straight-line relationship not only allows gas chromatography to be used clinically but can also in turn be used to check other methods, notably the much used UV-spectrophotometry after chloroform extraction. A correlation of this kind has been carried out by Bailey & Jatlow (1973) and is demonstrated in Fig. 9. Analysis by UV clearly gives values that are too high when compared to the other two methods, and it therefore should not be used for the analysis of drug levels in blood during therapy and even less so for forensic purposes.

The high values for methaqualone in the case just described was most likely due to a combination of a steady-state plasma level being established by prolonged administration and an incorrect high value given by UV analysis after chloroform extraction. Unfortunately UV analysis also requires such a large volume of blood that no material was left for mass fragmentographic or gas chromatographic control.

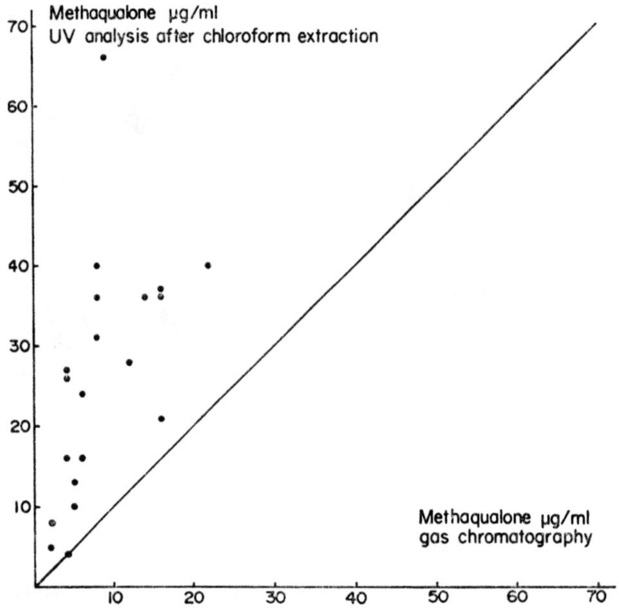

FIG. 9. Relationship between the concentration of methaqualone in plasma samples analysed with gas chromatography and ultraviolet absorption spectrophotometry.

RELATED ALTERNATIVE TECHNIQUES

Although GC–MS is by far the most powerful tool for both separation and identification there are alternative techniques (listed in Table 2).

For identification of compounds in gastric juice, urine, etc., the direct insertion probe to the mass spectrometer has been used both with low resolution EI (Law *et al.* 1971) and CI (Milne *et al.* 1971). In the latter case, most drugs gave only the $M + 1$ ion which can be used to identify the compound. In many cases, a follow-up by GC–MS using EI is needed.

The high resolution mass spectrometer (with which the composition of all ions can be determined) uses total extracts without prior separation and allows

TABLE 2

Related alternative techniques

(1) Direct inlet mass spectrometry	
(a) Low resolution:	EI, CI
(b) High resolution:	IIC (integrated ion current)
(2) Inlet through membrane separator	
(3) API (atmospheric pressure instrument)	

a relatively large number of heteroatoms to be surveyed quickly; this information is particularly important for the detection of halogen-containing or sulphur-containing drugs. This approach has found several applications in toxicological analysis (e.g. Althaus *et al.* 1970).

The high resolution instrument has also been used quantitatively with the so-called integrated ion-current technique (IIC) (Majer & Boulton 1973; Baughman & Meselson 1973). The cost of these instruments is often prohibitive and they seem to offer no better sensitivity than GC–MS.

Another approach to gas-phase analysis in toxicology is the introduction of samples via a *separator* without previous gas chromatography. Boerner *et al.* (1973) used this method to identify free drugs and metabolites in life-threatening overdose situations. The blood level of drugs in acutely poisoned patients is so high that gastric lavage, urine and blood specimens yield sufficient quantities of the unchanged offending agent to allow direct extraction and analysis. Quantification was not attempted.

Finally, equipment existing only as a prototype should be mentioned: the so-called *atmospheric pressure instrument* (API) (Horning *et al.* 1973*a*) seems to offer great promise for toxicological analysis in the low concentration range (Horning *et al.* 1973*b*).

CONCLUSIONS

The wide variety of compounds ingested in toxic quantities and the complexity of the mixtures often present in body fluids justify the use of gas chromatography–mass spectrometry–computer units. These units should preferably be located regionally, near large population centres. The variations in gas-phase analysis described in this article offer, simultaneously, the most sensitive and the most specific determination of toxic compounds in biological material.

ACKNOWLEDGEMENTS

Supported by the Swedish Medical Research Council B74-04X-4041-02B, B74-70E-3743-02, B74-40X-199-10C; the Swedish Environment Protection Board 7–1/73; the National Institute of Mental Health Grant MH 12007; the Wallenberg Foundation and the Tri-Centennial Fund of the Bank of Sweden 68/53:1.

We gratefully acknowledge the recording of chemical ionization mass spectra by Dr Evan C. Horning and co-workers, Baylor University, Texas.

References

Akagi, M., Oketani, Y. & Takada, M. (1963) Studies on metabolism of 2-methyl-3-o-tolyl-4

(3H)-quinazolinone. 1. The estimation of 2-methyl-3-o-tolyl-4 (3H)-quinazolinone in biological materials. *Chem. Pharm. Bull. (Tokyo) 11*, 62–67

ALTHAUS, J. R., BIEMANN, K., BILLER, J., DONAGHUE, P. F., EVANS, D. A., FÖRSTER, H.-J., HERTZ, H. S., HIGNITE, C. E., MURPHY, R. C., PRETI, G. & REINHOLD, V. (1970) Identification of the drug darvon and its metabolites in the urine of a comatose patient using a gas chromatograph-mass spectrometer-computer system. *Experientia (Basel) 26*, 714–717

ALVÁN, G., LINDGREN, J.-E., BOGENTOFT, C. & ERICSSON, Ö. (1973) Plasma kinetics of methaqualone in man after single oral doses. *Eur. J. Clin. Pharmacol. 6*, 187–190

ALVÁN, G., ERICSSON, Ö., LEVANDER, S. & LINDGREN, J.-E. (1974) Plasma concentrations and effects of methaqualone after single and multiple oral doses in man. *Eur. J. Clin. Pharmacol.* in press

BAILEY, D. N. & JATLOW, P. I. (1973) Methaqualone overdose: analytical methodology and the significance of serum drug concentrations. *Clin. Chem. 19*, 615–620

BAUGHMAN, R. & MESELSON, M. (1973) An analytical method for detecting TCDD (Dioxin): levels of TCDD in samples from Vietnam. *Environ. Health Perspect. 5*, 27–35

BERRY, D. J. (1969) Gas chromatographic determinations of methaqualone, 2-methyl-3-o-tolyl-4 (3H)-quinazolinone, at therapeutic levels in human plasma. *J. Chromatogr. 42*, 39–44

BOERNER, U., ABBOTT, S., EIDSON, J. C., BECKER, C. E., HORIO, H. T. & LOEFFLER, K. (1973) Direct mass spectrometric analysis of body fluids from acutely poisoned patients. *Clin. Chim. Acta 49*, 445–454

BORGÅ, O., PALMÉR, L., LINNARSON, A. & HOLMSTEDT, B. (1971) Quantitative determination of nortriptyline and desmethylnortriptyline in human plasma by combined gas chromatography–mass spectrometry. *Anal. Lett. 4*, 837–849

BORGÅ, O., PALMÉR, L., SJÖQVIST, F. & HOLMSTEDT, B. (1973) in *Problems of Therapy* (Okita, G. T. & Acheson, G. H., eds.) (*Pharmacology and the Future of Man*, vol. 3), pp. 56–68, Karger, Basel

BROWN, S. S. & SMART, G. A. (1969) Fluorimetric assay of methaqualone plasma by reduction to 1, 2, 3, 4-tetrahydro-2-methyl-4-oxo-3-o-tolylquinazoline. *J. Pharm. Pharmacol. 21*, 466–468

COSTA, E. & HOLMSTEDT, B. (eds.) (1973) Gas chromatography–mass spectrometry in neurobiology. *Adv. Biochem. Psychopharmacol. 7*

COSTELLO, C. E., SAKAI, T. & BIEMANN, K. (1972) Identification of drugs in body fluids, particularly in emergency cases of acute poisoning, in *20th Annu. Conf. Mass Spectrometry and Allied Topics, June 4–9, Dallas, Texas*, pp. 107–108, Am. Soc. Mass Spectrometry

ELKIN, K., PIERROU, L., AHLBORG, U. G., HOLMSTEDT, B. & LINDGREN, J.-E. (1973) Computer controlled mass fragmentography with digital signal processing. *J. Chromatogr. 81*, 47–55

FASS (1973) *Läkemedelsinformation AB*, p. 416, Almqvist & Wiksell, Uppsala

FINKLE, B., TAYLOR, M. & BONELLI, E. (1972) A GC/MS reference data system for the identification of drugs of abuse. *J. Chromatogr. Sci. 10*, 312–333

GOENECHEA, S., BROWN, S. S. & FERGUSON, M. M. (1973) Gas–chromatographische Bestimmung von Methaqualon in kleinen Mengen Serum nach Einnahme therapeutischer Dosen. *Arch. Toxikol. 31*, 25–30

HAMMAR, C.-G. (1971) Mass fragmentography and elemental analysis by means of a new and combined multiple ion detector—peak matcher device. Developments of new techniques in gas chromatography—mass spectrometry. Thesis. *Acta Pharm. Suec. 8*, 129–152

HAMMAR, C.-G., HOLMSTEDT, B. & RYHAGE, R. (1968) Mass fragmentography. Identification of chlorpromazine and its metabolites in human blood by a new method. *Anal. Biochem. 25*, 532–548

HAMMAR, C.-G., HOLMSTEDT, B., LINDGREN, J.-E. & THAM, R. (1969) The combination of gas chromatography and mass spectrometry in the identification of drugs and metabolites. *Adv. Pharmacol. Chemother. 7*, 53–89

HELLER, S. (1972) Conversational mass spectral retrieval system and its use as an aid in structure determination. *Anal. Chem. 44*, 1951–1961

HITES, R. A. & BIEMANN, K. (1968) Mass spectrometer-computer system particularly suited for gas chromatography of complex mixtures. *Anal. Chem. 39*, 1217–1221

HITES, R. A. & BIEMANN, K. (1970). Computer evaluation of continuously scanned mass spectra of gas chromatographic effluents. *Anal. Chem. 42*, 855–860

HÖHLEIN, H. (1966) Analysis of several medicinals. *Pharmazie 21*, 464–466

HOLMES, W. F., HOLLAND, W. H., SHORE, B. L., BIER, D. M. & SHERMAN, W. R. (1973) Versatile computer generated variable accelerating voltage circuit for magnetically scanned mass spectrometers. Use for assays in the picogram range and for assays of stable isotope tracers. *Anal. Chem. 45*, 2063–2071

HOLMSTEDT, B. & LINNARSON, A. (1972) in *Drug Abuse—Proceedings of the International Conference* (Zarafonetis, C. J. D., ed.) pp. 291–305, Lea & Febiger, Philadelphia

HOLMSTEDT, B. & PALMÉR, L. (1973) Mass fragmentography: principles, advantages and future possibilities. *Adv. Biochem. Psychopharmacol. 7*, 1–14

HORNING, E. C., HORNING, M. G., CARROLL, D. I., DZIDIC, I. & STILLWELL, R. N. (1973*a*) New picogram detection system based on a mass spectrometer with an external ionization source at atmospheric pressure. *Anal. Chem. 45*, 936–943

HORNING, E. C., HORNING, M. G., CARROLL, D. I., STILLWELL, R. N. & DZIDIC, I. (1973*b*) Nicotin in smokers, non-smokers and room air. *Life Sci. 13*, 1331–1346

JENDEN, D. J. & CHO, A. K. (1972) Applications of integrated gas chromatography/mass spectrometry in pharmacology and toxicology. *Annu. Rev. Pharmacol. 13*, 371–390

LAW, N. C., AANDAHL, V., FALES, H. M. & MILNE, G. W. A. (1971) Identification of dangerous drugs by mass spectrometry. *Clin. Chim. Acta 32*, 221–237

LINDGREN, J.-E., HAMMAR, C.-G., HESSLING, R. & HOLMSTEDT, B. (1969) The chemical identity of 'Hog'—a 'new' hallucinogen. *Am. J. Pharm. 141*, 86–90

MAJER, J. R. & BOULTON, A. A. (1973) Integrated ion-current (IIC) technique of quantitative mass spectrometric analysis: chemical biological applications. *Methods Biochem. Anal. 21*, 467–514

MILNE, G. W. A., FALES, H. M. & AXENROD, Th. (1971) Identification of dangerous drugs by isobutane chemical ionization mass spectrometry. *Anal. Chem. 43*, 1815–1820

MITCHARD, M. & WILLIAMS, M. E. (1972) An improved quantitative gas-liquid chromatographic assay for the estimation of methaqualone in biological fluids. *J. Chromatogr. 72*, 29–34

MORRIS, R. N., GUNDERSON, G. A., BABCOCK, S. W. & ZROSLINSKI, J. F. (1972) Plasma levels and absorption of methaqualone after oral administration to man. *Clin. Pharmacol. Ther. 13*, 719–723

MUNSON, M. S. B. & FIELD, F. H. (1966) Chemical ionization mass spectrometry. *J. Am. Chem. Soc. 88*, 2621–2630

PALMÉR, L. & KOLMODIN-HEDMAN, B. (1972) Improved quantitative gas chromatographic method for analysis of small quantities of chlorinated hydrocarbon pesticides in human plasma. *J. Chromatogr. 74*, 21–30

PHYSICIAN'S DESK REFERENCE (1970) (Baker, C. E. jr., ed.) vol. 24, p. 1137, Medical Economics, Oradell, N. J.

RÜCKER, G., BOHN, G. & FELL, A. F. (1971) Zur Identifizierung und quantitativen Bestimmung von Ureiden, Methaqualon und Barbituraten aus Organteilen durch NMR-Spektroskopie. *Arch. Toxikol. 27*, 168–172

RYHAGE, R. (1964) Use of mass spectrometer as detector and analyzer for effluents emerging from high temperature gas liquid chromatography columns. *Anal. Chem. 36*, 759–764

WALLER, G. R. (1972) *Biochemical Applications of Mass Spectrometry*, Wiley-Interscience, New York

WATSON, J. T. & BIEMANN, K. (1964) High resolution mass spectra of compounds emerging from a gas chromatograph. *Anal. Chem. 36*, 1135–1142

WATSON, J. T., PEISTER, D. R., SWEETMAN, B. J., FROLICH, J. C. & OATES, J. A. (1973) Display-oriented data system for multiple ion detection with gas chromatograph–mass spectrometry in quantifying biomedically important compounds. *Anal. Chem. 45*, 2071–2078

WAY, L. E. & ADLER, T. K. (1960) The pharmacologic implications of the fate of morphine and its surrogates. *Pharmacol. Rev. 12*, 383–446

[*For discussion see pp. 133–137*]

Determination of cannabis components in blood

STIG AGURELL

Faculty of Pharmacy, Stockholm, and Astra Läkemedel AB, Södertälje

Abstract For social and other reasons, e.g. traffic law enforcement, there has been an increasing need for a method that would identify a marihuana user. The obvious compound to look for would be Δ^1-tetrahydrocannabinol (THC)—the psychotomimetic compound of cannabis—or metabolites thereof. A quantitative method for THC might provide further useful information, such as an 'objective' measure of intoxication or pharmacokinetic data.

THC levels in blood are low and the major obstacles in measuring this compound appear to be interfering endogenous lipids. Possible methods have included the formation of dansyl derivatives followed by fluorometry; preparation of the heptafluorobutyryl derivative and the use of subsequent preparative and capillary column gas (electron capture) chromatography; the formation of the phosphate ester followed by gas chromatography with a special detector; and the use of pentafluorobenzoyl ester and electron capture detection.

However, the only human plasma levels reported so far seem to be those we determined by using gas chromatography–mass spectrometry after a clean-up with liquid chromatography.

The pharmacologically active constituents of cannabis have caused considerable scientific and social interest in recent years (cf. Paton & Crown 1972). It has been assumed that the physiological and psychological effects of cannabis are associated with the content of Δ^1-tetrahydrocannabinol (Δ^1-THC) in the drug. These assumptions, mainly based on investigations in the rhesus monkey by Mechoulam *et al.* (1970), have lately been verified in man by Perez-Reyes *et al.* (1973*b*), although the latter authors found slight activity also in cannabinol. Recently, fairly pure THC preparations have apparently been available occasionally on the illegal market.

In spite of social and scientific concern over the abuse of cannabis, toxicologically the drug has one 'asset'—it is comparatively non-toxic! It would seem that no fatal incident has been recorded as unquestionably due to smoking or eating cannabis, although intravenous injections of cannabis extract have sometimes been fatal.

Consequently, anyone wishing to trace the fate of the active cannabinoid or identify a cannabis smoker would look for the presence of Δ^1-THC or its metabolites in body fluids. The approach might differ according to the aims of the investigator. (1) For a forensic identification the unequivocally proven presence of either Δ^1-THC or its metabolites might have to be the criterion. (2) For a correlation of Δ^1-THC concentration in the blood with physiological and psychological parameters quantitative aspects—apart from the specific identification—would also be included.

The activity of Δ^1-THC is to some (a slight?) extent due to the formation of active metabolites such as the 7-hydroxy and 6β-hydroxy derivatives (Perez-Reyes *et al.* 1973*a*). The true contribution of these metabolites to the activity of cannabis in man is still being debated. Needless to say, it is difficult to evaluate these substances in animal models because metabolite patterns vary in different species and there is uncertainty about their formation, distribution and elimination.

POSSIBLE METHODS OF IDENTIFYING Δ^1-THC

A method of identifying and measuring Δ^1-THC in biological fluids has long been sought. The main obstacle appears to have been the presence of interfering lipophilic constituents in normal blood and the very low concentrations of Δ^1-THC in blood. However, Δ^1-THC has recently been detected in blood, according to a few reports, although it would appear that so far only our gas chromatographic–mass spectrometric method (Agurell *et al.* 1973) has yielded quantitative data in man.

Radioimmunoassay procedures have been thoroughly tested (e.g. Grant *et al.* 1972) but hitherto with no clearly encouraging results (Monique Braude, personal communication). The more recent development in immunoassay techniques—the enzyme-mediated immunoassay technique, or EMIT (Rubenstein *et al.* 1972)—has not yet been evaluated for use with cannabinoids. The formation of dansyl derivatives of Δ^1-THC extract from blood, urine and saliva of cannabis smokers was suggested by Just *et al.* (1972) as a means of detection.

An obvious technique to use for the detection of Δ^1-THC in body fluids would be gas chromatography, provided one could: (*a*) increase the sensitivity compared to ordinary flame ionization detection, and (*b*) decrease the background interference due to naturally occurring lipophilic components in blood.

Four possible solutions have been reported so far. Fenimore *et al.* (1973) prepared the heptafluorobutyrate of Δ^1-THC and used a dual column–dual oven gas chromatograph to separate Δ^1-THC and the internal standard from interfering compounds. The gas chromatograph contained, in series, a preparative column, a 'cold trap' for collecting the pertinent portion of the eluate, a capillary column for the final resolution, and an electron capture detector.

Garret & Hunt (1973) similarly used an electron-capture-sensitive derivative, namely, the pentafluorobenzoate ester of Δ¹-THC. The partitioning scheme designed to remove interfering compounds did not suffice for determination of Δ¹-THC in human blood but that scheme could be successfully replaced with a liquid chromatography clean-up (E. R. Garrett & C. A. Hunt, personal communication).

A quite different approach was taken by McCallum (1973) who, after an

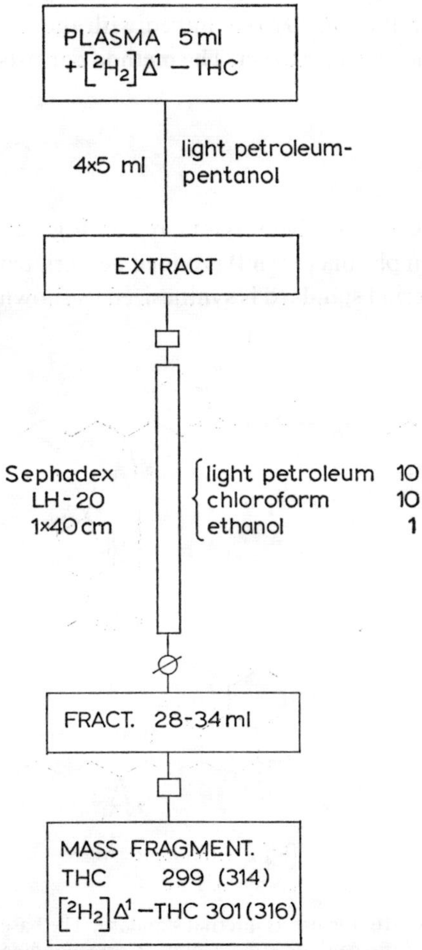

FIG. 1. Outline of procedure for measuring Δ¹-THC in blood.

initial purification of the plasma extract containing Δ¹-THC, converted Δ¹-THC into its diethyl phosphate ester. The specificity of the gas chromatographic detection was achieved with a flame photometric detector.

GAS CHROMATOGRAPHIC–MASS SPECTROMETRIC DETECTION OF Δ¹-THC

The further development of gas chromatography–mass spectrometry known as mass fragmentography (Holmstedt & Palmér 1973) is a possible method for the measurement and identification of low levels of Δ¹-THC in the plasma of cannabis smokers, and this has been investigated by several groups (Agurell 1970; Mikes *et al.* 1971; Skinner 1972). Our present success with mass fragmentography in measuring Δ¹-THC (Agurell *et al.* 1973) is linked with the use of a liquid chromatography clean-up of the plasma extract. The method consists of the steps outlined in Fig. 1.

Procedure

The procedure has been published in detail elsewhere by our research group (Agurell *et al.* 1973). To a sample of human plasma (5.0 ml) is added deuteriated Δ¹-THC (100–200 ng). The deuteriated internal standard is synthesized as shown

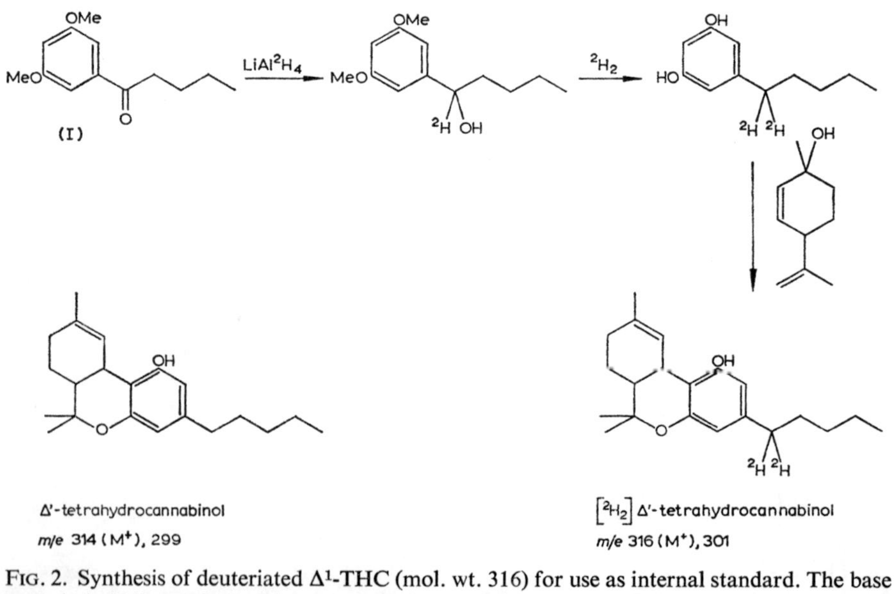

FIG. 2. Synthesis of deuteriated Δ¹-THC (mol. wt. 316) for use as internal standard. The base peak (*m/e* 301) was formed by removal of one of the *gem*-dimethyl groups. Corresponding fragments for unlabelled Δ¹-THC are *m/e* 314 and 299.

in Fig. 2. The plasma is extracted four times with 5 ml light petroleum (boiling range 40–60 °C; 1.5% pentanol v/v). The dried extract is chromatographed (0.2 ml/min) on a column of Sephadex-LH20 (1 × 40 cm) with light petroleum–chloroform–ethanol (10:10:1) as the eluent. The fraction containing Δ^1-THC (28–34 ml), determined by calibration—preferably with tritiated Δ^1-THC, is collected, dried and dissolved in 25 µl ethanol. This extract is subjected to mass fragmentography (3% OV-17 / Gas Chrom Q; LKB 9000) (Fig. 3). The intensity of *m/e* 299 from unlabelled Δ^1-THC in blood plasma was compared to the intensity of *m/e* 301 in the deuteriated Δ^1-THC used as internal standard (Fig. 3). We prepared standard curves by adding known amounts of Δ^1-THC and carrying out the procedure just described.

RESULTS AND DISCUSSION

The methods suggested previously for the determination of Δ^1-THC were all somewhat tedious. Our method may have some advantages. The gas

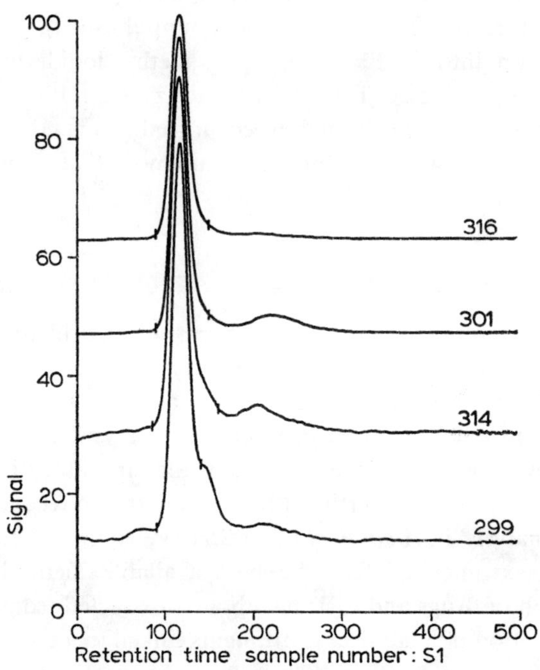

FIG. 3. Recording of Δ^1-THC (*m/e* 314, 299) present in plasma of a cannabis smoker. Internal standard [$^2H_2$]Δ^1-THC; *m/e* 316, 301. Plasma levels of Δ^1-THC 26 ng/ml. Retention time 3 min.

TABLE 1

Mean plasma levels of Δ^1-THC in three subjects who had smoked 10 mg Δ^1-THC

Time after smoking (min)	0	10	30	60	120
Plasma level of Δ^1-THC (mean value; ng/ml)	0	23	14	8	3

chromatogram (mass fragmentogram) is quite free from background and takes only a few minutes (Fig. 3). Furthermore, it is a quantitative procedure; the plasma levels in three tested subjects are shown in Table 1.

Disadvantages in our procedure include the need for a deuterium-labelled internal standard and the slow liquid chromatography clean-up. However, this latter step could undoubtedly be automated and speeded up by the use of high-pressure liquid chromatography. The deuterium-labelled standard can be synthesized by other routes than that described (Agurell *et al.* 1973), namely by reduction of the ketone, 1-(3,5-dimethoxyphenyl)-1-pentanone (I), with lithium aluminium deuteride, to the di-deuterium-labelled pentane (Fig. 2). Alternative routes include preparing [$^2H_4$] Δ^1-THC by exchanging the α-hydrogen atoms in the pentanone (I; Fig. 2) before reduction (K. Leander, unpublished), or introducing the C-7 methyl group into Δ^1-THC with [$^2H_3$]methyl iodide in Fahrenholtz's procedure for synthesizing Δ^1-THC (Fahrenholtz *et al.* 1967). In any case the use of internal standards in the published procedures is complicated, and the standards do not satisfy the common requirement that they should (*a*) not occur in nature, and (*b*) be crystalline.

CONCLUSIONS

Obviously, in certain types of biological analyses the necessary specificity, sensitivity and rapidity cannot always be provided. One may have to compromise. However, gas chromatography–mass spectrometry, as such and as mass fragmentography, is being increasingly used in biological analysis, often combined with data-handling systems. And since the role of the laboratory is the main theme of this symposium it may be pertinent to quote part of a recent editorial on 'GC/MS in drug analysis' in *Analytical Chemistry* (Petruzzi 1973): 'Gas chromatography/mass spectrometry offers the best available method for the unequivocal identification of drugs and their metabolites extracted from biological samples. This combination of analytical instruments linked to a computer programmed to identify any of more than 400 drugs, drug metabolites, natural body substances, and contaminants has been used for more than two years at Klaus Biemann's MIT laboratory in Cambridge, Mass., to examine blood and other body fluids from several hundred comatose patients in Boston hospitals'.

Similar programmes are going on elsewhere around the world and experience is rapidly increasing. It would appear that success in this area is still ahead!

References

AGURELL, S. (1970) in *The Botany and Chemistry of Cannabis* (Joyce, C. R. B. & Curry, S. H., eds.), Churchill, London

AGURELL, S., GUSTAFSSON, B., HOLMSTEDT, B., LEANDER, K., LINDGREN, J. E., NILSSON, I., SANDBERG, F. & ÅSBERG, M. (1973) *J. Pharm. Pharmacol. 25*, 554–558

FAHRENHOLTZ, E. E., LURIE, M. & KIERSTAD, R. W. (1967) *J. Am. Chem. Soc. 89*, 5934–5939

FENIMORE, D. C., FREEMAN, R. R. & LOY, P. R. (1973) *Anal. Chem. 45*, 2331–2335

GARRETT, E. R. & HUNT, C. A. (1973) *J. Pharm. Sci. 62*, 1211–1214

GRANT, J. D., GROSS, S. J., LOMAX, P. & WONG, R. (1972) *Nature (Lond.) 236*, 217–218

HOLMSTEDT, B. & PALMÉR, L. (1973) in *Gas Chromatography–Mass Spectrometry in Neurobiology* (Costa, E. & Holmstedt, B., eds.), pp. 1–14, Raven Press, New York

JUST, W. W., WERNER, C. & WIECHMANN, M. (1972) *Naturwissenschaften 59*, 222–223

MCCALLUM, N. K. (1973) *J. Chromatogr. Sci. 11*, 509–511

MECHOULAM, R., SHANI, A., EDERY, H. & GRUNFELD, Y. (1970) *Science (Wash. D.C.) 169*, 611–613

MIKES, F., HOFMANN, A. & WASER, P. G. (1971) *Biochem. Pharmacol. 20*, 2469–2476

PATON, W. D. M. & CROWN, J. (1972) *Cannabis and its Derivatives*, Oxford University Press, London

PEREZ-REYES, M., TIMMONS, M. C., LIPTON, M. A., CHRISTENSEN, H. D., DAVIS, K. H. & WALL, M. E. (1973*a*) *Experientia (Basel) 29*, 1008–1009

PEREZ–REYES, M., TIMMONS, M. C., DAVIS, K. H. & WALL, M. E. (1973*b*) *Experientia (Basel) 29*, 1368–1369

PETRUZZI, J. (1973) *Anal. Chem. 45*, 1213 A

RUBENSTEIN, K. E., SCHNEIDER, R. S. & ULLMAN, E. F. (1972) *Biochem. Biophys. Res. Commun. 47*, 846

SKINNER, R. F. (1972) *Proc. West. Pharmacol. Soc. 15*, 136–138

Discussion of the two preceding papers

Sunshine: Some UV techniques for the detection of methaqualone correlate well with the gas chromatography results.

Curry: Bailey & Jatlow (1973) studied differential solvent extractions followed by UV and showed that some of the figures are due to metabolites with the same UV spectra.

Brown: Bailey & Jatlow's paper (1973) gave relatively few clinical facts but quite a lot of analytical data. Fig. 1 (Brown), which has been derived from these

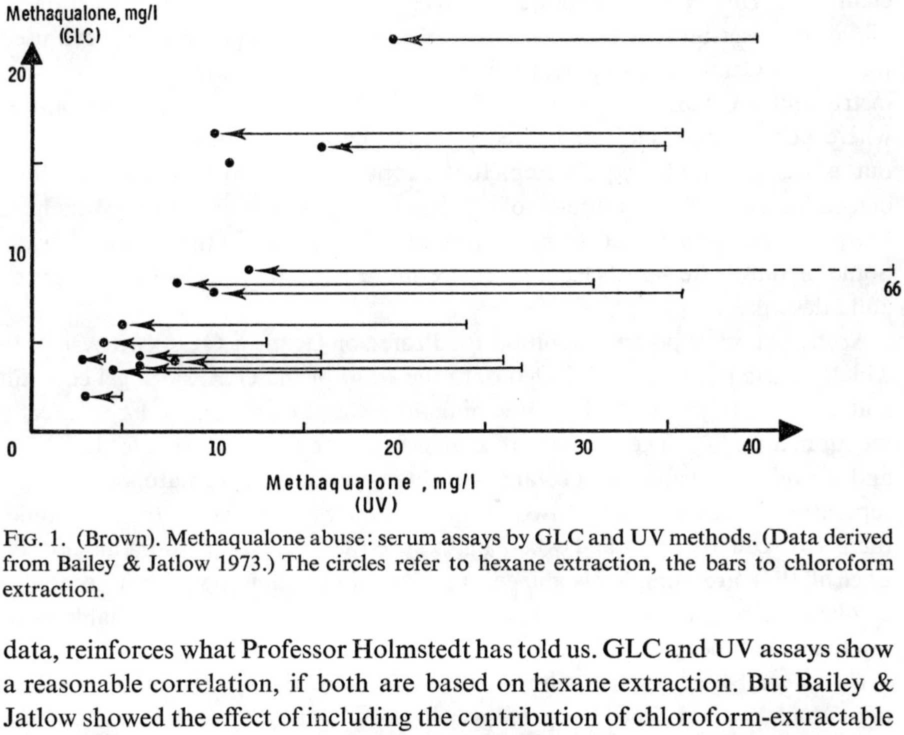

FIG. 1. (Brown). Methaqualone abuse: serum assays by GLC and UV methods. (Data derived from Bailey & Jatlow 1973.) The circles refer to hexane extraction, the bars to chloroform extraction.

data, reinforces what Professor Holmstedt has told us. GLC and UV assays show a reasonable correlation, if both are based on hexane extraction. But Bailey & Jatlow showed the effect of including the contribution of chloroform-extractable metabolites; there is a much poorer relationship between the results for GLC (hexane extraction) and UV (chloroform extraction). The validity of this UV method, like many others, depends heavily on the preliminary clean-up procedure.

Gee: As a morbid anatomist my idea of Utopia is the day when, after a post-mortem examination, I can send a body fluid to somebody for rapid screening for a vast number of toxic substances, and get an answer in a short time. Will this be possible in the foreseeable future?

Holmstedt: In some techniques that we use, one needs a work-up procedure, a chromatographic step for recording a spectrum, and computerization. Other laboratories, such as that of H. M. Fales at the National Institutes of Health, Bethesda, put gastric fluid directly into the mass spectrometer, with chemical ionization. That gives results quickly. But if there are still any doubts, this needs confirmation. Dr Fales tells me that mostly they have to use electron impact gas chromatography–mass spectrometry and establish the full spectrum. With direct inlet mass spectrometry a lower resolution instrument can be used with either electron impact or chemical ionization. A high resolution instrument can also be used to record molecular ions and integrate the area under a molecular ion. This can be used quantitatively as well as qualitatively. A technique for inserting gastric juice through a membrane separator has been used recently in California. Finally, for the future, there is the atmospheric pressure instrument of Horning *et al.* (1973). This is a kind of mass spectrometer where a compound is injected directly into a special ionization chamber, without a gas chromatographic step. It is supposed to be very sensitive. It can detect, for example, that non-smokers sitting in the same room as smokers have in their urine up to 5% of the amount of nicotine present in the smokers' urine. Some of these alternative techniques are more rapid than the ones Dr Agurell and I described.

Scott: Another possible solution for Professor Gee is a GLC–MS system in which gastric juice can be injected onto the front of the GLC silica gel column, and eluted progressively by something like the 12 solvents I have already mentioned (p. 80). The solutes are eluted from the column one after the other and a wide spectrum of substances is obtained on one chromatogram. If the separation is inadequate and two of the substances come out at the same time, these two can be identified when mass spectra are obtained simultaneously. Even if they are completely mixed, a subtraction technique with a computer can be used to give an either/or spectrum. Such a system is not available now, but the techniques you want are likely to be available soon.

Sunshine: Speed is not too important in forensic work, although the pathologists badger us at times for prompt responses. But 24 or 48 hours is not unreasonable and this time interval should be compared with the 24–48 minutes that the clinical toxicologists would like. One way to ensure faster and more reliable results, as funds become available, is to develop regional units for this work. As these demonstrate their value, because they can utilize more elegant techniques and because they have the necessary trained personnel, funding for them will be easier to obtain.

Gee: An answer in 24–48 hours is quick enough—anybody can hold off a funeral that long—but if it is going to take 48 hours to get the answer, the laboratory will soon have a backlog.

Scott: No, you can run through the complete polarity range in the chromatogram in 48 minutes. In these circumstances, you can use computer data handling, and as you do not want to spend time plotting the spectra a direct reproduction from an oscilloscope can be used. In this way you can cut the time down to something that might even be therapeutically satisfactory. These devices have already been shown to be practicable.

Beckett: I accept all that has been said about identification with mass spectrometry, but quantitatively there are dangers if we do not know exactly what is happening to a compound. For instance, most of the compounds that I work with have oxygen atoms on nitrogen, and in mass spectrometry many behave as though the oxygen atom was not there. So the metabolite gets measured as the drug. Oxygen atoms are also often lost from sulphur, so if we are working on quantitative aspects with mass spectrometry, we can easily go wrong with our pharmacokinetics unless we first adopt a separation technique.

Scott: This is what I am saying: it is unlikely that two compounds eluted at the same time will have the same mass spectrum.

Curry: I saw a machine demonstrated last year in the States which doesn't even have a print-out but just lights up when a sample has the appropriate mass numbers for, say, morphine.

Sunshine: It is like the old mass spectrometer with its phototube detector at a fixed mass. The new units utilize a form of chemical ionization mass spectrometry so that it records just when it hits one of several precalibrated points.

Scott: Once you have a mass spectrometer linked with a computer on the identification of a particular spectrum or ion mass, you can make it shine a light or shriek or do whatever you like!

Curry: Systems like that may have a place in the mortuary; if the lights don't come on, you needn't send anything on to the laboratory.

Holmstedt: I wouldn't rely on that!

Jackson: You still have to specify the poison you want to search for, haven't you?

Scott: Or the group of poisons.

Beckett: Techniques like Dr Moffat's (this volume, pp. 83–100) still have a big part to play in our total operation. A separation technique is involved in Dr Moffat's work and a separation technique linked with the newer techniques just described still means that detailed attention must be given to the separation part of the investigation.

Dole: Professor Holmstedt's methaqualone story is in some ways reminiscent of the situation with methadone, where therapy consists essentially of ensuring a stable pharmacological condition. In methadone maintenance programmes we obtain long-term stabilization of the patients by equilibrating a daily dose against the amount leached out of the tissue stores. This phenomenon makes chronic pharmacology different from acute pharmacology; certainly treating people with these drugs is different from treating acute poisoning.

When haemodialysis or some sort of wash-out technique was mentioned earlier (p. 12), Dr Newton said it was not a promising technique for the elimination of tissue-bound drugs. This is clear on theoretical grounds. If a removal operation diverts, say, 10% of cardiac output into a dialysis unit and completely removes the drug from this fraction, then if the drug is distributed between blood and tissues in a 1:100 proportion, the half-time of removal of drug from the body will be about 24 hours. With a tissue-bound drug that is toxic in itself or produces toxic metabolites, removal is therefore unlikely to be the strategy. If we are going to treat this kind of poisoning effectively, it has to be by an antidote that blocks cellular reactions or intercepts the production of toxic metabolites.

Prescott: I agree. If you know the pharmacokinetic characteristics, the distribution volume and the mechanisms of toxicity, you can predict fairly accurately which compounds you can remove in clinically significant amounts by artificial means.

Beckett: If a drug has to go from a tissue store to a site where it exerts its toxicity, the result depends on the rate at which it leaves the stores compared with the rate of elimination from the plasma. Therefore such a technique may protect the patient well enough, even though a fair amount of time is taken to remove the drug from the body.

Goulding: So, if one knows the pharmacokinetics, one can say what will work and, more often, what won't. But we have just heard that we don't know anything about the pharmacokinetics because our analyses are all wrong!

Holmstedt: Yes; there are beautiful formulae in a previous paper on the pharmacokinetics of methaqualone, but the authors were unable to measure the β-phase.

Beckett: If 99 molecules are in store and one molecule is at the site where it is doing the damage, you can still prevent most of the 99 from getting to that site by a suitable rate of elimination from the body. Thus the patient can be protected from the toxicity of that drug, even though there is a lot in the body.

Gillette: The problem is that some drugs are so highly localized in tissues that the rate-limiting step is the transfer of the drug to the blood from the tissues in which they act. For example, desipramine is so highly bound in the brain that dialysis is useless. On the other hand, with drugs that are not specifically localized in the tissues where they act but are present in other tissues, such as fat, dialysis may be useful in preventing the drug from reaching active sites. In that situation, I think you are right, Professor Beckett.

Dole: The store of toxic material is either in the neighbourhood of the susceptible cell, or it is being delivered there by the blood. Dialysis is obviously of no value in the first case, and it is of doubtful value in the second since the diffusion of drug from tissue stores to blood is likely to compensate for the removal of drug from the blood by dialysis.

Gillette: But I recall a case where the concept suggested by Professor Beckett does work. A patient took such a large overdose of thiopentone that he remained asleep even after the drug had distributed into fat. On dialysis he awoke, which indicated that the drug level in the brain had been markedly decreased. But when dialysis was stopped he went back to sleep because the dialysis had not been maintained long enough to remove the drug from adipose tissue.

Curry: A lot of people measure pentobarbitone in cases of thiopentone overdosage, because of the desulphurization during extraction.

Newton: There is no point in discussing methods of increasing drug elimination if the outcome is still the same for the patient. It can be argued for ever whether or not a drug comes out in significant quantities in urine, but if it is safer for the patient to be lying asleep, being adequately nursed, there is really no point in considering it.

Goulding: It depends how long they are asleep. A comatose patient is at risk the whole time, even in a very well-equipped specialized centre.

Newton: That is right, but one must remember that patients are comatose while they are being dialysed.

Goulding: You may reduce that period—that is the point.

Newton: This applies only to phenobarbitone, because there is no concrete evidence that the length of coma after poisoning with short- and medium-acting barbiturates can be substantially reduced.

References

BAILEY, D. N. & JATLOW, P. I. (1973) Methaqualone overdose: analytical methodology and the significance of serum drug concentrations. *Clin. Chem. 19*, 615–620

HORNING, E. C., HORNING, M. G., CARROLL, D. I., DZIDIC, I. & STILLWELL, R. N. (1973) New picogram detection system based on a mass spectrometer with an external ionization source at atmospheric pressure. *Anal. Chem. 45*, 936–943

Drug assay by radioactive reagents

W. RIESS

Research Department, Pharmaceuticals Division, CIBA-GEIGY Limited, Basle

Abstract The use of radioactively labelled reagents in analysing drugs and their metabolites in biological material is explained and the potential value of the technique is discussed.

In essence, the method consists of a sequence of analytical steps: isolation, formation of derivatives from the parent drug, separation, and detection. The reagent used in derivative formation is radioactively labelled, so allowing the derivative to be measured by radiometry. Since yields in the successive steps of the procedure are variable an internal standard is needed to indicate the overall yield of derivative. The ideal internal standard is the same compound as the one being analysed, labelled with a radioisotope different from that in the reagent. The specificity of the assay is achieved by two-dimensional thin-layer chromatography of the derivative before radiometry. Two or more compounds can be determined simultaneously if the appropriate labelled internal standards are added and an appropriate chromatographic system is used to separate the different derivatives.

Examples are given of the combined use of a ^{14}C-labelled internal standard, a ^{3}H-labelled reagent and liquid scintillation counting. An obvious advantage of the technique is that in commercially available β-spectrometers radiometry is fully automated, and optimum conditions for electronic data processing are thus provided. Special emphasis is paid to the need for apparatus that protects both operator and environment and that avoids contamination, so allowing low levels of drug to be measured reliably.

The increasing use of pharmacokinetic data in pharmacological research as well as in clinical therapeutics and toxicology has set new standards of quality and quantity for analytical methods of assaying drugs in biological material. Drugs in use today originate from many different chemical classes, and different chemical and physical principles need to be used for the detection and measurement of each class. Apart from the crucial conditions of specificity and sensitivity in the methods used, analytical laboratories have to process large numbers of samples in a short time as economically as possible. For optimum performance such laboratories must constantly look out for methods that fulfil all these demands.

In the analytical methods commonly used for drug assay, little use has been made of radioactively labelled reagents that allow derivatives to be formed from parent compounds and liquid scintillation counting to be used as a detector system. This technique looks especially attractive because commercially available liquid scintillation spectrometers operate fully automatically and produce an output ideal for electronic data processing. In biochemistry the isotope derivative method has long been applied, as shown in the review by Whitehead & Dean (1968), and one wonders why pharmacological chemistry has not profited more from this.

THE DOUBLE RADIOISOTOPE DERIVATIVE METHOD

When I was investigating radioisotope derivative methodology (Riess 1974), I found that precise and specific drug assays could be obtained by incorporating an internal standard and an appropriate separation process into the system. We therefore developed the radioisotope derivative assay and used exactly the same procedure for a number of drugs, as follows. A known amount of radioactively labelled drug of the same structure as the one to be assayed is dissolved in the biological sample containing that drug. The radioactive standard and the original drug are then isolated from the sample by solvent extraction, the work-up depending on the nature of the drug. The isolated material is next treated with an appropriate radioactively labelled reagent (carrying a different label from that in the internal standard) to form a derivative. The choice of reagent is based on the functional groups in the drug and on whether it is a practical source of radioactivity.

The product is separated from the excess of reagent and after enough unlabelled carrier of the same structure has been added, it is purified chromatographically. The derivative is then analysed for activity originating from the isotope in the internal standard and for that from the isotope of the reagent. The internal standard activity recovered equals the overall yield of the derivative and allows the activity introduced by the reagent to be corrected to the theoretical value equivalent to 100% yield. The concentration of the original drug in the biological material can then be calculated through the specific activity of the derivative, which in turn is obtained from reference samples of known concentrations of the drug. When a ^{14}C-labelled internal standard and a ^{3}H-labelled reagent are used, the radioactivity of the two isotopes can be discriminated conveniently with a Tricarb liquid scintillation spectrometer.

SYSTEMATIC DEVELOPMENT OF DOUBLE RADIOISOTOPE DERIVATIVE TECHNIQUES

When the double radioisotope derivative (DRID) assay was being developed for a number of drugs, we used a systematic scheme which allowed us to keep to a minimum both the time taken for setting up the method and the possibility of interference by drug metabolites or endogenous compounds. Experiments with benzoctamine (Tacitin, CIBA-GEIGY), which can be analysed as its [^{3}H]acetyl derivative, exemplify the general approach. Preliminary experiments to determine the best procedure should preferably be carried out with a ^{14}C-labelled drug, which gives the quickest possible evaluation of experiments and allows us to use concentrations within the expected *in vivo* range.

The first step is to isolate the drug from the biological material by solvent extraction. The pH dependence of the partition coefficient of the compound between aqueous and organic phase as well as between biological medium and organic phase should be measured (see Fig. 1) because the partition coefficients for the biological medium may differ. For acidic or basic compounds, re-extraction from the organic into the aqueous phase and back-extraction into the organic phase should be performed within the narrowest permissible pH range, so that coextraction of compounds that have a distinctly different dissociation curve can be prevented. This precaution ensures that disturbing background activity is drastically diminished.

The second stage is to optimize the conditions for the formation of the

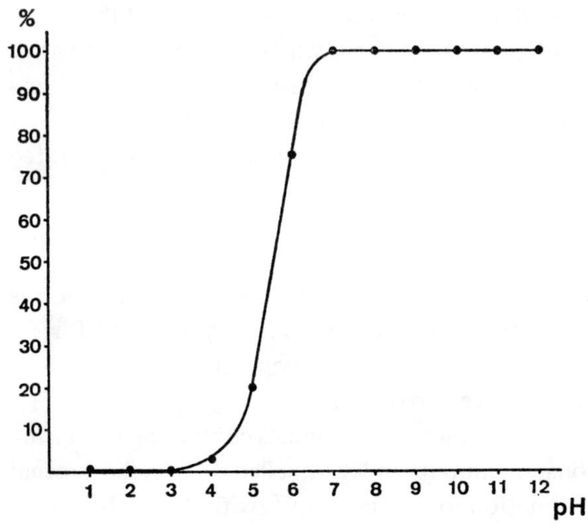

FIG. 1. Extraction of benzoctamine from aqueous phase (6 ml) into heptane (10 ml): % in organic phase which depends on pH of aqueous phase.

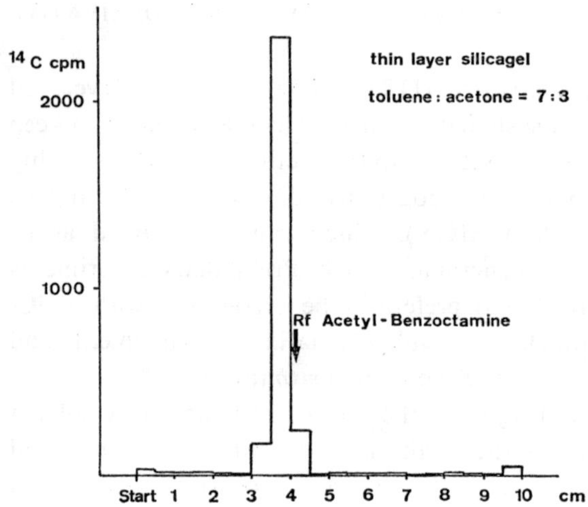

FIG. 2. Comparison of *N*-acetyl benzoctamine from analytical run with reference sample. Radioactivity distribution on thin-layer chromatogram of the acetate obtained from 200 ng [^{14}C]benzoctamine after base-specific extraction from human blood and reaction with 1 μmol unlabelled acetic anhydride.

derivative. The appropriate solvent, temperature, time of reaction, concentration and catalyst must be carefully established with the ^{14}C-labelled drug and unlabelled reagent. The product is then compared with authentic material, preferably by thin-layer chromatography (see Fig. 2).

The third step is to select two solvent systems for two-dimensional thin-layer chromatography. The appropriate solvent systems will separate the derivative of the unchanged drug from the derivatives that will form from known or expected metabolites. The main metabolites to be considered are those that differ very little in polarity from the parent drug. For benzoctamine, we have separated the *N*-demethyl metabolite.

The fourth step is to process aqueous and biological blank samples through the sequence of extraction and derivative formation using the ^{3}H-labelled reagent. When the carrier derivative has been added, the appropriate fraction is developed in the two selected chromatographic systems and analysed for ^{3}H activity, as shown for benzoctamine in Fig. 3. Only negligible amounts of ^{3}H activity should be seen near the reference derivative.

The next stage is to analyse a series of biological samples containing increasing concentrations of drug but a constant amount of ^{14}C-labelled drug as the internal standard. After extraction, formation of a derivative with the ^{3}H-labelled reagent, addition of carrier derivative and two-dimensional chromatography, the carrier spots are analysed in a dual-channel β-spectrometer for both ^{14}C and

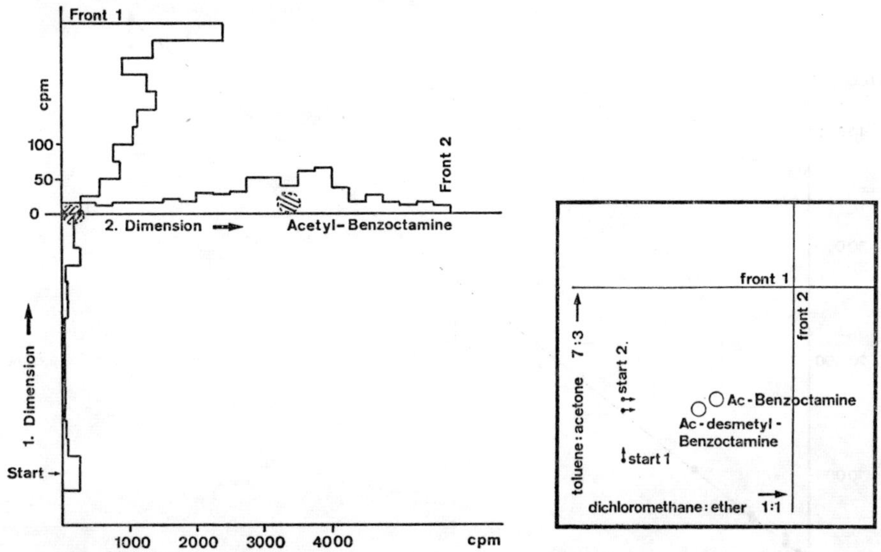

FIG. 3. Profiles of background ^{3}H activity on two-dimensional thin-layer chromatogram of [^{3}H]acetate from the extractable base fraction of 3 ml human 'blank' blood by acetylation with 1 μmol, 50 μCi [^{3}H]acetic anhydride and subsequent extraction before thin-layer chromatography.

Box: two-dimensional chromatographic scheme and locations of the acetyl derivatives of benzoctamine and its *N*-demethyl homologue.

^{3}H activities. The amount of ^{14}C activity from the internal standard is used to correct the ^{3}H activity to the equivalent of a 100% yield of derivative. When we plotted the corrected ^{3}H activity result for benzoctamine against the original concentration of cold drug in the biological samples, we obtained a strictly linear correlation (Fig. 4). The intercept of the straight line with the ordinate represents the ^{3}H activity attributable to the ^{3}H-labelled derivative of the ^{14}C-labelled internal standard, and the slope of the line represents the specific ^{3}H activity of the derivative (c.p.m. for each unit of original drug). When unknown concentrations of drug are being analysed the corrected ^{3}H activity can be converted into concentration units by reference to the slope and intercept of this correlation. The most convenient way to determine the slope and intercept for each analytical run is to analyse two sets of standard samples, representing two concentrations in suitable position along the abscissa in Fig. 4. We suggest calling this approach the two-point calibration mode.

The last step before samples of biological origin are analysed is analysis of biological material containing known concentrations of a drug, so that the analytical error of the final method can be assessed. Table 1 lists the results obtained with benzoctamine in 3 ml of human blood when ^{14}C-labelled benz-

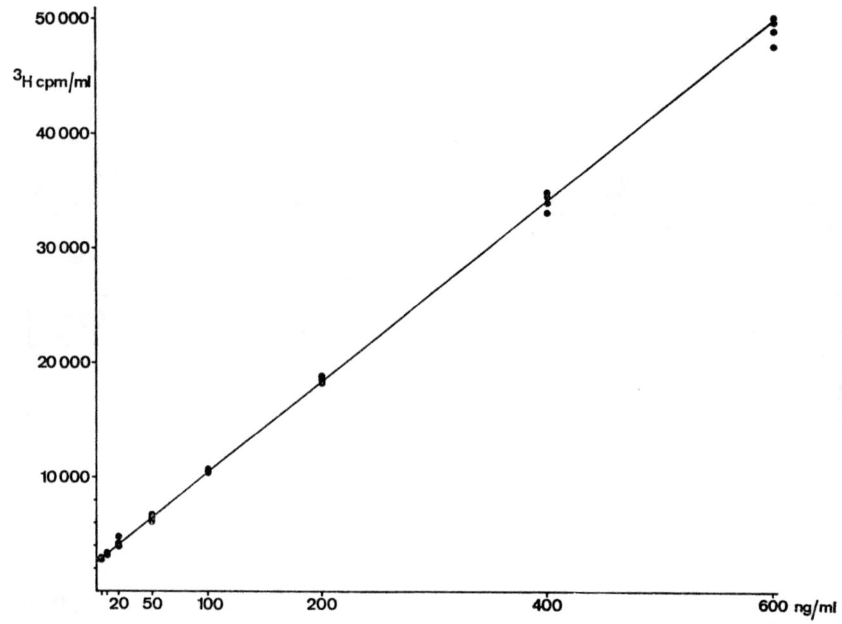

FIG. 4. Correlation of ^{3}H activity of the *N*-acetate of benzoctamine and the original concentration of unlabelled benzoctamine in human blood (3 ml of blood and 100 ng of ^{14}C-labelled benzoctamine were used as the internal standard for each analysis). Ordinate represents the ^{3}H activity measured and corrected by the yield of the internal ^{14}C standard.

octamine (100 ng, 2.9 μCi/μmol) was used as the internal standard for each sample. The [^{3}H]acetic anhydride was used at an activity of 50 μCi/μmol, with 1 μmol reagent per sample. The conditions were as described for maprotiline (Riess 1974) (and see Fig. 5). The precision of the DRID analysis of benzoctamine, especially with double determinations, is well within the limits needed for pharmacokinetic studies in man.

Using [^{3}H]acetic anhydride as the reagent, we have developed methods for assaying benzoctamine, maprotiline, demethylmaprotiline, hydroxymaprotiline, desipramine, nortriptyline, opipramol, de(hydroxyethyl)opipramol and oxprenolol (see Fig. 5). These ^{14}C-labelled standards were originally synthesized for metabolic studies in animals but for use as internal standards their synthesis can be greatly simplified since the label can be put into an accessible position in the side-chain with no regard for the metabolic stability of the drug.

PRACTICAL APPLICATION OF THE DRID METHOD

I shall now give an example of how the DRID method may be used, relevant

TABLE 1

Analysis of benzoctamine in human blood by double radioisotope derivative technique

Benzoctamine concentration in human blood		
Given (ng/ml)	*Found (ng/ml)*	*Mean ± standard deviation (ng/ml)*
5	5.9 6.4 4.1 6.9	5.8 ± 1.2
10	9.8 11.2 9.8 7.3	9.5 ± 1.6
50	47 47 52 45	47.8 ± 3.0
200	198 199 204 196	199.3 ± 3.4
600	588 606 598 570	590.5 ± 15.5

Four independent analyses per concentration
Volume of samples: 3 ml
Internal standard : [^{14}C] benzoctamine (100 ng, 2.9 μCi/μmol)
Reagent : [^{3}H] acetic anhydride (50 μCi/μmol)

to the context of this symposium. A patient who had been taking two 50 mg tablets of maprotiline daily attempted to commit suicide by taking a large number of four different kinds of tablets, among them an unknown quantity of maprotiline. The concentrations of the drug in the blood (Fig. 6) followed apparent first-order kinetics, with a half-life of about 30 hours. From previous experiments the distribution volume of maprotiline in man was known to be about 27 litres/kg; thus we were able to calculate the concentration that must have existed at the end of each dose interval during continuous treatment. The maximum concentration after the suicide attempt could be extrapolated roughly from Fig. 6, and the most likely amount of maprotiline ingested was thus estimated to have been about 300 mg, or six tablets.

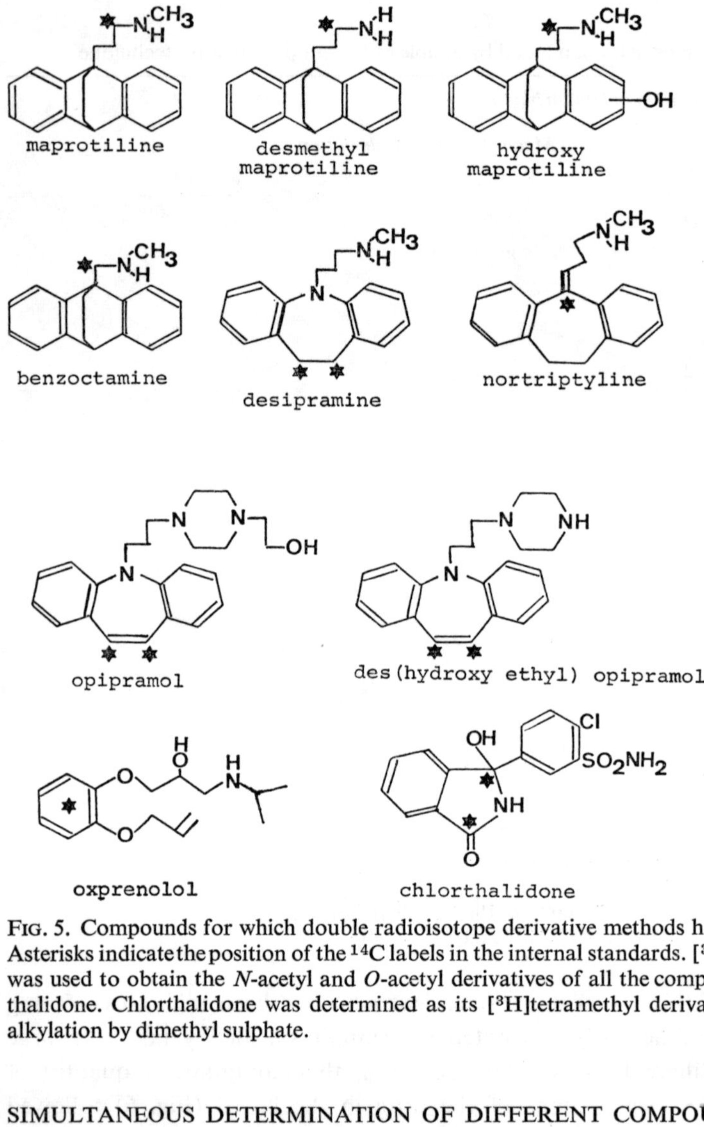

FIG. 5. Compounds for which double radioisotope derivative methods have been developed. Asterisks indicate the position of the ^{14}C labels in the internal standards. [^{3}H]Acetic anhydride was used to obtain the *N*-acetyl and *O*-acetyl derivatives of all the compounds except chlorthalidone. Chlorthalidone was determined as its [^{3}H]tetramethyl derivative after extractive alkylation by dimethyl sulphate.

SIMULTANEOUS DETERMINATION OF DIFFERENT COMPOUNDS

The DRID technique can be used to determine more than one compound at once if the appropriate ^{14}C-labelled internal standards are added simultaneously, and if chromatographic systems can be found that separate the mixture of derivatives that form when the ^{3}H-labelled agent reacts with them. Fig. 7*a* shows the separation, by a two-dimensional chromatogram, of a mixture containing acetyl derivatives of maprotiline and benzoctamine and the demethyl

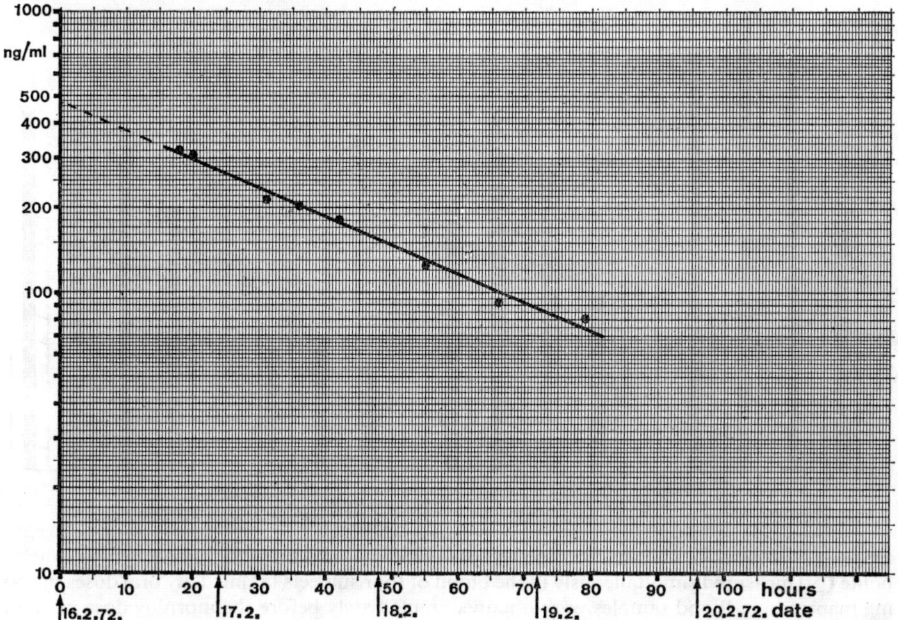

FIG. 6. Concentrations of maprotiline measured in human blood by double radioisotope derivative analysis in a suicide attempt by a person who took several different preparations, among them an estimated 300 mg maprotiline. Zero on the abscissa is the time the overdose was taken. Body weight of person 60 kg; estimated half-life of maprotiline: 29.7 hours.

metabolite of either compound. This system can be used when two drugs have been administered at the same time. A similar system (Fig. 7*b*) has been used to determine opipramol and its de(hydroxyethyl) metabolite simultaneously in

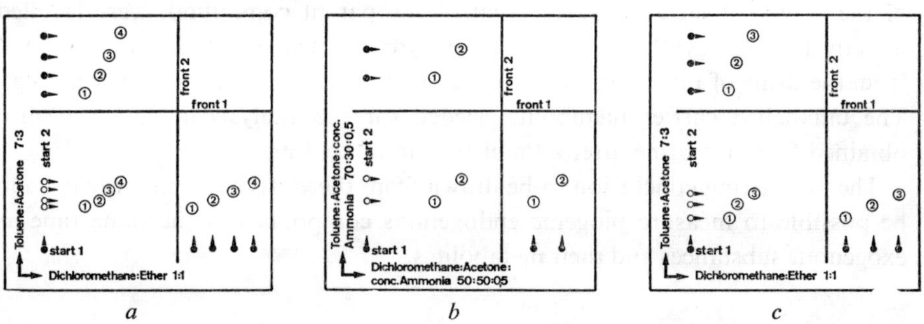

FIG. 7. Chromatographic systems on silica gel thin-layer that allow simultaneous determination of mixtures of (*a*) maprotiline (2), benzoctamine (4) and their respective *N*-demethyl homologues (1), (3), (*b*) opipramol (2) and its de(hydroxyethyl) metabolite (1), and (*c*) maprotiline and two of its metabolites.

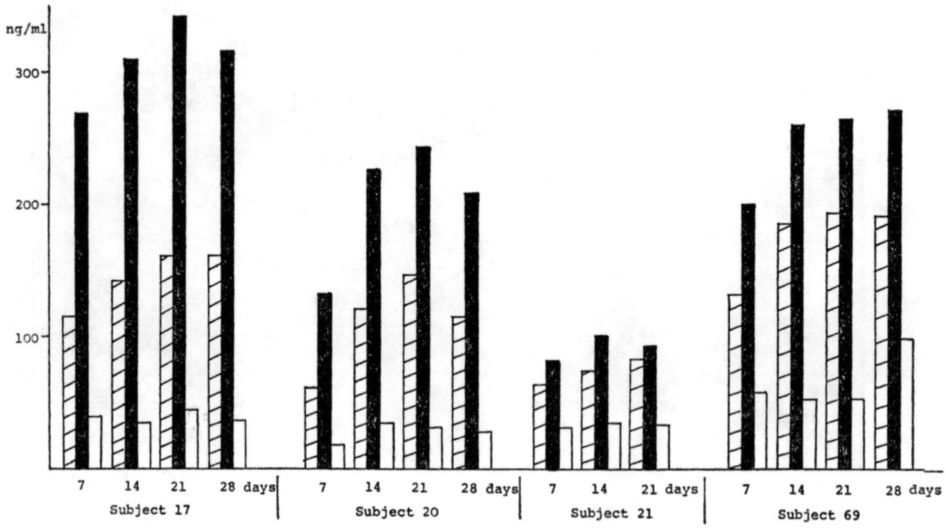

FIG. 8. Concentrations of maprotiline (■), its demethyl metabolite (▨) and hydroxy metabolite (□) measured simultaneously in the blood of four subjects taking daily oral doses of 150 mg maprotiline. Blood samples were obtained immediately before the morning dose on days 7, 14, 21 and 28 of treatment.

blood samples. If the extraction of the biological sample is modified so that phenolic amines as well as bases are isolated, the separation of derivatives, as shown in Fig. 7*c*, allows the parent compound, the demethyl metabolite and the phenolic metabolite to be determined simultaneously. Fig. 8 shows an example in which maprotiline and the two metabolites were determined simultaneously in the blood of patients on days 7, 14, 21 and 28 during continuous treatment with maprotiline (150 mg/day). The ^{14}C-labelled internal standards of the demethyl metabolite, like that of the parent compound, were labelled directly through synthesis, whereas the hydroxylated metabolite was isolated from the urine of rats after an oral dose of ^{14}C-labelled maprotiline (10 mg/kg). The unlabelled carrier metabolite needed for the analysis in man was also obtained from rat urine after administration of cold maprotiline.

The fascinating conclusion to be drawn from these studies is that it will soon be possible to measure biogenic endogenous compounds at the same time as exogenous substances and their metabolites.

TISSUE ANALYSIS

Because the internal standard is of the same structure as the drug to be analysed, the DRID technique is particularly suited for tissue analysis. If the

TABLE 2

Analysis of maprotiline in human tissue by double radioisotope derivative analysis (tissues were taken 3 days after death by suicide, supposedly from 300 mg maprotiline [Ludiomil])

Tissue	*Maprotiline found*	
	μg/g	*mean μg/g*
Liver	228.0 227.1	227.6
Lung	134.9 133.0	134.0
Kidney	87.4 87.4	87.4
Brain (thalamus)	80.6 83.7	82.2
Brain (medulla)	61.4 60.0	60.7
Adrenal gland	58.0 61.7	59.9
Heart	32.5 31.2	31.9
Muscle	10.5 10.1	10.3
Blood*	2.2	

Analytical conditions: Two independent determinations for each kind of tissue.
Aliquots of tissue homogenates ranging from 3.5 mg to 50 mg actual tissue weight per analysis.
200 ng (1 nCi) ^{14}C-labelled maprotiline internal standard per sample.
1 μmol (= 50 μCi) of [^{3}H]acetic anhydride per analysis.
* Blood sample taken 14 hours before death

tissue is ultrasonically homogenized directly in an aliquot of the internal standard solution and the homogenate is left to equilibrate overnight in the refrigerator, highly reproducible analyses can be obtained. Table 2 gives the double determinations of maprotiline in tissues from a person who had committed suicide by taking an overdose of maprotiline. From distribution studies with antidepressants in animals the organs analysed are known to carry higher concentrations of drug than blood does.

The principle of measuring parent compound and metabolites simultaneously can, of course, also be applied to tissue. Fig. 9 gives the concentrations of maprotiline, demethylmaprotiline and hydroxymaprotiline found in the tissues that had also been independently analysed for maprotiline alone (see Table 2).

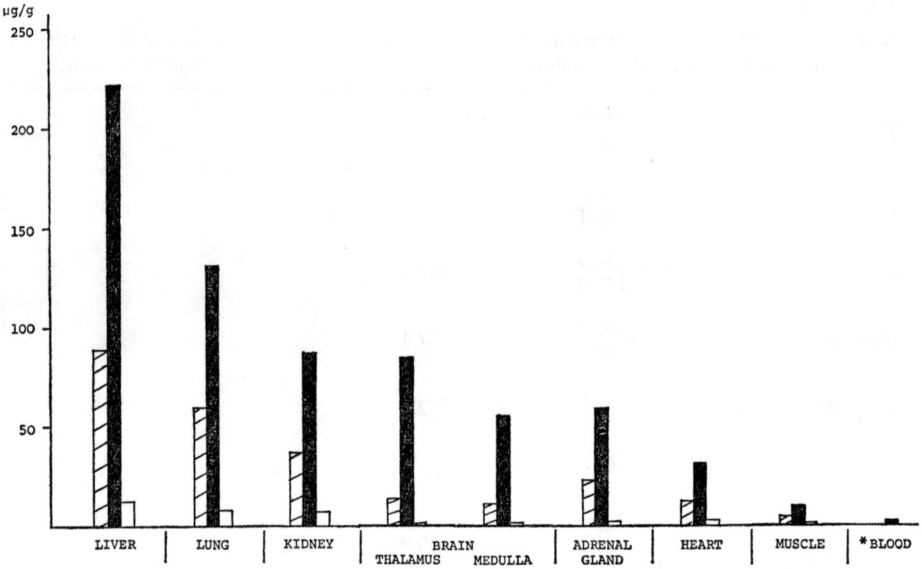

FIG. 9. Concentrations of maprotiline (■), its demethyl metabolite (▨) and hydroxy metabolite (□) measured simultaneously by double radioisotope derivative analysis in human tissue. The tissue samples were obtained 3 days after the death by suicide of a person who had supposedly taken a minimum of 300 mg maprotiline as well as previously administered repeated therapeutic doses. Concentration of maprotiline in blood 14 hours before death (*) was 2.2 µg/ml.

USE OF OTHER RADIOACTIVELY LABELLED REAGENTS

In all the examples given so far [^{3}H]acetic anhydride was the reagent of choice for primary and secondary amines as well as alcohols. However, other functional groups can be used for DRID analysis if the appropriate reagent is found.

Extractive alkylation has recently been introduced into analytical chemistry by Ervik & Gustavii (1974), who prepared a tetramethyl derivative of chlorthalidone (Hygroton) (see Fig. 10) suitable for gas chromatographic assay of the parent compound. Their method acts by extracting the compound as its tetrahexylammonium ion pair into dichloromethane. In this solvent, methyl iodide methylates the drug rapidly and quantitatively. This method seems very attractive for use with ^{3}H-labelled alkylating agents because it allows derivatives to be formed from carboxylic acids, C–H acids and phenols, as well as enols, alcohols and amides of weakly acidic nature.

Since [^{3}H]methyl iodide is inconvenient to handle, [^{3}H]dimethyl sulphate can be used instead. We used this reagent in the quantitative determination of chlorthalidone. Fig. 10 gives the plasma concentrations of chlorthalidone in

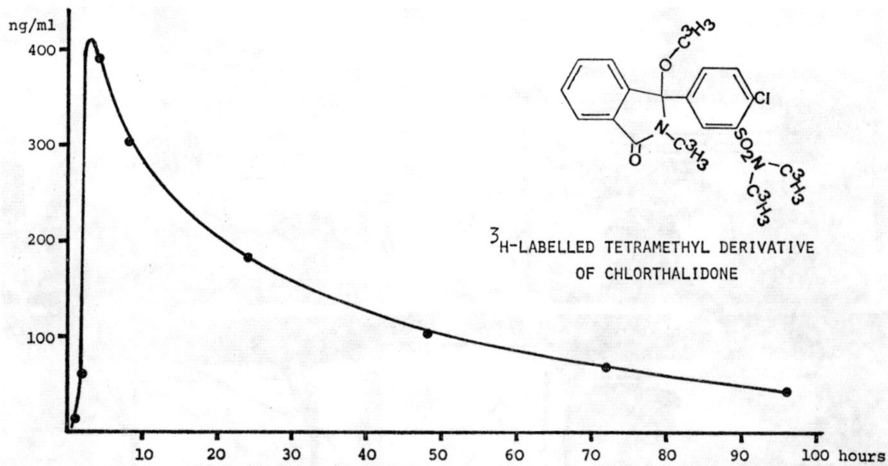

FIG. 10. Concentration of chlorthalidone in human blood plasma measured by double radioisotope derivative analysis after a single oral dose of 100 mg. The analysis is based on the formation of the [^{3}H]tetramethyl derivative from chlorthalidone by [^{3}H]dimethyl sulphate, using extractive alkylation.

human plasma after oral administration of 100 mg of the drug. For each analysis 1 ml plasma, 10 μmol tetrahexylammonium hydrogen sulphate, 200 ng (3.9 nCi) of ^{14}C-labelled chlorthalidone standard and 10 μmol (50 μCi) of ^{3}H-labelled dimethyl sulphate were used. Promising results have also been obtained in attempts to determine carboxylic acids by the same system.

It will be most interesting to examine other labelled reagents which may allow derivatives to be formed from other functional groups.

TECHNICAL PREREQUISITES OF DRID ANALYSIS

A major problem in radioisotope derivative methods is the safe handling of the radioactivity of the reagent. The excess reagent needs to be separated and trapped carefully so that all environmental contamination is avoided and low levels of drug can still be measured reliably. The operators must also be protected. For this reason I must say something about the technical prerequisites which are minimum technical requirements for any laboratory using the DRID technique. The radioactive reagent must always be handled in ventilated glove boxes (Fig. 11). Each box must, depending on the nature of the reagent and its hydrolysis products, be equipped with appropriate apparatus for absorbing or condensing the volatile radioactive material. In work with [^{3}H]dimethyl sulphate, [^{3}H]methanol should be condensed in cooling traps at the temperature of solid CO_2. In work with [^{3}H]acetic anhydride the acetic acid should be ab-

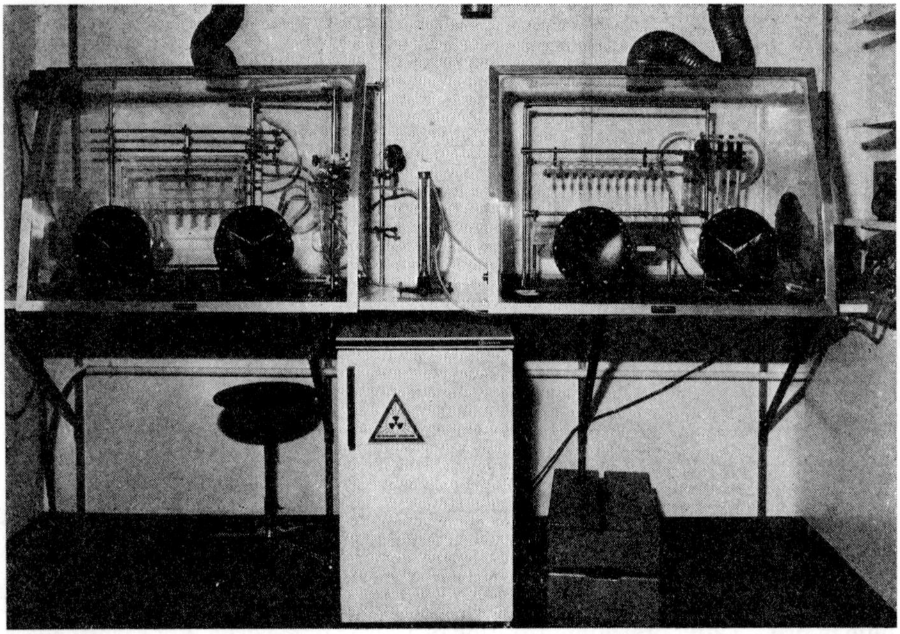

FIG. 11. Glove boxes used for the 'hot' stage of radioisotope derivative analysis.

sorbed into KOH. It is strongly recommended that the reagent should be stored in solvent ready for use and prepared in ampoules so that a fresh ampoule can be used for each analytical run. If appreciable amounts of volatile radioactivity enter the chromatographic process, thin-layer chromatography should also be done in a special ventilated box. It is advisable to use disposable glassware for routine analyses, to avoid even traces of contamination. Ordinary glass ampoules are suitable for most operations. The laboratory should routinely and frequently be checked for contamination. All analytical operations preceding the hot stage of the analysis must be done in a separate laboratory.

ACKNOWLEDGEMENTS

I am indebted to L. Dubey, G. Menge, H. H. Siegrist and H. Voisard for their valuable help during the development of the methods described. I am also grateful to my colleagues W. Kueng and K. Schmid for providing the ^{14}C-labelled compounds used as internal standards.

References

ERVIK, M. & GUSTAVII, K. (1974) Application of the extractive alkylation technique to the gas chromatographic determination of chlorthalidone in plasma in nanogram quantities. *Anal. Chem. 46*, 39–42

RIESS, W. (1974) The double radio-isotope derivative technique for the assay of drugs in biological material. Part 1. The determination of maprotiline. *Anal. Chim. Acta 68*, 363–376

WHITEHEAD, J. K. & DEAN, H. G. (1968) *Methods of Biochemical Analysis*, Interscience, New York

Discussion

Moffat: I imagine that in screening for unknown drugs, for example, the acetyl derivatives can be formed from secondary amines and phenols, and one could even perhaps use ketones which would react with primary amines. But a lot of the drugs we have to look at now are tertiary amines. Could you say more about the derivative you were looking at for tertiary amines?

Riess: We have used ethyl chlorocarbonate to degrade tertiary amines to the secondary amines and then go via the secondary amine to the acetyl product. If the tertiary amine is treated with ethyl chlorocarbonate we end up with the carbamate. If we used tritiated ethyl chlorocarbonate we would end up with tritiated carbamate which is a neutral product, very easy to separate from other compounds. This would allow tertiary amines to be determined. However, there is one snag. Secondary amines that form from the tertiary amine via metabolic processes would undergo the same reaction. We therefore need to run two separate analyses. In one we determine the secondary amine via acetylation, and in the other we determine the sum total of the tertiary amine and the secondary amine. Before we thought of using [^{3}H]ethyl chlorocarbonate we hydrolysed the 'cold' carbamate in KOH at 180 °C to form the secondary amine which can be acetylated with [^{3}H]acetic anhydride.

Holmstedt: Don't you find this procedure cumbersome, Dr Riess?

Riess: You mean it is not so efficient as GC–MS? The method with the hydrolysis step is certainly cumbersome. That is why we gave it up for routine analysis of large sample numbers. But it works nicely, even if the final yield of acetyl derivative is very low. Provided the recovered ^{14}C activity of the internal standard can be measured statistically reliably, one ends up with perfect analytical results. This is true also for straightforward acetylation of the secondary amines. Even if the overall yield of the derivative is below 10%, our analytical results agree perfectly with those of parallel samples that may have yielded 40 or 50% of derivative. This is because we are using an ideal standard which corrects the losses over all the processes involved.

Widdop: We have been measuring nortriptyline by a gas chromatographic method (Braithwaite & Widdop 1971). This will also determine the tertiary amine, amitriptyline, which my colleagues have shown to be of equal pharmacological importance in the context of therapeutic monitoring (Braithwaite *et al.* 1972). I am therefore sorry to hear that you do not intend to adapt your technique to cover the tertiary amines, Dr Riess.

Riess: Even though we have measured tertiary amines via their carbamates, we have also been developing GC–MS methods using a deuteriated internal standard, and I must admit that for large numbers of samples, as we usually analyse them, tertiary amines can be measured much more conveniently by mass spectrometry. However the investment in instruments is considerable there.

Widdop: To gain some idea of your analytical throughput, how many plasma nortriptyline samples can you handle in, say, one hour?

Riess: Of course the whole process of analysis takes several hours but one can analyse many samples at the same time and the output of the laboratory depends on how much has been invested in the system. With our electronic data processing system and the liquid scintillation counter running all through the night, we can do about 40 samples per person per day.

References

BRAITHWAITE, R. A. & WIDDOP, B. (1971) A specific gas-chromatographic method for the measurement of 'steady-state' plasma levels of amitriptyline and nortriptyline in patients. *Clin. Chim. Acta 35*, 461–472

BRAITHWAITE, R. A., GOULDING, R., THEANO, G., BAILEY, J. & COPPEN, A. (1972) Plasma concentration of amitriptyline and clinical response. *Lancet 1*, 1297–1300

An on-line liquid chromatograph–mass spectrometer system

R. P. W. SCOTT, C. G. SCOTT, M. MUNROE and J. HESS JR.

Chemical Research Department, Hoffmann-La Roche Inc., Nutley, New Jersey

Abstract An interface is described that permits the on-line operation of a liquid chromatograph and quadrupole mass spectrometer combination. The interface consists of two differentially pumped chambers through which a wire train system continually takes a sample of the column eluent, evaporates the solvent, and subsequently vaporizes the residual solute in the ionizing chamber of the mass spectrometer. The feasibility of the system has been confirmed and its use as an alternative method for probe injection has been demonstrated. Examples of its use with a liquid chromatograph are also given. The sensitivity of the present system is about 2×10^{-5} g/ml of solute, which is only just adequate for liquid chromatography separations. With relatively simple modifications, the ultimate sensitivity is predicted to be between 10^{-7} and 10^{-6} g/ml which would make the system generally applicable to most liquid chromatographic separations.

Most analytical methods incorporate three distinct processes: a separation procedure that removes the substance of interest from other contaminating materials, an identification procedure that confirms the identity of the substance separated, and a quantitative procedure which determines the amount of the substance present in the original mixture. Analysis can range, therefore, from a simple extraction procedure followed by titration to, for example, the highly sophisticated gas chromatography–mass spectrometry combination (GC–MS). In the latter, the direct combination of the two techniques provides simultaneous separation, quantitative estimation and identification. The gas chromatograph and the mass spectrometer are an ideal combination because the eluent of the chromatograph, usually helium, can be drawn directly into the mass spectrometer, together with the sample vapour, without seriously affecting the performance of the mass spectrometer. However, gas chromatography can only be effective for the separation of materials that are volatile, and many toxic materials and substances of biological interest are involatile; although some can be converted into derivatives sufficiently volatile for gas chromatography, these are a relatively small proportion of the substances of interest.

The ideal method for separating involatile materials of relatively high molecular weight is liquid chromatography (LC). Over the past five years or so there have been significant advances in this technique. These advances have been in both column technology and instrumentation. With suitable gradient elution systems (Scott & Kucera 1973*a*), relatively rapid separations (e.g. 45 min) of substances with widely different polarities can be achieved with only a few micrograms of material. However, where the mobile phase is a liquid, its association with an identification technique such as mass spectrometry is difficult because the liquid eluent from the column cannot be fed effectively into the mass spectrometer without impairing its operation. The liquid nature of the mobile phase also limits the combination of liquid chromatography with other spectroscopic techniques, particularly if the selection of solvents is not to be restricted so that complete versatility of the chromatographic technique can be maintained. Nevertheless, if the problem of introducing the eluted substance into the mass spectrometer without the solvent in which it is dissolved can be solved, mass spectrometry is ideal for use with liquid chromatography, as it can both provide a means of identification and at the same time be highly sensitive. A practical solution which has so far shown great promise lies in using the detecting principle of the wire transport detector (Scott & Lawrence 1970) devised for LC. In this detector a continuous wire passes through the eluent from the column and a thin film of liquid is left on the surface of the wire. The wire then passes through a heated air stream which evaporates the solvent so that only the solute originally present in the eluent is left on the wire surface. In its more customary use the wire passes into an enclosure at about 700 °C. The residue on the wire is burned to CO_2 and water; subsequently the CO_2 is drawn into a hydrogen stream and passed over a nickel catalyst that converts it into methane, which is then detected by a flame ionization detector.

Such a system could obviously lend itself to mass spectroscopic detection if the wire could be made to pass through the spectrometer and if the solute could be vaporized by suitable means in the ion source. Thus the wire transport system would remove a sample from the column eluent, evaporate the solvent, and carry the residue of eluted solute into the mass spectrometer. However, there are several difficulties to be overcome:

(1) The liquid chromatograph eluent leaves the column at atmospheric pressure whereas the pressure in the ion source of the mass spectrometer must be 10^{-5}–10^{-7} mmHg (13.33–1333 μPa). Thus an interface must be designed which will allow the wire to pass through the mass spectrometer while adequate low pressures are maintained in the ion source.

(2) For the low pressure to be maintained, the interface must carry small apertures for the wire to pass through, and these must be designed in such a way that the continual abrasive action of the wire on the walls of the apertures will not distort their shape and size.
(3) The wire must not interfere with the ion optics of the source during its passage through, or close to, the electron beam, otherwise the resolution of the mass spectrometer will be impaired.
(4) The interface must be designed in such a way that the wire can be heated when it is close to or actually in the electron beam, so that the coated solute will be volatilized and ionization can take place.

DESIGN OF THE INTERFACE

In the standard deflection mass spectrometer the ion optics are critically controlled by the potential gradients between the electrodes in the ion source. The ion optics would therefore be very sensitive to an earthed wire passing close to these electrodes. For this reason the mass spectrometer chosen was the Finnigan Quadrupole Mass Spectrometer, where the ion optics of the source are very simple and insensitive to the proximity of earthed conductors.

A diagram of the interface is shown in Fig. 1. The interfaces are made in pairs, one for the entry of the wire into the ion source and the other for its exit to the winding spool. Each interface consists of two small chambers separated and terminated by rubies with a central aperture 0.01 inches in diameter (0.254 mm). These jewels are standard watch jewels used for bearings in small time-pieces; they are 0.1 in (2.54 mm) in diameter and 0.014 in (0.356 mm) thick,

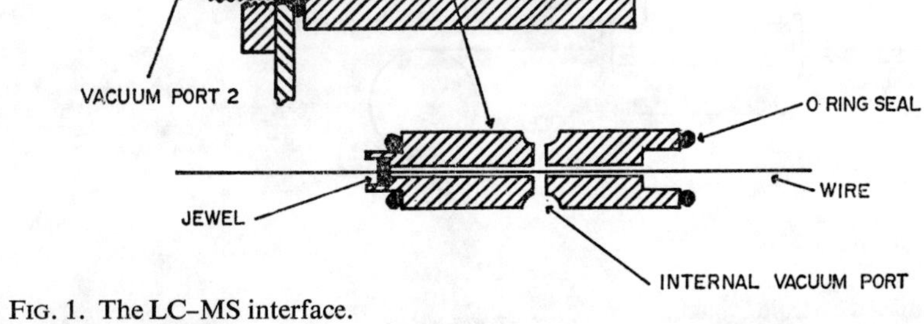

FIG. 1. The LC–MS interface.

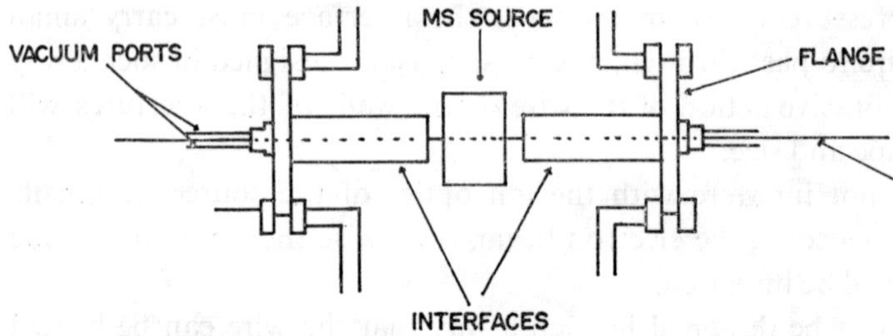

FIG. 2. Diagram of interfaces located in MS source.

and are set into the chambers with a high temperature epoxy resin cement. The wire cannot distort the hard surfaces of these jewels. Each chamber is connected to an evacuating port. The outside chambers directly in contact with the atmosphere are connected in parallel to a 300 litre/min rotary vacuum pump. The second chambers between the first chambers and the mass spectrometer source are also connected in parallel to a 2-in (5 cm) oil diffusion pump backed by a rotary pump with a capacity of 160 l/min. This system of differential pumps reduces the gas pressure in stages. In the first chamber it is reduced to about 0.2 mmHg (26.6 Pa) and in the second to about 2×10^{-3} mmHg (0.266 Pa). Fig. 2 shows the interfaces in the mass spectrometer head; they are arranged in a re-entrant design so that when the wire leaves the interface it is within 1 to 2 cm of the electron beam which will produce the ions.

The wire train we used was the standard unit from the Philips Chromatography moving wire detector and Fig. 3 shows a diagram of the complete arrangement. The wire from the train system passes around an insulated pulley, through the column eluent and directly into the first interface, and thence into the mass spectrometer. The wire leaves the mass spectrometer through the second interface, passes around another pulley and then to the capstan winding

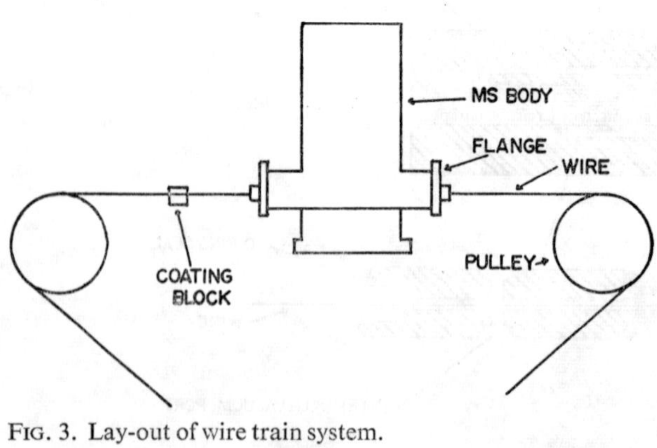

FIG. 3. Lay-out of wire train system.

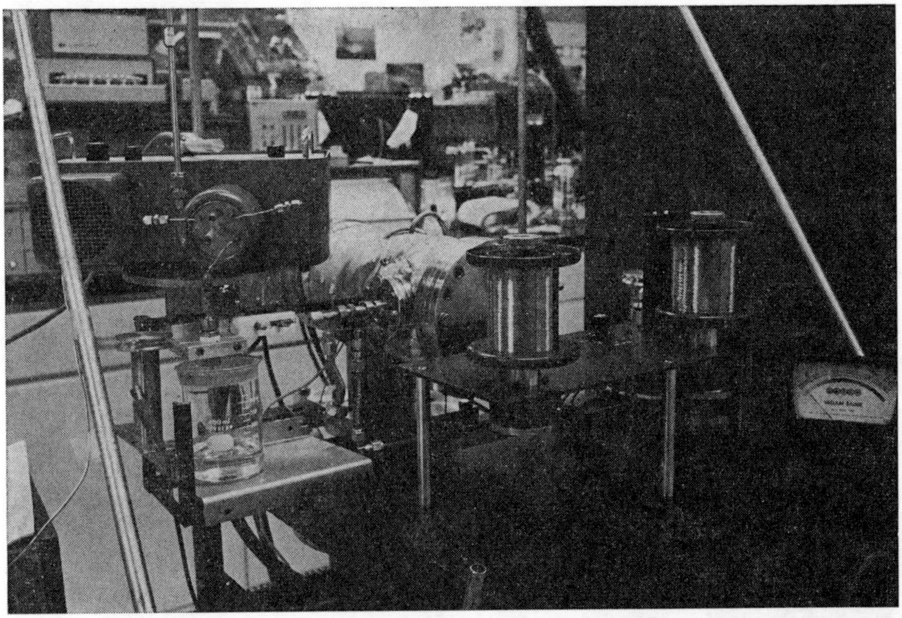

FIG. 4. First version of the LC–MS apparatus described here, with interfaces protruding from the mass spectrometer.

system of the wire train mechanism. The insulated pulleys were constructed using roller bearings and particular care was taken in their alignment to minimize friction.

Fig. 4 is a photograph of the first version of the apparatus, when the interfaces were not re-entrant in design. They are basically of the same form as the interfaces described and used in this paper but protrude outside the mass spectrometer. The general layout of the apparatus shown in Fig. 4, however, is identical to that used to provide the results given here. The feed spool mounted on the wire train system is near the centre of Fig. 4. The receiver spool is to the right and below this is the feed drive motor. The mass spectrometer analyser unit is behind the centre feed spool and the connections of the vacuum systems to the inlet interface are on the left of this. The wire passes from the feed spool to a pulley on the left and then through the coating block through which the eluent from the chromatography column passes, wetting the wire. From the coating block the wire passes through the inlet interface into the mass spectrometer, then through the second interface (not visible in the photograph) and around another pulley to the winding mechanism. Because of the insensitivity of the ion source to slight changes in potential in its neighbourhood, the wire could be heated to vaporize the solute by passing a current through it. The wire used was the standard wire supplied by Philips Chromatography for the wire transport detector and is made of stainless steel 0.005 in (0.127 mm) in diameter. When a current of 200 mA is passed through this wire in air, at atmospheric pressure, the surrounding air keeps the wire cool. However, when the wire is in the high vacuum of the mass spectrometer, heat can only be lost by radiation and with a 200 mA current its temperature rises to about 250 °C. The required volatilization can thus be obtained in the mass spectrometer. The current is applied to the wire between the left pulley and the coating block and to the pulley behind the receiver spool. In Fig. 4 the column is connected to the coating block through a refractometer detector. This detector was used as a reference in the development of the system.

The normal output from the mass spectrometer is usually taken to a UV chart recorder. However, with the recent developments in computer data-handling systems, the Finnigan Mass Spectrometer can now be associated with a computer that provides sophisticated data-processing procedures which will not be discussed in detail here. In essence, the computer stores all the mass spectra obtained during a chromatographic run and presents them either in the form of a reconstructed chromatogram or as any individual mass spectrum.

EXPERIMENTAL

The Finnigan Mass Spectrometer and its data-handling computer system are standard pieces of commercial instrumentation and their operation will not be discussed. After the interfaces have been connected to their respective pumps the pressure in their pump manifolds should be, for the first stage, 0.2 mmHg (26.6 Pa) and, for the second stage 2×10^{-3} mmHg (0.266 Pa). In these interface conditions the source pressure of the mass spectrometer should be between 10^{-6} and 10^{-5} mmHg (133.3–1333 μPa). The normal Finnigan GC–MS computer program can be used in an identical manner for the LC–MS system. The wire train mechanism has four speeds and these are selected to provide the desired range of sensitivity. For a given concentration of solute in the column eluent, the speed of the wire conditions the quantity of sample that enters the mass spectrometer per unit time; thus the faster the wire speed the higher the overall sensitivity. In most of the experiments discussed here the maximum speed ($\times$ 6 inches/s, or about 15 cm/s) was used; samples were coated on the wire by passing a solution of the substance in an appropriate solvent (or, for chromatographic separations, the column eluent) directly over the wire, using the standard Philips Chromatography coating block. During the run the data from the LC–MS system were continually stored in the disc memory associated with the computer and later they were processed by the computer. The results were then presented in the form of a reconstructed chromatogram or as mass spectra on a Houston Instruments plotter.

SAMPLE VOLATILIZATION

For mass spectra to be produced, the sample coated on the wire has to be volatilized in the ion source by a current passed through the wire, as already described. However, there is an optimum temperature and thus an optimum current that will provide optimum volatilization and maximum sensitivity. The optimum current was determined for three compounds: a diazepam metabolite, phenobarbitone (phenobarbital) and acetylsalicylic acid. They were coated individually (from a 0.1% v/v solution in methanol) onto the wire and, during a constant feed of sample, the current through the wire was progressively increased from 0 to 300 mA. The total ion current was measured and the results for the three substances investigated are shown in Fig. 5.

At wire speed ×6, the diazepam metabolite and phenobarbitone have similar optimum wire currents, of 160 and 190 mA respectively. However, due to the relatively high volatility of acetylsalicylic acid, the optimum current is much lower (50 mA) and the absolute sensitivity is less than one-fifth that for the

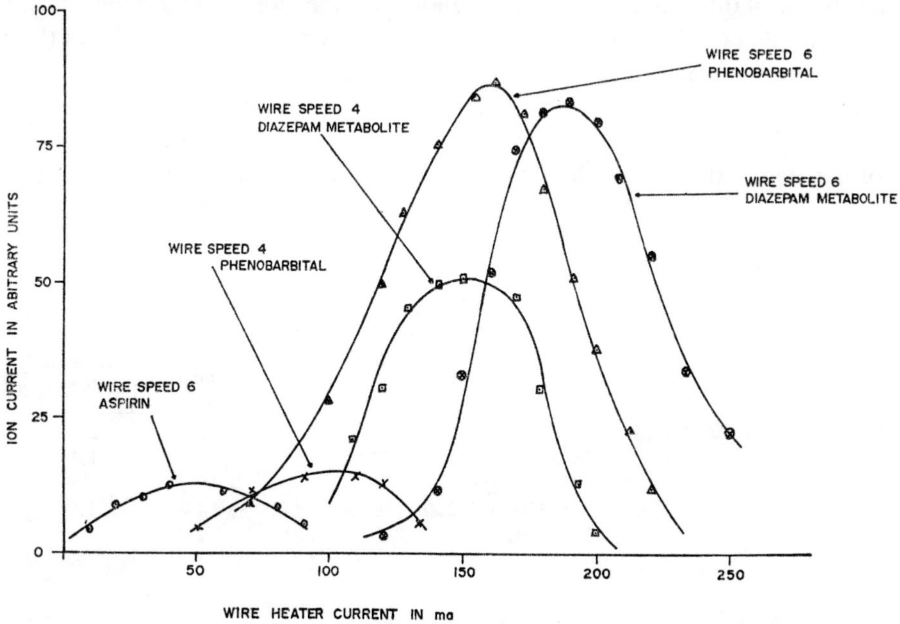

FIG. 5. Total ion current plotted against wire heater current.

other two compounds. The implication is that the system is more applicable to substances of low volatility. However, as the more volatile materials are likely to be amenable to elution by gas chromatography, volatility should not present a problem if the apparatus is used with a liquid chromatograph. Fig. 5 also shows that the lower wire speed has a significantly lower optimum wire current. This is because the wire starts heating in the interfaces and, if the temperature is too high and the movement of the wire too slow, the sample is therefore volatilized in the interface and probably lost through the second chamber pump before it can enter the mass spectrometer. It follows that the wire current must be adjusted to be appropriate to the wire speed.

DETERMINATION OF SENSITIVITY

The sensitivity of the system to the concentration of solute in a chromatographic eluent was determined by feeding a constant stream of solvent containing 1×10^{-4} g/ml solute onto the wire, then measuring the total ion current produced and comparing it with the noise level when no solute was present. To determine the effect of solvent polarity on response three steroids were used: 3β-cholestanol, a polar solute; cholesteryl acetate, a substance of intermediate polarity; and cholesterol, a relatively non-polar material. These were dissolved in solvents of different polarities, methanol being the most polar, acetone having intermediate polarity and chloroform relatively low polarity. The choice of these solutes and solvents permitted any effect of solute–solvent polarity on the wetting of the wire to become apparent. The most polar solute, cholestanol, was used in both the polar solvent methanol and the non-polar solvent chloroform, whereas the solutes cholesterol and cholesteryl acetate were used in solu-

TABLE 1

Sensitivity of the LC–MS system to different solutes

Solute	*Solvent*	*Scanning mass range (EMU)*	*Wire heater current (mA)*	*Mean signal (arbitrary units)*	*Noise (arbitrary units)*	*Sensitivity at a signal-to-noise ratio of 2 ($\times 10^{-5}$ g/ml)*
3β-Cholestanol	Methanol	215–220; 385–390	270	23.0	2.5	2.2
Cholesteryl acetate	Acetone	365–375	270	30.0	2.2	1.4
Cholesterol	Chloroform	365–370; 385–390	270	49.0	4.0	1.6
3β-Cholestanol	Chloroform	215–220; 385–390	270	29.0	2.9	2

Mass spectrometer conditions: Integration time, 100 ms; Attenuation, 3
Wire train conditions: Speed, × 6; Heater current, 250 mA

tions of chloroform and acetone, respectively. The results and the operating conditions are shown in Table 1. The sensitivity of the instrument to the solutes concerned lies between 1 and 2×10^{-5} g/ml. Also, all solutes in all solvents exhibit approximately the same sensitivity; thus the wetting characteristics of the wire do not appear to present a serious problem.

INJECTION OF SINGLE SAMPLES

The system can be used to simulate the more conventional procedure of solid probe injection. A solution of the material for which a mass spectrum was required was dropped on the wire and the spectra were recorded. This procedure was examined to provide spectra for racemethorphan, 3β-cholestanol, a diazepam metabolite, phenobarbitone, cholesterol, sulphamethoxazole, cholesteryl acetate, and nicotinic acid. The eight samples were manually placed on the wire (using 0.1% solutions of each substance in methanol) at 45 s intervals over a period of six minutes and spectra were obtained. The resulting peaks are shown in Fig. 6. The first curve represents the total ion current measured during the sampling procedure and shows a peak for each substance placed on the wire. The second and third curves demonstrate the selectivity of the mass spectrometer system. The second curve is a plot for the ion of mass 123, which is the base peak (the most abundant ion) for nicotinic acid. This gives a single peak for nicotinic acid, confirming its identification. In the third curve the molecular ion for cholesterol (*m*/*e* 386) was used; in this case the cholesterol peak is the only peak shown and again confirms the identity of the sample. From the individual peaks the mass spectra can be obtained, and two examples are also shown in Fig. 6. The system provides a rapid alternative method to normal probe sampling for obtaining spectra of involatile samples. The wire transport system at wire speed × 6 transports 10 μl of solution to the mass spectrometer/min. Thus, if the solution of the solute is at the maximum sensitivity level of 2×10^{-5} g/ml, the minimum mass of solute that can, at present, provide a spectrum is 0.15 μg. If an automatic injection system similar to that used in gas chromatography were used and if the samples were automatically dropped on the wire while it was being temperature-programmed, mass spectra of materials could be automatically obtained on a routine basis. Plotting each spectrum may still take several minutes, but with the computer system this could be automatically programmed with a queuing procedure and the spectra could be plotted for a large number of samples overnight. For a single sample the mass spectrum could be taken and spectra plotted in about five minutes.

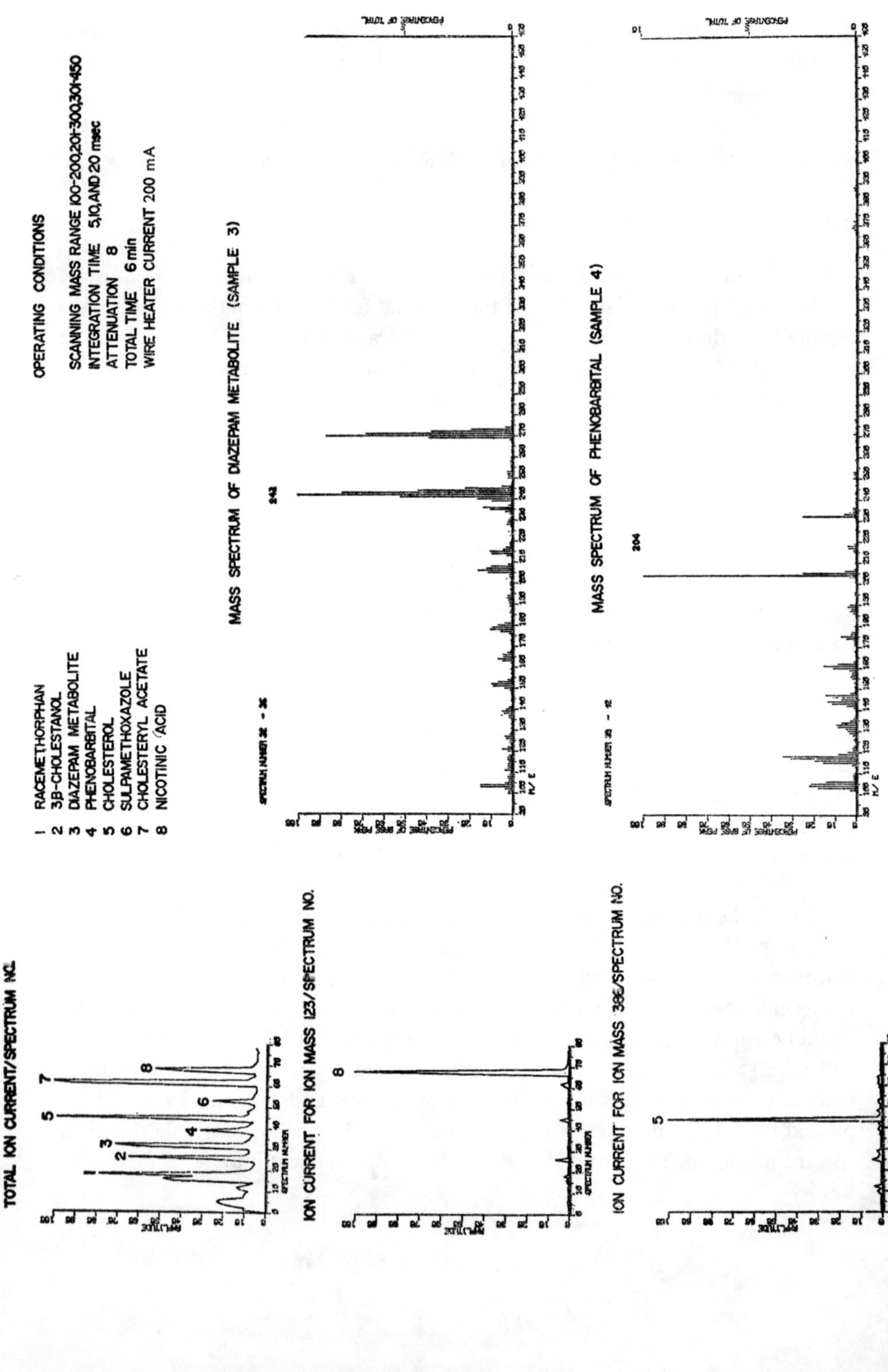
TOTAL ION CURRENT/SPECTRUM NO.
ION CURRENT FOR ION MASS 123/SPECTRUM NO.
ION CURRENT FOR ION MASS 386/SPECTRUM NO.
1 RACEMETHORPHAN
2 3β-CHOLESTANOL
3 DIAZEPAM METABOLITE
4 PHENOBARBITAL
5 CHOLESTEROL
6 SULPAMETHOXAZOLE
7 CHOLESTERYL ACETATE
8 NICOTINIC ACID
OPERATING CONDITIONS
SCANNING MASS RANGE 100-200,201-300,301-450
INTEGRATION TIME 5,10,AND 20 msec
ATTENUATION 8
TOTAL TIME 6 min
WIRE HEATER CURRENT 200 mA
MASS SPECTRUM OF DIAZEPAM METABOLITE (SAMPLE 3)
242
MASS SPECTRUM OF PHENOBARBITAL (SAMPLE 4)
204

THE LC–MS SYSTEM

The column we used was 25 cm long, 4.6 mm in internal diameter, and packed with 10 μm Partisil silica gel. The column was connected to a Waters 6000 pump which in turn was connected to the incremental gradient elution apparatus described by Scott & Kucera (1973*a*). The solvents used were those also described by Scott & Kucera (1973*b*) and the column flow rate was maintained constant at 2 ml/min. The sample contained *n*-triacontane (C_{30} *n*-alkane), cholesteryl laurate, cholesterol and phenobarbitone. This mixture was made up as a 0.6% solution of each component in a mixed solvent of heptane, acetone and methanol, and 150 μl was placed on the column. The mass spectrometry conditions used were the same as for the probe samples, except that the mass range scanned was from 50 to 600 mass units and the integration times for the mass ranges of 50 to 200, 201 to 400, and 401 to 600, were 8, 13 and 20 ms, respectively. The wire speed was set at × 6 and the heating current at 250 mA. During the development of the chromatogram each of the gradient elution solvents was used for 4 min; thus, as there are 12 solvents in the series, this resulted in a 48-min chromatogram with 8 ml of each solvent being used. The chromatogram is shown as curve 1 in Fig. 7. This is a monitor of the total ion current. The first peak is the *n*-alkane, the second cholesteryl laurate, the third cholesterol and the fourth phenobarbitone. The somewhat disappointing elution peak obtained for cholesteryl laurate is probably attributable to the wire current not being sufficiently high to vaporize the compound in the ion source. The conditions appear to be satisfactory for the three other components. The second chromatogram shown in Fig. 7 was plotted from the data collected during the run, using only the intensities for the molecular ion of cholesterol (*m*/*e* 386).

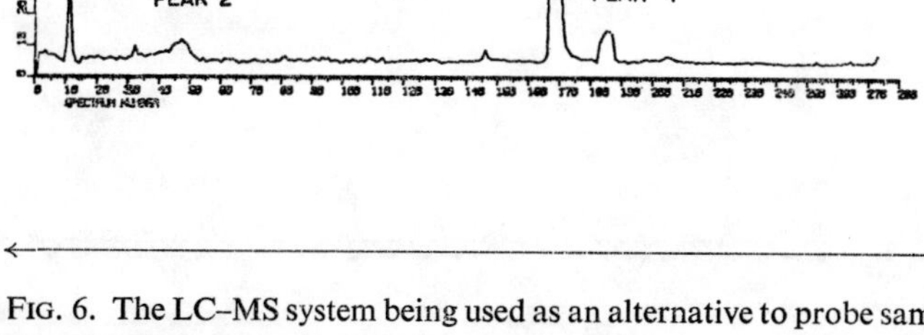

FIG. 7, continued overleaf

FIG. 6. The LC–MS system being used as an alternative to probe sampling.

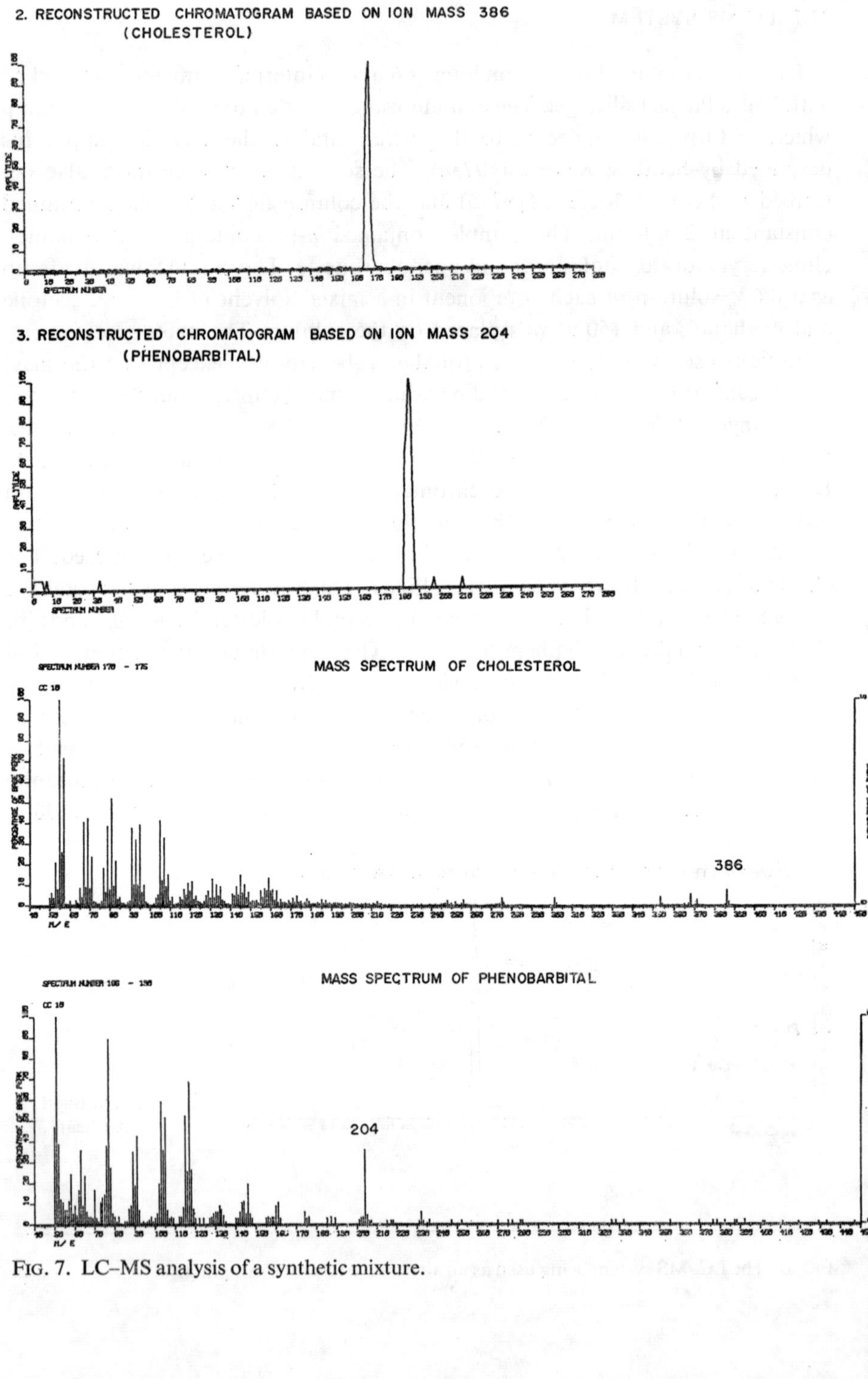

FIG. 7. LC–MS analysis of a synthetic mixture.

This chromatogram indicates that the third component is cholesterol. Similarly the third chromatogram, reconstructed on *m/e* 204, indicates that the fourth component is phenobarbitone. Mass spectra taken from these two peaks are included in Fig. 7. They confirm the identification and demonstrate the quality of the spectra that can be obtained from the peaks eluted from a liquid chromatographic column.

CONCLUSION

An interface has been described in this paper that permits the use of on-line mass spectrometric analysis with a liquid chromatograph, and the feasibility of the system has been confirmed.

In its present form the system can be extremely effective as an alternative method to probe sampling, permitting adequate sensitivity and at the same time lending itself to automatic operation. When used in conjunction with a liquid chromatographic column, the results are borderline, from a practical point of view. The combined system was shown to have a sensitivity of 2×10^{-5} g/ml, which is only just adequate for analytical liquid chromatography, as sample loads in excess of 1 mg can seriously impair resolution. However, the sensitivity of the instrument can be significantly increased by reducing the pressures in the interface; this will require a slightly modified interface system. Reducing the interface pressures will allow the ion source to be operated at 10^{-7} to 10^{-6} mmHg (13.33–133.3 μPa) instead of 10^{-5} to 10^{-6} mmHg (133.3–1333 μPa) as it is with the present apparatus. Such pressures will not only improve the resolution obtained from the mass spectrometer but also significantly increase the signal-to-noise ratio. Another source of loss of sensitivity is the evaporation of the sample from the wire in the second chamber of the interface before it enters the mass spectrometer. This can also be reduced by modifying the geometry of the second chamber and could possibly be eliminated by using a different heating procedure to volatilize the sample from the wire. The mass spectrometer we used for this work was of an early design and does not include magnetic focusing, which can also significantly improve the overall sensitivity of the instrument. Modification of the interfaces and possibly the use of an alternative method for heating the wire, together with a magnetic focusing ion source, should increase the sensitivity by one to two orders of magnitude. A sensitivity of 10^{-7} to 10^{-6} g/ml would make the LC–MS system widely applicable to the analysis of involatile or high molecular weight substances. Work on increasing the sensitivity of the apparatus on the lines suggested is now being done.

ACKNOWLEDGEMENTS

We wish to thank Mr T. Z. Chu of the Finnigan Corporation for the loan of the Quadrupole Mass Spectrometer and Mr T. Filipi of Philips Chromatography for the loan of the wire train mechanism.

References

SCOTT, R. P. W. & KUCERA, P. (1973*a*) An apparatus for use with incremental gradient elution. *J. Chromatogr. Sci. 11*, 83–87

SCOTT, R. P. W. & KUCERA, P. (1973*b*) A rational series of solvents for use in incremental gradient elution. *Anal. Chem. 45*, 749–754

SCOTT, R. P. W. & LAWRENCE, J. G. (1970) An improved moving wire liquid chromatography detector. *J. Chromatogr. Sci. 8*, 65–71

Discussion

Leach: Do you have any problems with contamination or scraping of material off the wire?

Scott: No, there is virtually no carry-over at all. Even if the wire touches a jewel orifice, it only touches at one point and contamination will be very small indeed.

Holmstedt: How long have you been able to run this system without deterioration, such as the holes getting bigger?

Scott: The first model with the external ports was run for about three months. Then we took it apart, not because the jewel apertures had deteriorated but to put in the re-entrant design of interface so that we could get closer to the electron beam. Under the microscope the jewels showed no wear at all. One wouldn't expect any, if one remembers how hard rubies are, compared with stainless steel.

Holmstedt: Have you estimated the layer of substance on the wire?

Scott: Its sensitivity is 10^{-5} g/ml and the wire takes 10 μl/min into the system. Thus 1.7×10^{-9} g/s enters the main spectrometer.

Holmstedt: Does part of the inner surface of the interface become contaminated with one substance which interferes with the following one?

Scott: No; as I said, there is no indication of wear or deposit on the jewels. I don't think one would expect it with this system. A carry-over of two or three seconds may occur, but this really doesn't matter in liquid chromatography. There is no permanent contamination.

Holmstedt: What sensitivity have you reached?

Scott: At the moment it is 10^{-5}, or 10 μg/ml. Later we should reach 10^{-6} or 10^{-7}, but at present I can't predict much further than that.

Holmstedt: That may not be sensitive enough for the analysis of modern drugs in blood.

Scott: It depends on the column we use with it. If a peak on the chromatogram is 1 ml wide and the sensitivity is 10^{-5} g/ml, then there will be 5 μg in that peak. In modern microparticle columns the peak may be less than 0.1 ml wide and there will be 500 ng in the peak at a sensitivity of 10^{-5} g/ml. That is the present sensitivity of our system.

Holmstedt: That is fair enough. You should be able to analyse polar compounds, for example glucuronides.

Scott: This depends on the chromatography of course. With the right chromatographic system, you can get virtually anything out in a single separation.

Holmstedt: Were the single ion detections you demonstrated carried out by on-line monitoring of an *m/e* value? That is, were they mass fragmentograms or mass chromatograms?

Scott: They were on-line mass chromatograms.

Moffat: How much sample could you actually put in?

Scott: With our present sensitivity about 0.15 μg. The peaks in Fig. 7 are each 120 ng.

Gillette: Could you increase the amount of material on the wire by adding several drops and evaporating the solvent between the additions?

Scott: You could, but it makes it more involved.

Moffat: What volume can you put at the top of the column?

Scott: You can put in as much as 250 μl. With gradient elution you can use a lot. It may deactivate a small part of the front of the column but this doesn't matter. The sample is adsorbed and piles up on the front of the column and as you go through the gradient you lift each solute off one by one. Using the wire just as a detector, we have put in, for instance, 150 μl of a fermentation broth with all its cells and everything else. Then we can carry out a gradient elution procedure and pick out the solute peaks we are interested in.

Curry: Would glucuronides be volatilized off that wire? You showed us examples of steroids.

Scott: We will always be faced with the limitations of the mass spectrometer. For anything that we can get into the mass spectrometer from a solid injection we should be able to obtain spectra from the wire system. We may sometimes not obtain parent ions but we will get quite a lot of information.

Jackson: Did you have to determine the optimum wire current for each compound?

Scott: No, we only did that to see how it changed. For compounds with molecular weights of about 250 the optimum temperature seems to be obtained from wire currents of 175–200 mA.

Luminescence methods in drug analysis

J. W. BRIDGES

Department of Biochemistry, University of Surrey, Guildford, Surrey

Abstract The present status of fluorescence and phosphorescence assays of drugs is briefly reviewed and the future prospects of these methods examined. Studies of the relationship between chemical structure and luminescence properties of the barbiturate drugs are described. Barbiturates able to form a di-anion in alkaline solution typically display a strong fluorescence at 420 nm which is sufficient to enable barbiturates extracted from serum to be determined in submicrogram concentrations. *N*-Substituted and thio-barbiturates only fluoresce weakly. Barbiturates possessing a 5-phenyl group, such as phenobarbitone (phenobarbital), also emit an intense phosphorescence, attributable to the phenyl ring, which allows compounds of this type both to be distinguished from other barbiturates and to be assayed. Examples are given of some other commonly used drugs whose inherent phosphorescence properties are sufficient for analytical purposes, including phenothiazines, tricyclic antidepressants, central nervous system stimulants and monoamine oxidase inhibitors.

A novel phosphoroscope is described which extends the scope of luminescence assays by permitting the fluorescence and phosphorescence of drugs and their metabolites on thin-layer chromatography (TLC) plates to be estimated, and its application is illustrated by the phosphorescence analysis of sulphonamide mixtures.

The use of fluorescent derivative formation, followed by separation and estimation on TLC plates, is also discussed with reference to the synthesis and assay of dansyl derivatives.

Assay techniques based on light emission from excited drug molecules are not used widely in clinical and forensic laboratories, despite the obvious prospective assets of high sensitivity, non-destructive nature, ease of automation and ready interfacing with most separation techniques. Potentially, fluorometric and phosphorometric techniques are of comparable sensitivity to other methods of photon counting such as scintillation counting. In practice the limits of detection of the luminescence method for a particular compound are usually governed by the

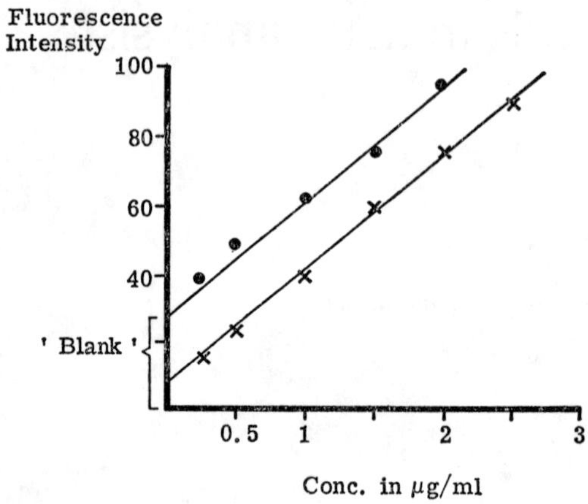

FIG. 1. Influence of the 'biological blank' on barbitone fluorescence calibration curve (λ_e 265 nm λ_f 410 nm in 0.1M-NaOH)
x——x calibration curve of barbitone extracted from water
●——● calibration curve of barbitone extracted from serum

ability of the instrument to discriminate between the luminescence properties of the sample and those of the 'biological blank' (control sample). The luminescence of the blank may be attributable to contaminants arising from either the biological sample or the solvents and chemical reagents used in the sample work-up procedure (see Fig. 1). Many spectroscopic grade and analar solvents and reagents contain significant amounts of unidentified contaminants which luminesce, particularly in the blue region of the spectrum. Where high sensitivity is demanded from an assay it may be necessary to purify some of the chemicals by washing or distilling them first (Udenfriend 1962). Some chemicals of fluorometric grade can be obtained commercially but so far their range is limited.

Because the results obtained on a fluorometer or phosphorometer are instrument-dependent, the presence of a significant 'biological blank' poses a problem in the reporting of sensitivities of luminescence assays. A valid way of overcoming the difficulty of comparing results achieved on different instruments is to record the concentration of compound which gives a reading of twice the blank value and that which gives a full-scale deflection (usually 100 units). If these figures are quoted, together with the concentration of a known luminescence standard which gives a reading of 50 units, then comparisons between instruments can readily be made (Bartos & Pesez 1972). Recommended fluorescent standards for this purpose include quinine sulphate (in 0.1M-sulphuric acid), fluorescein or eosin (in 0.1M-sodium hydroxide), and tryptophan or tyrosine (in water). A rapid check on instrumental performance can be obtained either by measuring the Raman spectra of water at selected wavelengths

(Parker 1959) or by scanning the spectra of some luminescent plastic samples.

Despite the limitations imposed on luminescence assays by interference from the 'biological blank', the sensitivity of light emission methods is still frequently of the order of 100 to 1000 times better than that obtainable with UV and visible spectrophotometry, and it is generally more specific. The likelihood of enhanced specificity arises because only a small number of light-absorbing compounds (about 2%) luminesce and because of the advantage of two defining wavelength maxima, namely the excitation (λ_e) and emission wavelengths (λ_f or λ_p). It is a popular misconception that the optimal luminescence assay conditions are necessarily at the peak excitation and emission wavelengths. In practice, by careful selection of these wavelengths above or below their maxima, interference from the 'biological blank' can often be minimized without undue loss of sensitivity.

An often-quoted disadvantage of luminescence techniques is that they are generally more prone to interference (e.g. quenching) from external agents than light absorption methods, since they depend on the formation of a chemically reactive state (excited singlet state) from which light emission occurs. However, this susceptibility of the light output of the excited molecules to changes in their environment can often be used to increase the specificity of an assay. Significant

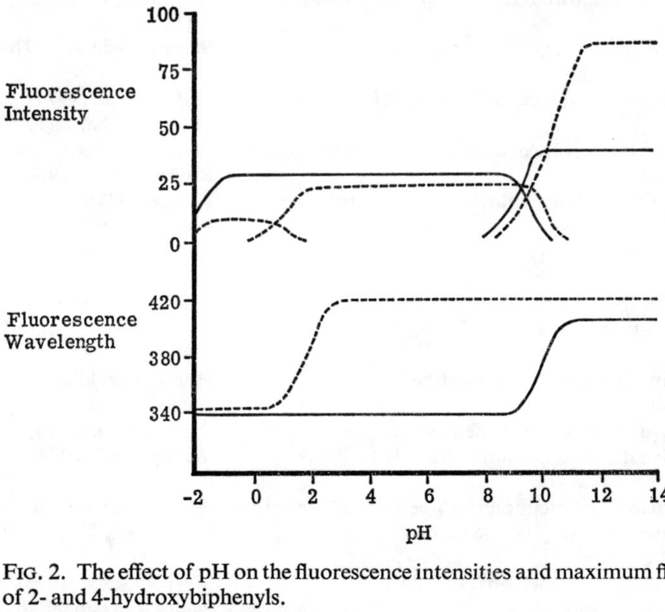

FIG. 2. The effect of pH on the fluorescence intensities and maximum fluorescence wavelengths of 2- and 4-hydroxybiphenyls.

----- 2-hydroxybiphenyl

——— 4-hydroxybiphenyl

improvements may often be brought about by a change in solvent viscosity or polarity (Van Duuren 1963) or by careful pH selection. For example, the fungistat biphenyl produces two major metabolites, 4-hydroxybiphenyl and 2-hydroxybiphenyl, which have similar light absorption properties. However, they differ in their fluorescence characteristics in that the 2-isomer but not the 4-isomer is ionized in the excited state (Fig. 2). If the fluorescence emissions are measured at pH 6 these two compounds can be individually estimated without further separation (Bridges *et al.* 1965). Other ways of improving an assay include the addition of selective quenching agents (Duggan & Udenfriend 1956) to enable a drug to be measured in the presence of its metabolites. Luminescence measurements are usually made after chromatographic separation, selective solvent extraction or differential chemical reaction. A promising approach has been the development of fluorescent reagents which can serve as a counter ion for the extraction of ionizable drugs. With 8-methoxyanthracenesulphonate as

TABLE 1

Some fluorometric methods for assay of drugs

Compound	*Method*	*Sensitivity*	*Reference*
Reserpine	Treatment with HNO_2	0.2 μg	Haycock *et al.* (1966)
Quercetin	Complexing with tetraphenylboron	1.0 μg/ml	Gugler & Dengler (1973)
Salicylate	Native fluorescence in chloroform–acetic acid		Miles & Schenk (1970)
Barbiturates	Native fluorescence in 0.1M-NaOH		Gifford *et al.* (1974) Miles & Schenk (1973)
LSD (lysergide)	Native fluorescence in acid	0.003 μg/ml	Dal *et al.* (1966)
Phenothiazines	Oxidation		Ragland *et al.* (1969)
Imipramine	Reaction with formaldehyde and acetylacetone	0.15 μg/ml	Hayes (1973)
Morphine	Conversion into pseudomorphine		Nadeau & Sobolewski (1958)
Quinine	Native fluorescence in acid	0.001 μg/ml	Udenfriend (1962)
Librium (chlordiazepoxide)	Formation of a lactam		Koechlin & D'Arconte (1963)
Indomethacin	Native fluorescence in alkaline solution		Holt & Hawkins (1965)
Sulphonamides	Native fluorescence at neutral pH		Bridges *et al.* (1974)
Methapyrilene HCl	Native fluorescence at neutral pH		Wilson *et al.* (1973)
Heroin	Formation of pseudomorphine	0.2 μg/ml	Sansur *et al.* (1972)
Pyrimethamine	Treatment with $(NH_4)_2SO_4$ on TLC plate	0.005 μg	Simmons & De Angelis (1973)
Trimethoprim	Native fluorescence on TLC plate		Sigel & Grace (1973)
Oxytetracycline	Alkaline degradation	0.1 μg/ml	Scales & Assinder (1973)

the reagent, propantheline bromide can be estimated with a high degree of selectivity, provided that the solvent extraction conditions are carefully chosen (Westlund & Borg 1973*a*, *b*). Light scattering is also a problem in fluorometric though not in phosphorometric assay. However, scattering also interferes in light absorption methods, although it is commonly ignored because it is not readily identifiable. It has been reported that the use of a single light polarizer (e.g. Polarcoat 105 UV polarizing filter) in the exciting light path of the fluorometer can often be used to suppress scatter without any great loss of sensitivity (Chen 1966).

LUMINESCENCE PROPERTIES OF BARBITURATES

The development of luminescent procedures for new drugs has until recently been limited by the scarcity of information about the predictability of the relationship between luminescence and molecular structure. Despite this, many commonly used drugs can be estimated by fluorometric or phosphorometric assay procedures (see Table 1 and Bridges 1969). Luminescence studies on barbiturates (Gifford *et al.* 1974*a*) demonstrate the relationship between struc-

TABLE 2
Luminescence characteristics of some oxybarbiturates

Compound	λ_e (*nm*)	λ_f (*nm*)	λ_p (*nm*)	*Phosphorescence decay half-life (s)*	*Detection limit (µg/ml)* *Fluorescence*	*Phosphorescence*
(Rutonal) (5-methyl-5-phenyl-barbituric acid)	266	395	395	3.0	0.3	0.5
Phenobarbitone	266	395	395	4.1	0.2	0.3
Mebaral (methyl-phenobarbital)	260	395	395	3.6	0.5	0.5
Diphenylbarbituric acid	260	395	395	2.4	—	—
Barbitone	265	410	NP	—		
Butabarbitone (secbutabarbital)	266	410	NP	—	0.2	—
Pentobarbitone	266	410	NP	—	0.2	—
Seconal (secobarbital)	—	WF	NP	—	—	—
Heptabarbitol (heptabarb)	—	WF	NP	—	—	—

Fluorescence was only observed in 50% ethanediol–water containing 0.1M-NaOH.
Phosphorescence was measured in neutral solution.
WF: weak fluorescence
NP: no phosphorescence

ture and luminescence which is an important criterion in defining the specificity of an assay, and these studies provide a useful illustration of the application of conventional methods of fluorometry and phosphorometry to drug analysis (see Table 2).

Most barbiturates are fluorescent in alkaline solution in the di-anion form (I) but not as the mono-anion (II) or in the un-ionized state (III).

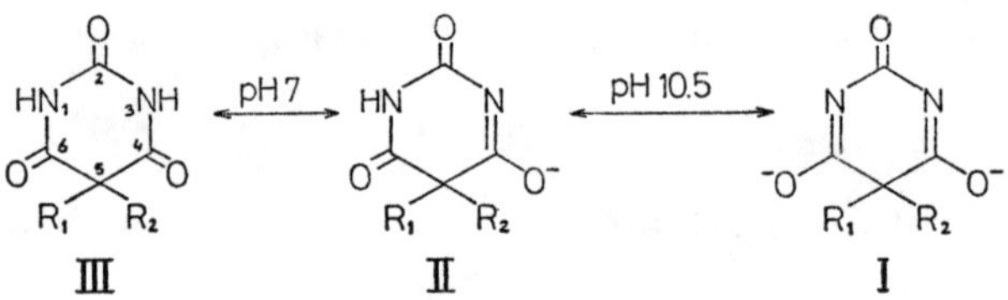

N-Substituted barbiturates such as hexobarbitone (hexobarbital) and Mebaral (methylphenobarbital) which are unable to form di-anions are generally non-fluorescent. The excitation and emission wavelength characteristics of each barbiturate in 0.1M-sodium hydroxide are similar, although there are considerable differences in fluorescence intensity. Di-anions derived from 5,5-di-substituted barbiturates are the most highly fluorescent and can be readily determined after suitable solvent extraction from plasma. In those compounds, for example phenobarbitone (phenobarbital) and Seconal (secobarbital), where one of the 5-substituents is aromatic or another unsaturated group, the fluorescence intensity is considerably reduced. Despite the fact that all the barbiturates are excited and emit at similar wavelengths, this approach gives better specificity than light absorption spectroscopy methods, since no interference is found from drugs such as diphenylhydantoin (phenytoin) and bemegride. The flexibility of the fluorometric barbiturate assay could probably be considerably increased by the use of microcells rather than the conventional 1-cm^2 cells; this would allow smaller samples to be used and reduce the possibility of concentration quenching. For the 5-phenyl-substituted barbiturates and those substituted with an unsaturated group, the fluorescence intensity can also be enhanced by making measurements at low temperatures, when energy losses due to lack of rigidity in the molecule are minimized (King *et al.* 1974). A more selective approach to assaying phenyl-substituted barbiturates, however, is to estimate them phosphorometrically for, unlike their non-phenyl-substituted analogues, they emit a strong phosphorescence signal at 420 nm. This phosphorescence, which is very unusual in that it is emitted at a lower wavelength than the prompt fluorescence, appears to be attributable to the phenyl group rather than to the heterocyclic ring, for a similar phosphorescence is also shown by toluene (see Fig. 3). To achieve a quantitative measurement of the phosphorescence emission in a con-

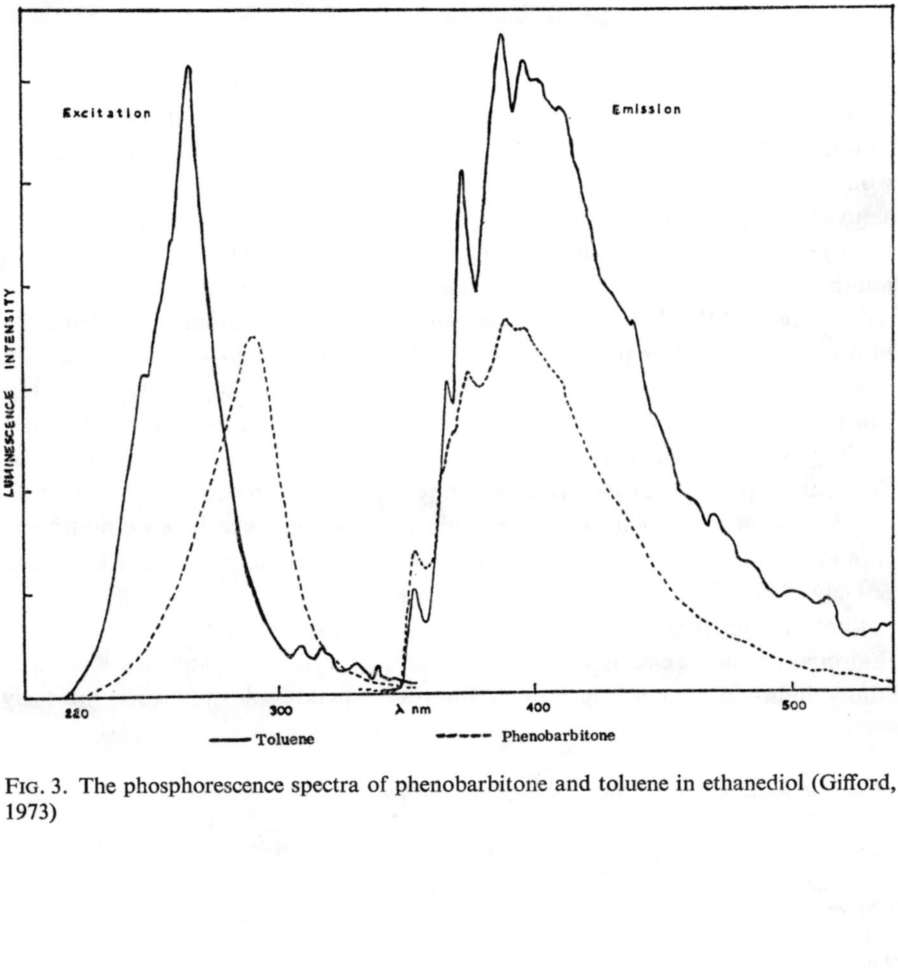

FIG. 3. The phosphorescence spectra of phenobarbitone and toluene in ethanediol (Gifford, 1973)

ventional phosphorometer attachment for a spectrofluorometer it is necessary to dissolve the sample in a solvent, such as ethanediol, ethanol or isopentane, which does not crack at liquid nitrogen temperatures. The reproducibility of this type of phosphorometric analysis can be improved if the apparatus is modified to allow the sample to rotate and open-ended sample tubes to be used that are not prone to fracturing. With this approach, a detection limit of 0.5 μg/ml (S.D. < 6%) can readily be obtained for samples of serum phenobarbitone extracted in chloroform, then evaporated and re-extracted in ethanediol. A high instrumental reading for control samples containing solvent alone prevented a greater sensitivity from being achieved in these studies, but careful purification of solvent should lead to considerably improved sensitivity.

METHODS OF IMPROVING PHOSPHOROMETRIC ANALYSIS

Recently, Winefordner and his colleagues (Lukasiewicz *et al.* 1972) have shown that with micro sample tubes a wide range of solvents, including water, can be used for assay purposes without any loss of accuracy. This modification would seem to overcome one of the principal limitations of phosphorometric assay, namely the narrow range of solvents it is normally possible to use. A particular advantage of phosphorometric analysis is that the light scatter is minimized by the relatively slow speed of the phosphoroscope. A second potential asset is that the decay half-life can sometimes be used either as an identification criterion or, by careful selection of phosphoroscope rotation speed, as a means of separately estimating the constituents of several component mixtures. For example, on this basis it should be easy to distinguish the phosphorescence of drugs such as demethylimipramine (desipramine) from that of drugs of the diazepam type without having to use any separation procedure (see Table 3). The increased availability of pulsed light sources and pulsed photomultipliers should encourage wider use of this approach (Harbaugh *et al.* 1973; Hamilton & Naqvi 1973).

Phosphorometry can in many ways be regarded as a complementary method to fluorometry, and it clearly offers considerable promise as an analytical method. Many light-absorbing drugs which fluoresce weakly phosphoresce intensely

TABLE 3

Phosphorescence characteristics of some common drugs (data from Gifford 1973)

Compound	λ_e *(nm)*	λ_p *(nm)*	*Phosphorescence decay half-life (s)*
Chlorpromazine	335	495–510	0.072
Triflupromazine	345	510, 520	0.072
Thioridazine	335	500	0.066
Perphenazine	330	495–510	0.072
Trifluoperazine	340	515	0.071
Thioxanthene	280	460	0.2
Chlorprothixene	260, 310, 385	470	0.2
Desipramine	300	433	0.95
Chlorimipramine (clomipramine)	305	450–470	0.12
Iprindole	310	425, 450, 485	5.3
Benzedrine (amphetamine)	270, 355	385	10.6
Chlordiazepoxide	310, 320	450, 470	0.16
Diazepam	290, 325	440, 470, 510	0.070
Sulphamerazine	310	412	0.8
Sulphapyridine	350	410, 440	0.6, 1.3
Iproniazid	300, 370	440	0.2

Measurements were made in 50% ethanediol–water

enough for phosphorometry to be considered seriously for their analysis (see Table 3). Phosphorometric assay can be carried out quickly and should be capable of dealing with many samples in a relatively short time. Perhaps the most useful prospect is that the fluorescence: phosphorescence ratios of drugs could be determined, which would significantly improve the criteria of identification in many instances.

PHOSPHORESCENCE DETERMINATION ON TLC PLATES

Improved specificity and marked reductions in the readings from the 'biological blank' can also be achieved by TLC separation followed by extraction of drug and metabolite from the plate into the sample tube. Alternatively, a novel attachment for a conventional fluorometer makes it possible (Gifford *et al.* 1974*b*) to estimate drugs fluorometrically and phosphorometrically directly on plastic or metal-backed TLC plates, cellulose acetate strips or paper chromatograms (see Fig. 4). The attachment consists of two parts, a single disc phosphoroscope (*a*) and a sample compartment. In use the TLC plate is clipped after development to the outside of a copper drum which contains liquid nitrogen so that the samples on the plate are cooled by conduction. The drum is placed in a dry airtight box which prevents water from condensing on the plate. The drum is rotated slowly in the path of the exciting light, which is interrupted by the variable-speed single disc phosphoroscope as it rotates. The light emitted at 90° to the incident light also passes through the phosphoroscope to the

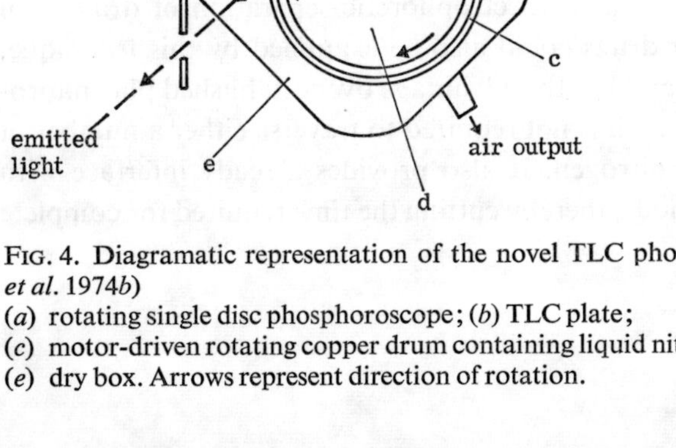

FIG. 4. Diagramatic representation of the novel TLC phosphorometer from above. (Gifford *et al.* 1974*b*)
(*a*) rotating single disc phosphoroscope; (*b*) TLC plate;
(*c*) motor-driven rotating copper drum containing liquid nitrogen (*d*);
(*e*) dry box. Arrows represent direction of rotation.

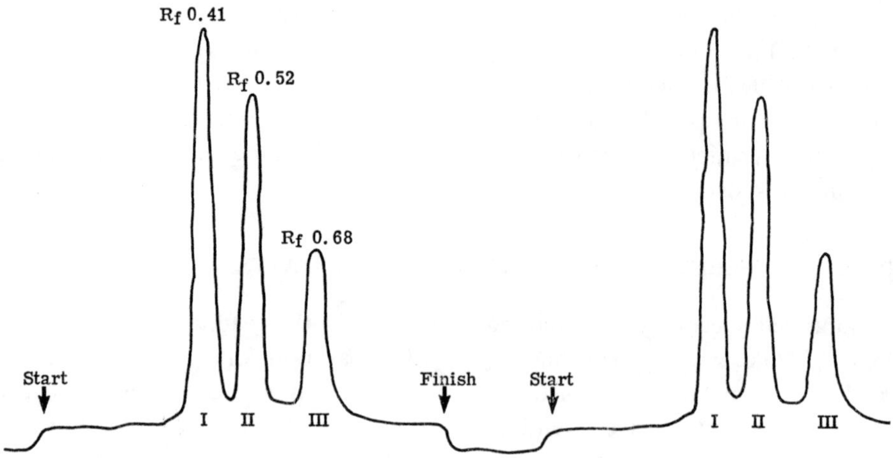

FIG. 5. Repeat scan at λ_p 410 nm of a chromatogram of a mixture of sulphadiazine (I), sulphamerazine (II) and Sulphamezathine (III) in the novel thin-layer phosphorometer (Gifford *et al.* 1974*b*).
Each spot represents 2 μg of sulphonamide on an aluminium-backed silica gel TLC plate developed in $CHCl_3$–MeOH–NH_4OH (30:12:1 v/v).

receiving monochromator system. The liquid nitrogen in the drum is maintained at a constant level from a reservoir. The phosphoroscope disc has three equally spaced rectangular slots which, on rotation, allow the sample to receive and transmit light alternately. The drum can be stopped in any position so that the spectral characteristics and R_f of samples on the plate can be ascertained.

We evaluated this device by analysing developed chromatograms of a mixture of three sulphonamides: sulphadiazine, sulphamerazine and Sulphamezathine (sulphadimidine) (see Fig. 5). Plastic or aluminium-backed plates were prewashed in the chromatography solvent. The intensities were reproducible within $\pm$ 6% and submicrogram quantities of each sulphonamide could be readily determined. Mixtures of 5-phenyl-substituted barbiturates have also been satisfactorily estimated, using a similar approach. Electrophoretic separation of drug from its metabolites or from other drugs could also be examined by this technique. The method is simple to use and has the advantage over established phosphorometric methods that the light path is not required to traverse either a number of silica windows or the liquid nitrogen. It also provides a ready interface with suitable TLC separation methods, thereby cutting the time required for complete analysis.

PROCEDURES BASED ON THE FORMATION OF DERIVATIVES

So far I have been discussing the use of native luminescence properties for drug assays. Frequently, however, the sensitivity and specificity can be considerably enhanced by preparing suitable derivatives (termed chemically induced fluorescence or functional fluorescence). Derivative formation appears to have gained recognition recently as a means of improving the fluorometric assay of drugs (Udenfriend 1969; Bartos & Pesez 1972; White & Weissler 1972; White & Argauer 1970) (see Table 4), although it appears not to have been used for phosphorometric assays. The slow acceptance of derivative formation for this purpose, compared with its widespread use for GLC and light absorption techniques, presumably stems from lack of information about the relationship between luminescence properties and chemical structure. Nonetheless, particular success has been achieved by preparing derivatives from drugs and their metabolites after simple extraction followed by TLC separation and fluorometric estimation of the derivatives directly on the plate. For this purpose, conventional

TABLE 4
Some reagents used to improve the sensitivity of fluorescence assays

Functional group	*Reagent*	*Compound estimated*	*References*[a]
Hydroxy	5-Dimethylamino-1-naphthalene-sulphonyl chloride (dansyl chloride);	Hashish	Just *et al.* (1972);
	4-(Dichloro-s-triazinyl) -1-ethoxy naphthalene	Tolalamol[b]	D. Stopher (1974, unpublished work)
Amino	9-Isothiocyanatoacridine	Amphetamine	De Leenheer *et al.* (1973)
	4-Chloro-7-nitro-2, 1, 3-benz-oxadiazole	*N*-methyl- and *NN*-dimethyl-carbamate	Lawrence & Frei (1972)
	Fluorescamine	Amino acids	Böhlen *et al.* (1963)
	o-Phthaldehyde	Indolylalkylamines	Maickel & Miller (1968)
	Dansyl chloride	Barbiturates	Dünges & Peter (1972)
Aldehydes and ketones	3, 5-Diaminobenzoate	Acetaldehyde	Velluz *et al.* (1949)
	2-Phenylacetyl-1, 3-indandione 1-hydrazone	Various aldehydes and ketones	Pretrzyk & Chen (1970)

[a] See also White & Argauer, 1970; Udenfriend (1969); Bartos & Pesez (1972); White & Weissler (1972)
[b] Tolalamol (Pfizer) is a β-blocking drug.

densitometers may be more effective than the TLC attachments provided for commercial spectrofluorometers, where extensive light losses due to the attachment design often severely reduce the potential assay sensitivity. Dansylation (treatment with 5-dimethylaminonaphthalene-1-sulphonyl chloride) is at present the most widely used method for derivative formation, although a number of other promising reagents, such as 4-chloro-7-nitro-2,1,3-benzoxadiazole, 4-(dichloro-*s*-triazinyl)-1-ethoxynaphthalene and fluorescamine, are now available. The sensitivity obtained in this approach is often in the nanogram range, with reproducibility in the $\pm$ 5–10% range. However, for such reliable results to be achieved at these concentrations, meticulous chromatographic procedures and an appropriate internal standard are mandatory. Prewashing of plates to remove luminescent contaminants, the incorporation of an antioxidant such as butylated hydroxytoluene (BHT) in the support material and minimum exposure to ultraviolet light (to minimize photodecomposition of samples) may often improve reproducibility. Sensitivity is usually enhanced by spraying the plate after development with a solvent such as triethanolamine, liquid paraffin or a buffer.

Formation of the dansyl derivatives of barbiturates after their extraction from serum and subsequent chromatographic separation allows amounts as low as 4 ng to be determined with a standard error of less than 8%. New equipment permitting more reproducible formation of derivatives from very small quantities of drug should considerably enhance the accuracy of this procedure (Dünges 1973). Drugs can of course also be estimated accurately in many instances if one makes use of their ability to quench on fluorescent plates or if the derivatives are made on the plates after development of the chromatogram (Simmons & De Angelis, 1973). In these instances an internal standard is again advisable. Luminescence measurements on TLC plates clearly have some advantages over drug or metabolite estimations made in 1-cm^2 cells in a liquid medium, not only because they incorporate a separation method, thus enhancing specificity, but also because they allow several samples to be handled at the same time. The introduction of a means of rapid scanning of wavelengths would allow spectral determination and luminescence intensity to be measured simultaneously, which would clearly enhance the specificity of this type of measurement and enable changes in luminescence characteristics due to abnormalities in the blank to be detected.

Other recent developments of particular interest for the future include the use of fluorescent detectors linked to continuous methods of separation, such as GLC and high pressure liquid chromatography, which have been used successfully for the estimation of pesticides and aromatic hydrocarbons (Bowman & Beroza 1968; Freed & Faulkner 1972; Pellizzari & Sparacino 1973; White &

Argauer 1970). The use of computer links to phosphorometers and fluorometers should enable instrumental variables to be corrected and provide rapid and efficient resolution of complex spectra; this would be valuable for the analysis of multicomponent mixtures (Shepherd 1973; Holland *et al.* 1973). Methods based on the induction of chemiluminescence have yet to find a place in drug analysis but could prove useful in some instances. Luminescence techniques are also likely to play an important future role in enzyme-mediated immune assay techniques (EMIT), both as a means of improving the sensitivity of enzyme activity measurements and in protein-binding estimations (such as saturation analysis) where changes in the fluorescent properties (polarization and solvent effects) of drugs such as warfarin could be monitored automatically as they bind to or dissociate from proteins.

ACKNOWLEDGEMENTS

I am indebted to my colleagues at the University of Technology, Loughborough, Dr D. Thorburn-Burns, Dr J. Miller, and Dr L. A. Gifford (now at St Bartholomew's Hospital, London), for allowing me to report some of our unpublished collaborative research findings.

References

BARTOS, J. & PESEZ, M. (1972) *Talanta, 19*, 93

BÖHLEN, P., STEIN, S., DAIRMAN, W. & UDENFRIEND, S. (1973) *Arch. Biochem. Biophys. 155*, 213

BOWMAN, M. C. & BEROZA, M. (1968) *Anal.Chem. 40*, 535

BRIDGES, J. W. (1969) in *CRC Handbook of Analytical Toxicology* (Sunshine, I., ed.), CRC Press, Cleveland, Ohio

BRIDGES, J. W., CREAVEN, P. J. & WILLIAMS, R. T. (1965) *Biochem. J. 96*, 872

BRIDGES, J. W., GIFFORD, L. A., HAYES, W. P., MILLER, J. N. & THORBURN-BURNS, D. (1974) *Anal. Chem. 46*, 1010

CHEN, R. F. (1966) *Anal. Biochem. 14*, 497

DAL, L. A., BROICH, J. R., DIHRBERG, A. & NEWMAN, B. (1966) *Anal. Chem. 38*, 1959

DE LEENHEER, A., SINSHEIMER, J. E. & BURCKHALTER, J. H. (1973) *J. Pharm. Sci. 66*, 1370

DUGGAN, D. E. & UDENFRIEND, S. (1956) *J. Biol. Chem. 223*, 313

DÜNGES, W. (1973) *Anal. Chem. 45*, 963

DÜNGES, W. & PETER, H. W. (1972) (Meijer, J. W. A., Meinardi, H., Gardner-Thorpe, C. & Van der Kleyn, E., eds.) in *Methods of Analysis of Anti-Epileptic Drugs*, pp. 126–133, ICS No. 286, Excerpta Medica, Amsterdam

FREED, D. J. & FAULKNER, R. (1972) *Anal. Chem. 44*, 1194

GIFFORD, L. A. (1973) Ph. D. Thesis, University of Loughborough

GIFFORD, L. A., HAYES, W. P., KING, L. A., MILLER, J. N., THORBURN-BURNS, D. and BRIDGES, J. W. (1974*a*) *Anal. Chem. 46*, 94

GIFFORD, L. A., MILLER, J. N., THORBURN-BURNS, D. & BRIDGES, J. W. (1974*b*) *Anal. Chim. Acta* in press

GUGLER, R. & DENGLER, H. J. (1973) *Clin. Chem. 19*, 36

HAMILTON, T. D. S. & NAQVI, K. R. (1973) *Anal. Chem. 45*, 1581

Harbaugh, K. F., O'Donnell, C. M. & Winefordner, J. D. (1973) *Anal. Chem. 45*, 948
Haycock, R. P., Sheth, P. B., Connolly, R. J. & Mander, W. J. (1966) *J. Agric. Food Chem. 14*, 437
Hayes, T. S. (1973) *Clin. Chem. 19*, 390
Holland, J. F., Teets, R. E. & Timnick, A. (1973) *Anal. Chem. 45*, 145
Holt, L. P. J. & Hawkins, G. F. (1965) *Br. Med. J. 1*, 1354
Just, W. W., Werner, G. & Weichmann, M. (1972) *Naturwissenschaften, 59*, 222
King, L. A., Miller, J. N., Thorburn-Burns, D. & Bridges, J. W. (1974) *Anal. Chim. Acta 68*, 205
Koechlin, B. A. & d'Arconte, L. (1963) *Anal. Biochem. 5*, 195
Lawrence, J. F. & Frei, R. W. (1972) *Anal. Chem. 44*, 2046
Lukasiewicz, R. F., Rozymes, R. A., Sanders, L. B. & Winefordner, J. D. (1972) *Anal. Chem. 44*, 237
Maickel, R. P. & Miller, F. P. (1968) *Adv. Pharmacol. 6* (Pt.A), 71
Miles, C. I. & Schenk, G. H. (1970) *Anal. Chem. 42*, 656
Miles, C. I. & Schenk, G. H. (1973) *Anal. Chem. 45*, 130
Nadeau, G. & Sobolewski, G. (1958) *Can. J. Biochem. Physiol. 36*, 635
Parker, C. A. (1959) *Analyst 84*, 446
Pellizzari, E. M. & Sparacino, C. M. (1973) *Anal. Chem. 45*, 378
Pietrzyk, D. J. & Chan, E. P. (1970) *Anal. Chem. 42*, 37
Ragland, J. W., Kinross-Wright, V. J. & Ragland, R. S. (1965) *Anal. Biochem. 12*, 60
Sansur, M., Buccofuri, A. & Morgenstein, S. (1972). *J. Assoc. Of. Anal. Chem. 55*, 880
Scales, B. & Assinder, D. A. (1973) *J. Pharm. Sci. 66*, 913
Sigel, C. & Grace, M. J. (1973) *J. Chromatogr. 80*, 111
Simmons, W. S. & De Angelis, R. L. (1973) *Anal. Chem. 45*, 1538
Shepherd, T. M. (1973) *Chem. Ind. (Lond.)* 332
Udenfriend, S. (1962) *Fluorescence Assay in Biology and Medicine*, vol. 1, Academic Press, New York
Udenfriend, S. (1969) *Fluorescence Assay in Biology and Medicine*, vol. 2, Academic Press, New York
Van Duuren, B. L. (1963) *Chem. Rev. 63*, 325
Velluz, L., Amiard, G. & Bartos, J. (1949) *J. Biol. Chem. 180*, 1137
Westlund, D. & Borg, K. O. (1973*a*) *Anal. Chim. Acta 67*, 89
Westlund, D. & Borg, K. O. (1973*b*) *Anal. Chim. Acta 67*, 99
White, C. E. & Argauer, R. J. (1970) *Fluorescence Analysis—a Practical Approach*, Dekker, New York
White, C. E. & Weissler, A. (1972) *Anal. Chem. 44*, 182R
Wilson, D. L., Witz, D. R. & Schenk, G. H. (1973) *Anal. Chem. 45*, 1447

Discussion

Brown: I can't see how you can use an internal standard with luminescence methods unless you use a different activation or emission wavelength, either of which would tend to defeat the purpose of the exercise.

Bridges: One way is to use a different fluorescent substance with similar excitation and emission wavelengths to the sample but different pH fluorescence characteristics. If quenching is a likely problem an internal standard approach similar to that used in scintillation counting can be used (e.g. Bridges *et al.*

1967). With a TLC plate system quenching is generally not a major problem. With dansyl derivatives we use hydroxybiphenyls as internal standards. For TLC plate procedures it is imperative to have such an internal standard to get good quantitative results.

Beckett: I accept that when the parent drug makes a single derivative all is well. But in most cases metabolism will lead to the formation of several derivatives by the reagent. Unless we can separate these selectively on TLC the choice of the reagents will be critical. At present dansyl derivatives are being used a lot in work with phenothiazines. This has been looked upon as measuring the ring hydroxylation but reactions may occur with the hydroxylamine metabolites. These seem to me to present great problems in terms of reaction with metabolites.

Bridges: I agree. Future developments in derivative formation should be towards more specific reagents. Forming derivatives with dansyl chloride is rather a 'blunderbuss' technique, since NH and OH groups both react. We have used it mainly as a model in order to identify the problems of quantitative measurements on TLC plates.

Gee: Some luminescence or fluorescence techniques can be used in histological studies for localizing particular substances. Is there any possibility that these techniques can be used on histological material to determine the amounts present?

Bridges: Yes, if the drug has different luminescence characteristics from those of the tissue. Possibly phosphorescence is better but I remain to be convinced.

Leach: Some years ago several microfluorometers had microscope optics. Their main limitations stemmed from the electronics which were available at the time. Now the problems are more manageable and with better methods of measuring low light levels—photon counting for example—this type of instrument should be a practical proposition.

Bridges: They have been used in a limited context already. For example C. A. Parker (unpublished) has measured oil residues in marine algae using a scanning microspectrofluorometer.

Sunshine: We have had some experience with 4-chloro-7-nitro-2,1,3-benzoxadiazole and phenylacetaldehyde and ninhydrin sprays (Valentour *et al.* 1974). The sprayed plates produce a series of spots in glorious technicolour. How you identify one particular spot and then get some data from that is quite a challenge.

Bridges: It depends on the nature of the sample. Obviously you may have to carry out several separation processes before either direct estimation or derivative formation and subsequent assay.

Scott: Your technique might have an even greater potential with lasers. Have you tried that?

Bridges: No, but others have. It is a possible way of improving sensitivity although one may get photodecomposition problems (Fraser & Winefordner 1972).

Scott: It tremendously improves the sensitivity in Raman spectra. When you wash the plates and increase the sensitivity by spraying them with polar material, you are probably displacing material from the surface of the silica gel, bringing it out of the pores by displacing it from the surface with the more polar solvent.

Bridges: That is one possibility.

Scott: Is the increase greater with a polar spray like water than with hexane?

Bridges: Yes, in general, but it depends on the particular compound. The problem with water is that it evaporates too quickly, so a more viscous solvent is often preferable.

Moffat: Some of my colleagues have developed fluorescent methods for estimating morphine and primary amines (Blackmore *et al.* 1971; Hayes 1973). These have lately been converted into automated methods using Autoanalyser equipment and differential extraction procedures so that the machine can estimate four different kinds of drugs—methaqualone, barbiturates, amphetamine and morphine. Would automation increase the usefulness of a technique like fluorescence?

Bridges: Undoubtedly it can often help, providing you ascertain what you are measuring in the first place.

Moffat: Would this cut out some of the unknowns you had? It would give a standardized extraction every time.

Bridges: It certainly improves things. For example, calcium estimations using calcein reagent can be enormously improved by using an Autoanalyser.

Holmstedt: You mentioned that dansylation had been used with cannabinol. Have you tested cannabinol under practical conditions with your more refined technique?

Bridges: Not yet.

Parker: As you know, when dansyl derivatives in aqueous solutions are treated with specific antibody, fluorescence increases in intensity by up to 100-fold, which would make the measurement much more sensitive. However, I suppose it would be just as easy and certainly cheaper simply to dissolve the dansyl derivative in a hydrophobic solvent.

Bridges: One interesting effect of changing the solvent is that the wavelength and intensity of fluorescence often also changes and this can be useful analytically. For example we have used warfarin as a fluorescence probe. When it binds to protein (serum albumin), warfarin changes its fluorescent wavelength characteristics from those of an aqueous solution. With a drug that competes with warfarin for protein binding sites, the warfarin fluorescent wavelength characteristics are again changed. Potentially this might be a very quick screen for possible warfarin-displacing agents (J. W. Bridges & A. G. E. Wilson, unpublished).

References

BLACKMORE, D. J., CURRY, A. S., HAYES, T. S. & RUTTER, E. R. (1971) Automated analysis for drugs in urine. *Clin. Chem. 17*, 896–902

BRIDGES, J. W., DAVIES, D. S. & WILLIAMS, R. T. (1967) The fate of ethyltin and diethyltin derivatives in the rat. *Biochem. J. 105*, 1261–1267

FRASER, L. M. & WINEFORDNER, J. D. (1972) Laser excited atomic fluorescence flame spectrometry as an analytical method. *Anal. Chem. 44*, 1444–1451

HAYES, T. S. (1973) Automated fluorometric determination of amphetamine in urine. *Clin. Chem. 19*, 390–394

VALENTOUR, J. C., MONFORTE, J. R. & SUNSHINE, I. (1974) Fluorimetric determination of propoxyphene. *Clin. Chem. 20*, 275–277

General discussion I

Prescott: A major problem with analytical techniques concerns the discrepancies between the amounts of drug extracted from biological material and from simple aqueous solutions. It was implied that this was due merely to a shift in the recovery due to changes in pH. But this is not my experience. Recently we looked at a new anti-arrhythmic drug which we could extract from simple aqueous solutions with a variety of non-polar solvents; when we used plasma buffered to the same pH, there were enormous discrepancies. In fact, some solvents which took 95% of the drug out of an aqueous solution removed only 5–10% from plasma at the same pH. Each solvent behaved differently. I feel uncomfortable using plasma standards for calibrating the system, because I do not understand what is happening.

Scott: The discrepancy is due, of course, to the solubility characteristics of plasma being quite different from those of water. Even the presence of a lipid will give the plasma a non-polar characteristic. But this doesn't matter. The plasma composition remains fairly constant in terms of physical distribution, providing that the same solvent is used in standard conditions and that the patient's blood is not full of something like liquid paraffin.

Prescott: But the plasma often becomes white and full of fat particles after a meal. In other words, the blood composition does change.

Scott: It is fairly easy to determine what levels would be significant.

Beckett: That depends on how long the sample has been stored before it is analysed.

Scott: I don't think so. Isn't there between 90 and 100% water in blood?

Leach: There is about 7% protein and I would say whole blood was only about 85–90% water.

Scott: Therefore 85–90% of the solubility characteristics of that fluid will be conditioned by the water content, and up to 15% may have individual variations. Could that 15% show a 50% variation within itself?

Leach: There is also the effect of protein binding; some drugs are bound to albumin, for example.

Scott: They may be bound to albumin, but albumin is always in the blood. How much does the concentration of albumin in blood vary?

Prescott: There can be marked quantitative and qualitative changes in the distribution of different protein fractions in different disease states. For example, the albumin concentration can vary by 200–300%.

Leach: We could discuss this for a long time but we seem to be missing the point. Partition coefficients of many drugs, particularly at low concentrations, can readily be determined using labelled compounds. The pharmaceutical companies are the only ones who, without any difficulty, have labelled compounds at their disposal for various investigative purposes. They determine partition coefficients and recoveries from aqueous and biological solutions, often for a number of solvents. All this information is available but we seldom see it and may have to re-determine these factors ourselves under far less favourable conditions.

Riess: The companies are in fact obliged to document all the properties of new drugs and also provide details of the analytical procedures. You can always ask us these things about new drugs.

Leach: This is true, but we are seldom looking for a single drug. We often do not know what the drug may be. What we really want is sufficient exchange of information so that we can choose a reasonably effective solvent for extraction. Once we have decided on a probable identity of the drug it is fairly easy to know what to do.

Gee: Everybody is talking about blood from a live person. Blood from a dead body is quite different.

Prescott: There is another complication. Very small amounts of polar substances like isoamyl alcohol are often added to non-polar solvents to increase recovery, which they do. They may reduce adsorption onto glass. But again the effects are very different in simple aqueous solutions and in plasma. Protein binding, to me, does not explain this at all.

Scott. One should never expect to get the same extraction characteristics from plasma as from water, and you should never even consider a comparison.

Prescott: But many workers do! You can get the same results with plasma and aqueous solutions with some drugs and some solvents.

Scott: Yes, but not in general. Hexane will dissolve some substances to the same extent as another solvent. But this is irrelevant for plasma, which has its own characteristics. Something may have the same solubility in both ethyl acetate and hexane but this is not a good basis for comparison. If you work out a system on water and then hope it will work with plasma, you are being optimistic, to say the least.

Prescott: But we do need help, because these problems occur in practice.

Curry: The problem goes very deep. We may get a drug which is very soluble in ether and chloroform, and has a distribution coefficient compared to water of 99.9% in either solvent. Blood may be 85% water but if you break it down with concentrated acid, destroy the protein binding, then make it alkaline and shake it with chloroform, the recovery may be nil. With an ether recovery it may be 100%. There are dramatic changes. Blood would seem to be a biological medium even after we have done this strong chemistry.

Scott: Adsorption can certainly be eliminated but I am talking about solubility characteristics. Blood is not pure water so it will not give the performance of pure water. The change may indeed be dramatic.

Leach: A point sometimes overlooked is that we do not always compare like with like. At microgram and submicrogram levels, a drug in a non-polar solvent may be lost because it is adsorbed on the surface of the glass. It can be recovered if alcohol is added, and the effect can be prevented by use of a polar solvent.

Scott: I agree, but that is another phenomenon. As a physical chemist I would use water just as a model. If I was trying to get distribution coefficients between a solvent and blood, or plasma, the characteristics of blood *must* be very different to those of water and I would use either blood or plasma.

Beckett: You have mentioned what I think is a key variable. It is not the partition coefficient that is variable but an apparent coefficient, because finally you measure something that you get out of the blood. If you work with a small amount, relative adsorption onto the surface of the glass vessel is altered and that is a more important variable than the characteristics of the fluid.

Scott: At nanogram levels, an absorption effect will obviously be important but at microgram levels I would have thought it would have no effect.

Beckett: It is still there at microgram levels.

Riess: The influence of that effect depends on how much sensitivity you need, and what concentrations you actually measure. In any case, we have to live with the phenomenon that extraction from plasma is not the same as from water. It needs to be very carefully tested, preferably with labelled compounds. As soon as you reach concentration ranges at which your results vary intolerably, you must compensate for the variation. The only answer I can see is to use an internal standard of the same structure as the one you are analysing.

Curry: We are beginning to realize the snags of all these analytical techniques. Dr Dole, in view of these, do you think we can help the patients?

Dole: There is progress in the fact that we are asking questions that would have been meaningless ten years ago. With poor and insensitive methods we were dealing only with massive poisonings. Now we are concerned with much smaller concentrations, either the early phases of poisoning with very potent compounds, or the late phases of poisoning with less potent substances.

Clinically, the first problem is the overwhelmed patient who has absorbed an enormous quantity of poison. He needs immediate supportive treatment. The laboratory is not of critical importance at this early stage, since the treatment needed in the emergency (artificial respiration, maintenance of circulation and body temperature) cannot be delayed for laboratory diagnosis and would be the same whatever the diagnosis. However, for the patient who has survived the acute stage, it becomes important for us to understand the dynamics of the intervening processes. The laboratory in these later stages of poisoning is very important. Have the analysts reached the ultimate limits of detectability with the techniques described here? It may well be that critical questions remain to be asked when detection goes down to picogram quantities.

Leach: I think you probably could detect femtogram quantities, or 10^{-15} g, in very favourable circumstances.

Holmstedt: According to international conventions, it all stops at 10^{-18}, or attograms!

Curry: The analysts are asking for a bit more time to answer the questions. I hope also that toxicologists reading this book will take to heart the point about aqueous solutions being different from other biological media.

Immunoassay of drugs

IRVING SUNSHINE

Cuyahoga County Coroner's Laboratory, Cleveland and Institute of Pathology, Case Western Reserve University School of Medicine, Cleveland, Ohio

Abstract Four immunological techniques used in assaying drugs are described. In these immunoassays a labelled (known) drug is displaced from a drug–antibody complex by an unlabelled drug in the sample being tested. The concentration of drug in the sample can then be measured. The techniques are sensitive, fairly specific, and quick and easy to perform. Their great advantage lies in their capacity for screening large numbers of samples for a given substance such as morphine or methadone, although they are also valuable clinically when rapid analyses are needed for the diagnosis or treatment of poisoning. One method (radioimmunoassay) can be used with serum, so providing a new order of sensitivity. On the other hand, equipment, reagents and antisera are often expensive, and positive results usually need to be confirmed by another method.

This paper is concerned with an ingenious innovative approach to the assay of drugs and other important biologically active substances. It introduces the analyst to a new ally, immunoassay, whose future contributions will be significant as well as unusual. The assays at present in common use are based primarily on chemical reactions and physical measurements of the reaction products. In these new techniques a physical measurement is made of a chemical substance, but the primary reagent is a substance synthesized by a cooperating animal (not man). Although the methods used for synthesizing the reagents are commonplace to immunologists, most chemists are unfamiliar with them.

Before I describe the methods it may be helpful if I consider their potential value and proper place in the analyst's armoury. Immunoassay techniques are sensitive and relatively specific, can be performed easily and rapidly by personnel with modest scientific training, and most of them provide objective results. These attributes are best suited to those laboratories which have to screen large numbers of samples for a given substance. The ability to deal with many samples is the great advantage of these immunoassay techniques. Many other elegant procedures which satisfy a similar need possess one or more of the attributes just listed, but few others combine them all, as these do. Furthermore, these procedures can be used effectively in any clinical chemistry laboratory, whatever the size of its toxicology workload.

GENERAL PRINCIPLES OF IMMUNOASSAY

Immunoassay of drugs is based on classical immunochemical procedures and utilizes an antigen–antibody reaction as an analytical tool. This may be a meaningless definition to some and a brief explanation is warranted. An antigen is any substance capable of eliciting an immune response when injected into a host animal. Generally the best antigens are high molecular weight proteins, polysaccharides or lipoproteins. Low molecular weight compounds such as those of interest to clinical chemists—steroids and drugs, for example—will usually not elicit an immune response. However, if these compounds are coupled to a large carrier protein or polysaccharide, they may then be antigenic.

Antibodies are immunoglobulins formed in an animal as part of its immune response to an antigenic stimulus. The antibodies thus formed have a highly specific ability to react with the antigen that stimulated their formation. Thus in a suitable analytical system they can act as detectors for a drug in the antigen.

The first step in producing drug-specific antibodies is to couple the drug to a suitable carrier protein. Many synthetic pathways can be used for this purpose. These include the use of diazonium salts for primary aromatic amines and phenols, carbodiimide for carboxylic acids, and dihalodinitrobenzenes or diisocyanates for aliphatic amines. Synthesis of the antigen is critical because the specificity of the antibody depends on the result. In several instances alternative pathways may be used; the resulting antigens will be different and have properties affecting the sensitivity and specificity of the antibody.

When the antigen has been synthesized and purified, a mixture of the antigen and Freund's adjuvant (a suitable carrier vehicle) is injected into an animal (usually a rabbit, but goats, sheep and horses have been used when larger volumes of antisera are required) to form the antibody. Some animals are better than others for this purpose because, among other reasons, they have a better ability to recognize the antigen as a foreign body and thus generate a better antiserum. The site and frequency of injection varies with each preparation. Usually the animal is bled three to six months after the first injection and the serum is checked for its sensitivity (titre) and its specificity for the antigen. The titre is determined by measuring the ability of different dilutions of the antiserum to react with a given small amount of antigen. Specificity is determined by observing to what extent chemically similar substances react in the same way as the antigen. When a suitable antiserum has been prepared, the probability is great that the animal used will continue to produce it for a reasonable time afterwards. Thus some animals literally become worth their weight in gold. But just as gold veins become depleted, so may an animal's antisera. And just as the probability is high that other gold strikes will occur in a region where one mine exists, so is the probability high that other animals of the same species will generate a similar antiserum. Yet there is no guarantee of this, and continual vigilance is required if a desired titre and specificity are to be maintained. Once a suitable antiserum has been obtained it can be stored frozen at –80 to –20 °C or it can be lyophilized and stored at –20 to +4 °C. After it has been thawed or reconstituted it is undesirable to refreeze or relyophilize any unused material. Hence small amounts are preferred for storage.

All immunoassays are based on a simple principle—the competitive displacement of a labelled drug from the antibody complex by the unlabelled drug in the sample. The concentration of the drug in the sample can then be determined by measuring the amount of displaced labelled drug or, alternatively, by measuring the amount of labelled drug still bound to antibody. In some immunoassays this involves separating the free and bound drug forms, which is usually accomplished easily by standard techniques. In other procedures this separation step is not required and these procedures need fewer manipulations.

FREE RADICAL ASSAY TECHNIQUE (FRAT)

Now that the general principles have been elaborated, I shall discuss specific applications. The first major application of immunoassay to drug problems was the FRAT system, or free radical assay technique. In this procedure a stable free radical, a nitroxide, is attached to morphine. The free radical contains unpaired electrons which may be observed and measured by an electron spin resonance (ESR) spectrometer. This instrument measures the energy absorbed by unpaired electrons as they flip from a stable to a metastable position in a magnetic field.

The FRAT system was developed for the detection of morphine in urine, and it was and is successfully used for this purpose. A drop of sample is mixed with a drop of antibody and nitroxide-labelled morphine in a capillary tube, the tube is inserted in the ESR spectrometer and the resulting signal is measured. The components do not have to be separated before measurement because a high (positive) signal is obtained only when the labelled drug in the antiserum is displaced by the unlabelled drug in the sample. If no morphine is present in the sample, no increase in the basic response is noted.

The FRAT technique has been extended to amphetamine, methadone and barbiturates as well as morphine. It is simple to use, rapid (one sample per minute) and objective, needing just the measurement of the recorded response, and it finds application in laboratories where a large number of samples—1000 or more a day—are routine. However it is expensive, with equipment costing $25 000 and reagents $0.50–$0.60 per test, and it is subject to interference from chemically related compounds, particularly from codeine in the opiate analysis. Hence a positive result is equivocal and needs corroboration. On the other hand, a negative result is definitive. FRAT sensitivity is not the highest available but it is usually more than adequate for most applications.

ENZYME-MEDIATED IMMUNOASSAY TECHNIQUE (EMIT)

The group that developed FRAT have made another significant contribution to drug detection—the EMIT system, or enzyme-mediated immunoassay technique. The label attached to the drug here is the enzyme lysozyme. This enzyme catalyses hydrolysis of the mucopolysaccharide components in the cell walls of certain bacteria. When the antibody binds morphine attached to lysozyme, the enzyme is inactivated. In the presence of drug the enzyme is released, and hydrolysis takes place and can be measured. There is no need to separate the components of the reaction because a negative sample will not displace the enzyme label, hence no activity will ensue. If the drug is present the released enzyme is active; its activity and hence the drug concentration can be measured by measuring the rate of clearing of the suspension of bacterial cell walls (seen as a decrease in absorbance) which the enzyme hydrolyses into small soluble pieces. Three measurements are needed: of the initial and subsequent optical density and of the time between these measurements. Instruments are available which can do this automatically and they are part of the semiautomated EMIT system. The procedure takes one minute to complete and is simple to perform. Its primary advantage over the FRAT system is the moderate cost of the equipment: $6000. Of course the cost of the antiserum is significant—$0.50–$0.60 a test—but when prompt results are required this system can provide individual results very quickly. Another advantage is its applicability to many drugs—morphine, amphetamine, barbiturates, cocaine and methadone. Thus this system can be valuable in clinical situations which require rapid analysis to aid in the diagnosis of poisoning. A drawback of the EMIT system is that the lysozyme naturally present in some samples can be a source of false positive results. One can easily check for this interference by adding the urine sample to the bacteria suspension and noting whether any activity results. This is inexpensive because no antibody is needed to obtain a result.

RADIOIMMUNOASSAY (RIA)

A third technique, which has become very popular and has been applied to many substances other than drugs of abuse, is radioimmunoassay (RIA). The antigen is labelled with a suitable radioactive isotope, most often ^{125}I, ^{3}H or ^{14}C, and when the usual drug–antibody reaction has taken place the mixture is separated and either the bound or the displaced radioactive drug is then measured. Usually it is the latter, and the measuring device used depends on the label. ^{125}I-labelled products are measured in a γ-counter while a scintillation counter is needed for ^{3}H-labelled compounds. ^{125}I can also be counted in a scintillation counter but this imposes additional costs and effort that are seldom warranted.

The inherent advantage of the RIA technique is that, because the radioactively labelled drug has a high specific radioactivity, its concentration can be determined with great sensitivity and precision. As a matter of application, if quantitative data are desired one usually has to dilute the sample to obtain a reasonable reading. The standard curves are obtained by plotting counts per minute against concentration. Usually these curves have a limited linear section and above certain concentrations, unless the sample is diluted, all that can be determined is that the reaction is positive. One advantage of RIA over FRAT and EMIT is that it is applicable to serum and thus opens a whole new sensitivity horizon still unattainable by the other procedures.

The general objections to immunoassays also apply to RIA, plus a few additional ones. Since radioactive substances are involved additional precautions and safety measures, all reasonable and easily met, are required. Licensing requirements exist and can be annoying. Shelf-life may also be a problem, particularly for ^{125}I-labelled compounds. The time for one determination is relatively long, maybe 40 minutes, but when many samples are analysed together, as they can be, the time per sample decreases significantly. One person can do about 400 tests a day without unusual stress. Of course this is also true of FRAT, whereas EMIT probably allows for about 300 a day.

The applications of RIA are many and growing. This combination of radioactive measurement and immunology has many adherents who testify to the great potential of this technique. Many analyses, previously unobtainable, have become commonplace. One has only to read the journals to realize how the list has grown.

HAEMAGGLUTINATION INHIBITION

For those who prefer less elaborate procedures and who cannot afford the costly equipment needed for the three techniques just described, the classical immunological procedures can be, and are being, used. Haemagglutination inhibition is one of these. In this technique the label to which the drug molecules are attached is a red blood cell which has been stabilized by treatment with formaldehyde. Since antibodies are bivalent, they may bind more than one red blood cell and agglutination occurs. When the test sample contains antigens, which compete for the active sites on the antibody, agglutination is inhibited. This classical test is performed using small plastic dishes containing many conical wells in which the reagents are placed. The reagents are added in proper sequence and allowed to stand until agglutination occurs in the control samples, the entire unit is then inspected and the results are noted. The sensitivity of this procedure is high and this may produce many false positive results. However, the sensitivity can be adjusted easily to satisfy the needs of a given situation.

If all the proper reagents are available and properly prepared, this system has high potential—it is cheap, it has a high throughput for a large number of samples even though the time for one sample is long, and it has selective sensitivity which can be used for semiquantitative data. However, this 'if' is a large one, and commercial suppliers at present have difficulty in ensuring that reagents are reliable. Of course, immunologists who prepare their own material in their own laboratories can better ensure the quality of the reagents and so obtain reliable results. Those who depend on the commercial companies may have problems.

CONCLUSIONS

These immunological techniques are clearly here to stay and we have to decide to what extent we can use them. I have mentioned many of the attributes of several immunoassays (see Table 1) and a few of their faults. The greatest defect is their specificity or lack of it. Very few antisera are specific for one compound, although some have been prepared with very high specificity when cost was no object. Hence the need to confirm all positive results by some other procedure, if specificity is important. If one doesn't care whether morphine, codeine or another opiate-like drug is the basis for a positive opiate reaction, the need for confirmation is minimal. If this distinction is important, when a job may be in jeopardy or when a parolee may be incarcerated, or in any of several other vital situations, then confirmation is essential. One experiment we did was very popular and I have had many requests to repeat it: I purchased a coffee cake well filled with poppy seeds and several of our staff ate some of it with their morning coffee. For 24 hours thereafter their urines gave a positive result when assayed with opiate antisera. Were a new group of addicts thus uncovered?

TABLE 1

Sensitivity of some immunoassays and other established techniques

	Sensitivity (μg/ml)			
	Morphine	*Amphetamine*	*Barbiturate*	*Methadone*
RIA	0.1	1.0	0.1	n.d.
EMIT	0.5	3.0	1.0	0.5
Fluorometry (10 ml sample)	0.5	n.d.	n.d.	n.d.
UV	n.d.	250	3.0	n.d.
TLC (5 ml sample)	0.5	2.5	1.5	1.0
GC (5 ml sample)	0.2	0.1	0.1	0.5

n.d. = not done

Those who perform such tests have a responsibility to those who request the analyses. This entails a clear definition of what the analytical results mean so that no misinterpretation will ensue.

The future holds great promise for this field. There is talk of polyvalent immunogens—a mixture of antisera that will respond to any one of several drugs. Such an immunogen will have great potential in situations where the expected incidence of a positive reaction is low and the test is being used primarily as an exclusion tool. Positive samples will have to be retested but, *a priori*, the number repeated will be small because past experience has indicated that the incidence of positives will be about 7–10% of those tested. When automation is applied to these immunoassays their value for mass screening will increase significantly. This has already been realized with the EMIT system, resulting in a throughput of at least 80 samples an hour, and requiring less reagent and fewer personnel.

On that bright prospect I shall end my discussion of the new approaches to drug analysis.

Selected bibliography

ADLER, F. L. & LIU, C. T. (1971) Detection of morphine by hemagglutination inhibition. *J. Immunol. 106*, 1684

ADLER, F. L., LIU, C. T. & CATLIN, D. (1972) Methodology and application of a hemagglutination inhibition test for the detection of morphine. *Clin. Immunol. Immunopathol. 1*, 53

BASTIANI, R., PHILLIPS, R., SCHNEIDER, R. & ULLMAN, E. (1973) Homogeneous immunochemical drug assays. *Am. J. Med. Technol. 39*, 211

BASTOS, M., JUKOFSKY, D., SOFFER, E., CHEDEKEL, M. & MULÉ, S. (1972) Modification of the XAD-2 resin column method for the extraction of drugs of abuse from human urine. *J. Chromatogr. 71*, 549

BLACKMORE, D. J., CURRY, A. S., HAYES, T. S. & RUTTER, E. R. (1971) Automated analysis for drugs in urine. *Clin. Chem. 17*, 896

CATLIN, D., CLEELAND, R. & GRUNBERG, E. (1973) A sensitive and rapid radioimmunassay for morphine and immunologically related substances in urine and serum. *Clin. Chem. 19*, 216

DAVIDOW, B., LI PETRI, N. & QUAME, B. (1968) A thin-layer chromatographic screening procedure for detecting drug abuse. *Am. J. Clin. Pathol. 50*, 714

DUBOWSKI, K. (1971) Free radical assay technique for drugs. *Ann. Clin. Lab. Sci. 1*, 199

FOLTZ, R. & CLARK, P. (1974) Quantitative analysis of morphine in urine by gas chromatography—chemical ionization mass spectrometry. *Clin. Chem. 20*, 465

KUPFERBERG, H., BURKHALTER, A. & WAY, E. L. (1964) A sensitive fluorometric assay for morphine in plasma and brain. *J. Pharmacol. Exp. Ther. 145*, 247

LEUTE, R. K., ULLMAN, E. F., GOLDSTEIN, A. & HERZENBERG, L. A. (1972) Spin immunoassay technique for determination of morphine. *Nat. New Biol. 236*, 93

MULÉ, S. & HUSHIN, P. L. (1971) Semiautomated fluorometric assay for submicrogram quantities of morphine and quinine in human biological material. *Anal. Chem. 43*, 708

MULÉ, S., SUNSHINE, I., BRAUDE, M. & WILLETTE, R. (eds.) (1974) *Immunoassay of Drugs*, CRC Press, Cleveland, Ohio

RUBENSTEIN, K. E., SCHNEIDER, R. S. & ULLMAN, E. F. (1972) 'Homogeneous' enzyme immunoassay. A new immunochemical technique. *Biochem. Biophys. Res. Commun. 47*, 846

SKELLY, D. S., BROWN, L. P. & BESCH, P. K. (1973) Radioimmunassay. *Clin. Chem. 19*, 146

SPECTOR, S. & PARKER, C. W. (1970) Morphine: radioimmunassay. *Science (Wash. D.C.) 168*, 1374

SUNSHINE, I. (1973) Stand up and be counted. *J. Chromatogr. 82*, 125

[*For discussion see pp. 213–217*]

Immunological methods for detecting drugs: their application in the detection of digitoxin, digoxin and morphine

CHARLES W. PARKER

Washington University School of Medicine, St Louis, Missouri

Abstract In the past few years immunological techniques have come into increasing use for the detection and quantification of drugs in body fluids. Immunoassays utilize anti-drug antibodies obtained by immunizing animals with covalent drug–protein conjugates, and these assays can in principle be applied to virtually any drug. As a rule immunological analysis is carried out by radioimmunoassay, in which a drug or antibody (usually the former) is labelled and an unlabelled drug is measured by its ability to inhibit binding of the labelled drug by antibody. Other labels which can be applied to immunological measurements include enzymic activity, fluorescence, haemagglutination and electron spin resonance. In the development of immunoassays a knowledge of the mode of evolution of the immune response, genetic factors in the response, the structural basis for antibody specificity and cross-reactivity, and the kinetics and thermodynamics of antigen–antibody reactions, is very helpful. These topics are discussed, together with the procedures followed in this laboratory in the development of immunoassays for digitoxin and morphine.

Satisfactory physicochemical methods are generally available for the detection and quantification of drugs that reach high concentrations in body fluids during ordinary pharmacological usage. When pharmacological levels are low, standard methods tend to be marginal in sensitivity and cumbersome or unreliable, and the use of immunochemical procedures deserves serious consideration. The knowledge that antibodies can be produced to drugs has existed since the classical studies of Landsteiner, Eisen and others which showed that antibodies were obtainable to a seemingly endless list of aromatic, aliphatic, heterocyclic and polycyclic organic molecules of low molecular weight (Landsteiner 1936; Eisen 1959). Antibodies were applied to the measurement of polypeptide hormones in the late 1950s (Yalow & Berson 1960) but it was not until 1966, when our laboratory described a practical radioimmunoassay for digitoxin, that the feasibility of developing highly sensitive immunochemical measurements for drugs was clearly established (Oliver *et al.* 1966; Oliver *et al.* 1968). Since that time immunoassays have been evolved for other digitalis preparations and for opiates, barbiturates, cannabinoids, the prostaglandins, cyclic nucleotides, steroids, LSD (lysergide), serotonin, normetanephrine and gentamicin as well as for a wide variety of proteins and polypeptides. There is no doubt that the list will continue to grow as new immunoassays are developed.

As a rule, immunoassays for drugs are based on the ability of an unlabelled drug (D) (the unknown) to inhibit the binding of a labelled drug (D^*) by antibody (Ab):

$$D - Ab \underset{}{\overset{D}{\rightleftarrows}} Ab \qquad \overset{D^*}{\rightleftarrows} D^* \cdot Ab$$

The process may be visualized as a simple competition in which D reduces the amount of free Ab, decreasing the availability of Ab to D^* and the amount of $D^* \cdot Ab$ complex which is formed (Parker 1972). D^* is usually radioactively labelled but, as discussed below, fluorescent or electron spin resonance labels may be used, and it is even possible to apply the label to the antibody rather than the drug. When the assay is performed, D^* and Ab are incubated together in the presence or absence of tissue samples containing unlabelled D. After equilibration free D^* and $D^* \cdot Ab$ are separated. Commonly used separation procedures include the use of a solid-phase absorption (for example, charcoal) or the precipitation of $D^* \cdot Ab$ complexes with either a second antibody or a salt. D^*—Ab (or free D^*) is then determined by radioactive counting (or whatever measurement is appropriate). The concentration of drug in the sample is calculated by relating the diminution in binding of D^* to a standard drug-inhibition curve obtained by adding graded, known amounts of D to D^* and Ab. A new standard curve is determined in each assay to allow for variation in binding of D^* from assay to assay. In optimum conditions, a single technician using semiautomated equipment can process up to 1000 samples in a day.

Competitive binding assays utilizing tissue-binding proteins rather than antibodies will not be discussed. These methods are very similar in principle to immunoassays and where a receptor protein of high affinity and specificity is available they are equally applicable to the measurement of hormones or drugs.

A necessary first step in developing an immunoassay is the preparation of a suitable antiserum. Most drugs have a molecular weight of less than 1500 daltons and exhibit little if any immunogenicity. However, if they are covalently attached to an immunogenic carrier, such as a protein, an immune response is obtained. Molecules which are non-immunogenic as such, but which produce an immune response when they are attached to an immunogenic carrier, are termed haptens. As a rule the carrier is a protein and is chosen on the basis of commercial availability, foreignness to the species being immunized, number of functional groups for conjugation, and potency as an immunogen (Parker 1971). Synthetic polyamino acids with suitable functional side-chains have also been used for this purpose, although this approach is sometimes unsuccessful. The hapten is added to the carrier *in vitro* in conditions in which covalent bonds are formed. Unless the drug has intrinsic protein reactivity, which is unusual, the reaction requires an activating agent. Commonly used activating agents include water-soluble carbodiimides, mixed anhydrides and diisocyanates.

More frequently than not, conjugation to protein cannot be accomplished directly, either because the drug does not contain appropriate functional groups or because these groups must be left unsubstituted if maximum specificity for the unaltered drug is to be obtained. Groups with a formal charge at neutral pH exert an important influence on antibody specificity and the antibody must recognize the drug itself as well as the drug–protein conjugate used for immunization. In addition to the importance of charged groups in immunological specificity, it should be noted that in hapten–protein conjugates involving complex organic molecules the immunodominant region of the hapten is likely to be in its most distal portion (e.g. penultimate to its point of attachment to protein). Thus immunological specificity and cross-reactivity will be governed partly by where on the haptenic molecule the functional group for attachment to protein is placed. A new functional group can usually be introduced at a non-critical site on the hapten by organic synthesis and this is the procedure that has been followed in the production of antibodies to digitoxigenin (Oliver *et al.* 1966), morphine (Spector & Parker 1970), oestrogen (Abraham 1969), testosterone (Midgley *et al.* 1971), aldosterone (Oliver *et al.* 1971*a*), cyclic AMP and cyclic GMP (Steiner *et al.* 1969, 1972). Where a drug has several therapeutic forms or metabolites, the level of immunological discrimination may be increased if antibodies to more than one kind of conjugate are prepared and simultaneous assays are run.

The reason why an immunogenic carrier is required in the induction of antibodies to drugs is uncertain. It is not a simple matter of delaying the excretion of the drug or rendering it multivalent. Much of the current speculation centres on an apparent ability of the carrier to interact with and stimulate thymus-dependent (T) lymphocytes as a necessary first step in the activation of bone marrow-dependent (B) lymphocytes (antibody-producing cells). There is also evidence that in association with T cells the carrier helps to modulate the switchover from IgM to IgG antibody formation and aids in the development of immunological learning (in which antibody affinity for hapten increases with time after immunization) (Katz & Benacerraf 1972).

In addition to properly selected conjugation procedures being important, the immunization protocol that is followed is important in the development of highly sensitive immunoassays. (*a*) There are major genetic influences on immune responsiveness which result in marked variations in antibody affinity and specificity, even in animals of the same species; therefore, a large number of animals should be immunized and the antisera evaluated individually. Thus the sensitivity of immunoassays for cyclic AMP (cAMP) may vary by at least three orders of magnitude, depending on the antiserum, and the cross-reactivity for ATP and other non-cyclic nucleotides may vary from 1 in 2000 to 1 in 1 million (e.g. the concentration of ATP required for 50% inhibition of precipitation of radiolabelled cAMP is as much as 1 million times that of cAMP). (*b*) As a rule, antibody affinity is maximized by administering the immunogens in complete adjuvant and giving the animals booster doses for many months. (*c*) Aside from the adjuvant itself, the immunogen should be as free of immunologically active contaminants as possible, to avoid antigenic competition (by immunization with structurally unrelated substances capable of non-specifically reducing the response to the designated immunogen) or immunological cross-reactivity (by immunization with congeners which coexist with the drug in body fluids).

In optimal circumstances as little as 2–5 picograms of a drug can be detected by immunoassay but practical sensitivities are usually in the 100–400 pg range. Depending on the drug and how it is administered, immunoassay sensitivity may be critical in determining whether the assay is clinically useful. Four factors exert an important influence on immunoassay sensitivity:

(1) *Antibody affinity:* The interaction between a radiolabelled drug and antibody is described mathematically by the Law of Mass Action:

$$K_a = \frac{D^* \quad — \quad Ab}{(D^*) \quad (Ab)},$$

where K_a is the association constant (in litres mole^{-1}) and (D^*—Ab), (D^*) and (Ab) are the molar concentrations of antibody-bound drug, free drug, and free antibody sites, respectively. In sensitive immunoassays using serum from hyperimmunized animals, the antibody responsible for D^* binding will be largely of the IgG class. If, for purposes of simplicity, it is assumed that enough antibody will be used to produce 50% binding of D^* in the radioimmunoassay (in the absence of inhibitor), the terms (D^*—Ab) and (D^*) in the above equation cancel each other out, and the required molar concentration of free antibody sites is the reciprocal of the association constant. (In most immunoassay systems the level of antigen binding is maintained in the 25–40% range.) For an antibody with an association constant of less than 1×10^6 l mol^{-1} the concentration of antibody required to obtain substantial binding of D^* will be large (> 0.1 mg/ml, using 75 000 as the equivalent weight of IgG). With such large amounts of antibody present the concentration of unlabelled drug needed to inhibit the binding of D^* will be high and the immunoassay will be insensitive. Even where a high affinity antibody is obtained it must be used in limiting concentrations if a sensitive immunoassay is to be obtained.

Whether practical immunoassays can be developed to every commonly used drug remains to be established. The interaction between an antibody and a drug apparently involves a summation of binding energies, including ionic, hydrogen bonding and hydrophobic forces. It may be that relatively aliphatic molecules will be unable to undergo a high affinity interaction with antibody because they lack sufficient antigenic complexity.

(2) *Interfering substances in serum or tissue:* Normal tissue constituents which competitively bind or metabolize the drug or cross-react immunologically may have to be eliminated for the apparent maximum sensitivity of the assay to be attained (e.g. the sensitivity indicated by standard inhibition curves based on measurements in simple buffer solutions). In tissues that have been extracted with acidic solutions or concentrated, the non-specific effects of pH and ionic strength on antibody binding must be considered.

(3) *Immunoassay conditions:* The rate at which an antigen reacts with an antibody depends on the concentrations of the reacting species. Immunoassays for polypeptide hormones take at least a few days to attain maximum sensitivity, which reflects the very low concentration of the reactants and a possible need for re-equilibration before complexes of maximum stability can be obtained. Equilibration occurs more rapidly in antibody–hapten systems but even here somewhat greater sensitivity is likely to be obtained with an incubation time of 18–24 h than with an incubation time of only a few hours. Immunoassay procedures are available in which the measurements can be completed within 5–30 min, but some diminution in sensitivity is inevitable in these conditions. For many immunoassay systems this will not be a serious drawback and adequate sensitivity will be achieved, even in a short incubation assay. The sensitivity of the assay will also depend on the order of mixing of D^* and D, inhibition of D^* binding being more marked if the antibody is exposed to D first (provided the subsequent incubation is not so long that complete re-equilibration occurs).

(4) *The specific activity of the marker:* As already mentioned, the indicator or marker molecule in the immunoassay is usually the drug itself, although radiolabelled antibody may also be used. Molecules of drug may be labelled by radioactivity or by attachment to an enzyme, spin label, or fluorescent molecule.

^{3}H, ^{14}C, ^{125}I, ^{131}I, ^{32}P, ^{35}S are among the radioactive markers which may be used. In general, radioiodinated markers are preferred to ^{3}H or ^{14}C markers because they have a much higher specific activity (unless an organic molecule with many carbon atoms is involved) and counting is easier (Hunter 1967). The preparation of a satisfactory radioiodinated hapten has been possible in immunoassays for digitoxin, cyclic AMP, cyclic GMP and testosterone, with specific activities in excess of 150 Ci/mmol being obtained (Parker 1972). In the preparation of an iodinated hapten, the hapten is first conjugated to tyrosine (Oliver *et al.* 1968) or to a tyrosine-containing protein or polyamino acid (Van Vunakis *et al.* 1972). The conjugate is then iodinated with chloramine T, as in the procedure Hunter & Greenwood (1962) originally described for protein and antigens. Difficulties in obtaining a satisfactory radioiodine marker for a haptenic system have arisen with haptens that are altered chemically during iodination or where the iodotyrosine moiety is bound non-specifically to glassware or other components of the incubation mixture; in these circumstances ^{14}C or ^{3}H labels may be more desirable.

Haptens conjugated to enzymes of high specific activity may also be used as markers in immunoassays (Van Weeman & Schuurs 1972). Enzymes that have been used for this purpose include horseradish peroxidase, alkaline phosphatase and β-galactosidase. With enzymes of high specific activity and a sensitive method for measuring substrate or hydrolysed substrate, the theoretical sensitivities of enzyme immunoassays and of radioimmunoassay are similar. One interesting recent development in enzyme immunoassays is the use of a hapten-substituted preparation of lysozyme which undergoes a change in catalytic activity in the presence of antihapten antibody. In this system there is no need to separate antibody-bound from free haptenated enzyme and the analysis of samples is thereby simplified (Rubenstein *et al.* 1972).

Antigen- or antibody-containing particles can be used for immunological assays, agglutination occurring when there is immunological bridging between particles (due to the multivalence of antibody) and inhibition when bridging is prevented by hapten. The procedure is rapid but only semiquantitative, and non-specific agglutination is sometimes a problem.

In two other procedures for marking the hapten so that its interaction with antibody can be followed electron spin resonance (ESR) or fluorescence polarization are used. When a nitroxide spin label is attached to hapten a change in the ESR spectrum occurs when anti-hapten antibody is added (Stryer & Griffith 1965; Leute *et al.* 1972). Unlabelled hapten can be detected by its ability to inhibit the change. The advantage of the spin immunoassay method over most other methods is that samples of whole serum can be used without the need to separate antibody-bound and unbound labelled hapten. This disadvantage of the method is that with existing ESR detection systems the level of sensitivity is low (in the μmolar range).

Fluorescence polarization utilizes the change in vertically and horizontally excited fluorescence that occurs when a fluorescent molecule of low molecular weight becomes bound by a much larger, more slowly moving macromolecule such as an antibody. Since most drugs are not fluorescent in conditions in which antibody binding occurs, the drug has to be attached to a highly fluorescent organic molecule such as fluorescein or dansyl (Dandliker & de Saussure 1970). The procedure is rapid, convenient and sensitive but in whole serum or extracts of tissue the maximum theoretical sensitivity will not be achieved because of interfering fluorescence and the susceptibility of highly fluorescent molecules to non-specific binding (Parker 1973).

Apart from their usefulness in measuring overall drug levels, antibodies can be used to determine the subcellular localization of drugs in tissue. Thus antibodies to cAMP have been used in combination with a fluoresceinated second antibody for visualizing local deposits of cAMP in intact cells exposed to agents that stimulate adenylate cyclase (Bloom *et al.* 1973). Antibodies are also useful in studies of the mechanism of drug action, where they help to determine whether the drug is acting on extracellular receptors or inside the cell. Antibodies to digoxin have been shown to partially reverse the cardiotoxic effects of the drug *in vivo* and *in vitro*, which suggests that the agent acts at the cell surface (Butler *et al.* 1973). The ability of anti-digoxin antibodies to reduce cardiac toxicity provides a possible approach to the treatment of digitalis toxicity. The antibodies could be injected as a solution of purified antibody or attached to a solid-phase immunoadsorbent such as a nylon catheter (Lyle *et al.* 1973) which could be cycled through the venous system or used extracorporeally. The amount of antibody required is substantial but not prohibitive, and if extracorporeal catheters were used they could perhaps be regenerated and used again. In man, toxic levels of digoxin usually are in the 2–5 ng/ml range, which represents a total of about 28–70 μg of the drug in extracellular fluids (assuming even distribution in the body). This quantity of digoxin can theoretically be neutralized by 3–16 mg antibody, but unless antibodies of exceptionally high affinity were available more antibody would be needed. Even if this approach proves to be applicable to drugs such as digoxin which are toxic at low molar concentrations, it will not be useful for drugs which are toxic only at much higher serum concentrations, are sequestered in tissue, or have already produced irreversible toxicity.

DIGITALIS

Digoxin, digitoxin and related digitalis preparations have been used extensively in the treatment of congestive heart failure. In the past the administration of these drugs has been based on empirical dosage schedules. The clinical diagnosis of digitalis toxicity has sometimes presented serious difficulties because of similarities between the manifestations of drug toxicity and those of the underlying cardiac condition. The diagnosis of digitalis toxicity is so difficult that individuals have sometimes been given graded amounts of ouabain, a short-acting digitalis preparation, as a diagnostic test, the end-point being the development of multifocal ventricular premature contractions. This practice has now been discontinued but the fact that it was used at all illustrates the difficulties that sometimes arise in clinical decisions about the use of digitalis. The non-immunological methods available for measuring digitalis in blood have been too cumbersome or non-specific for routine clinical use. Recently, radioimmunoassays have become available for a number of digitalis derivatives, including digitoxin and digoxin. The first practical immunoassay for a cardiac glycoside was developed by Oliver *et al.* (1966, 1968). Antibodies to digitoxin were prepared by immunizing rabbits with a 3-*O*-succinyl-digitoxigenin–protein conjugate. With a radioiodinated marker of very high specific activity (obtained by coupling 3-*O*-succinyl digitoxigenin to tyrosine and iodinating with ^{125}I by the chloramine T method [Hunter & Greenwood 1962]), as little as 100 pg of digitoxin could be measured. The average serum concentrations in patients receiving the drug corresponded closely to the values obtained with the accurate but laborious isotope dilution method. Individuals with a clinical diagnosis of digitalis toxicity (established by an independent prospective evaluation) had increased concentrations of digitoxin in their blood, establishing the value of the serum immunoassay in difficult decisions about further digitalis use. This conclusion has subsequently been confirmed for digoxin as well as digitoxin by studies in a number of laboratories. In the original immunoassay for digitoxin a preliminary extraction step was carried out with chloroform to eliminate digitoxin binding to albumin. Assays for digitoxin and digoxin have now been shortened to one or two hours by the use of antibodies of higher affinity (eliminating the need for albumin extraction) and by using dextran-coated charcoal to separate bound and free marker (Smith *et al.* 1969; Oliver *et al.* 1971*b*). Immunoassays for these two cardiac glycosides are now sensitive enough to permit cardiac glycoside determinations on less than 0.5 ml blood, an important advantage in studies in infants and small children.

MORPHINE

In recent years opium addiction has become a leading cause of death in the United States in teenagers and young adults, so creating an urgent need for convenient and reliable techniques for the detection of morphine and its congeners. Spectrophotometric and spectrofluorometric methods of identifying the opium alkaloids are relatively insensitive and laborious, requiring both extraction and chromatographic separation. In 1970 Spector & Parker described a radioimmunoassay for morphine which has the specificity and sensitivity needed in large-scale screening studies for morphine addiction. Antibodies to morphine were obtained by immunizing rabbits with a 3-*O*-carboxymethylmorphine–bovine serum albumin conjugate; inhibition of binding of marker ([^{3}H]dihydromorphine) was obtained at concentrations of morphine and its surrogates of less than 1 ng/ml. Antibody-bound [^{3}H]dihydromorphine was separated from unbound marker by precipitation with ammonium sulphate and counted by liquid scintillation. The assay was applicable to the measurement of opiates in unextracted serum. The molar concentration of codeine (morphine 3-methyl ether) required for 50% binding of marker was less than that for morphine itself, presumably because codeine has greater structural similarity to the immunizing 3-carboxymethylmorphine group than morphine itself. Sensitive measurements were possible with heroin (3,6-diacetylmorphine) as well as with codeine and morphine. Antibodies to morphine have subsequently been prepared by conjugation through the OH group at position 6 of the morphine molecule (morphine 6-hemisuccinate) or through an azo linkage at position 2 (Van Vunakis *et al.* 1972; Spector *et al.* 1973). Antibodies to morphine 6-hemisuccinate bind morphine 3-glucuronide, an *in vivo* conjugation product of morphine, almost as effectively as morphine itself—in contrast to antibodies to 3-carboxymethylmorphine, which display a marked decrease in binding affinity for molecules of morphine which contain the hydrophilic glucuronide group (Spector *et al.* 1973). Nalorphine, dextromethorphan and levallorphan have exhibited relatively little cross-reactivity with all three antibodies. Methadone, which is currently being used for the treatment of morphine addiction, is essentially not cross-reactive, making it possible to use the immunoassay to detect morphine in patients undergoing methadone treatment.

Binding measurements similar to those used in the morphine immunoassay have been used to detect antibodies to morphine in the serum of opiate addicts (Ryan *et al.* 1972). There has been speculation about the possible role of these antibodies in morphine tolerance and in acute, life-threatening reactions to heroin, but no conclusions are possible yet.

Antibodies to 3-carboxymethylmorphine have also been used to develop haemagglutination inhibition and spin label immunoassays for morphine. In the haemagglutination assay, tanned erythrocytes sensitized with a 3-carboxymethylmorphine conjugate were agglutinated by anti-morphine antibody, with inhibition of the agglutination by morphine, codeine and heroin (Adler & Liu 1971). The assay is suitable for the rapid screening of large numbers of samples, although it is less quantitative than the conventional radioactive morphine immunoassay. The spin label assay for morphine (Leute *et al.* 1972) is even more rapid but is of marginal sensitivity in terms of routine clinical application.

As performed at present, immunoassays for opiates do not critically distinguish between major opiate derivatives. Thus antibodies to 3-carboxymethylmorphine provide a sensitive means of detecting morphine, codeine or heroin. A given level of inhibition could be due to small amounts of codeine (the best inhibitor) or slightly larger amounts of morphine or heroin. Further discrimination by immunoassay could be made by analysing samples after a preliminary chromatographic separation or by carrying out a simultaneous immunoassay with antibodies to 6-succinylmorphine which will bind codeine less well than morphine. This approach could also be used to exclude the rare false positive inhibition reactions for morphine which are due to cross-reacting substances in special types of foods.

CONCLUSIONS

Because of their versatility, sensitivity, simplicity and specificity, immunoassay methods have broad applicability in the measurement of toxins, hormones, macromolecules and drugs. Over the next decade the already widespread use of immunological assays is likely to increase, with these methods being used to measure many substances now being quantified by other techniques. The major value of an immunoassay is its adaptability to rapid screening, which makes it of potential value in the differential diagnosis of the poisoned patient, in the detection of drug abuse, and in the routine monitoring of blood and urinary drug levels. The extent to which these procedures can be applied on a routine basis clinically will depend on the development of very simple, inexpensive methods of analysis in which extensive handling of tubes and repeated recalibration of reagents is avoided and sophisticated counting equipment can be by-passed. There is good reason to believe that this goal can be achieved.

ACKNOWLEDGEMENT

This work was supported by National Institute of Health Research Grant AI04646.

References

ABRAHAM, G. E. (1969) Solid phase radioimmunoassay of estradiol-17β. *J. Clin. Endocrinol. 29*, 866–870

ADLER, F. L. & LIU, C. (1971) Detection of morphine by hemagglutination inhibition. *J. Immunol. 106*, 1684–1685

BLOOM, F. E., WEDNER, H. J. & PARKER, C. W. (1973) Use of antibodies to study cell structure and metabolism. *Pharmacol. Rev. 25*, 343–358

BUTLER, V. P., WATSON, J. G., SCHIDT, D. H., GARDNER, J. D., MANDEL, W. J. & SKELTON, C. L. (1973) Reversal of the pharmacological and toxic effects of cardiac glycosides by specific antibodies. *Pharmacol. Rev. 25*, 239–249

DANDLIKER, W. B. & de SAUSSURE, V. A. (1970) Fluorescence polarization in immunochemistry. *Immunochemistry 7*, 799–824

EISEN, H. M. (1959) Hypersensitivity to simple chemicals, in *Cellular and Humoral Aspects of the Hypersensitive States*, pp. 89–122, Hoeber-Harper, New York

HUNTER, W. M. (1967) The preparation of radioiodinated proteins of high activity, their reaction with antibody in vitro: the radioimmunoassay, in *Handbook of Experimental Immunology*, pp. 608–654, Blackwell Scientific Publications, Oxford

HUNTER, W. M. & GREENWOOD, F. C. (1962) Preparation of iodine^{131} labeled human growth hormone of high specific activity. *Nature (Lond.) 194*, 495–496

KATZ, D. H. & BENACERRAF, B. (1972) The regulatory influence of activated T cells on B cell responses to antigen. *Adv. Immunol. 15*, 1–94

LANDSTEINER, K. (1936) *The Specificity of Serological Reactions*, pp. 156–197, Dover Publications, New York

LEUTE, R. K., ULLMAN, E. F., GOLDSTEIN, A. & HERZENBERG, L. A. (1972) Spin immunoassay technique for determination of morphine. *Nat. New Biol. 236*, 93–94

LYLE, L., PARKER, C. W. & PARKER, B. M. (1973) The use of nylon catheters for selective immunoadsorption in vivo. *J. Clin. Invest. 52*, 53

MIDGLEY, A. R., NISWENDER, G. D., GAY, V. L. & REICHERT, L. E. (1971) Use of antibodies for characterization of gonadotropins and steroids. *Recent Prog. Horm. Res. 27*, 235–285

OLIVER, G. C., BRASFIELD, D., PARKER, B. M. & PARKER, C. W. (1966) A sensitive radioimmunoassay for digitalis. *J. Lab. Clin. Med. 68*, 1002

OLIVER, G. C., PARKER, B. M., BRASFIELD, D. L. & PARKER, C. W. (1968) The measurement of digitoxin in human serum by radioimmunoassay. *J. Clin. Invest. 47*, 1035

OLIVER, G. C., BAHL, O. P. & PARKER, C. W. (1971*a*) Characterization of antialdosterone antibodies. *Circulation 64*, 122

OLIVER, G. C., BAHL, O. P. & PARKER, C. W. (1971*b*) Characterization of antialdosterone antibodies. *Circulation 44*, 446

PARKER, C. W. (1971) in *Principles of Competitive Protein-Binding Assays* (Odell, W. D., & Daughaday, W. H., eds.), pp. 25–48, Lippincott, Philadelphia

PARKER, C. W. (1972) Radioimmunoassays. *Prog. Clin. Pathol. 4*, 103–141

PARKER, C. W. (1973) Spectrofluorometric methods, in *Handbook of Experimental Immunology*, pp. 14.1-14.25, Blackwell Scientific Publications, Oxford

RUBENSTEIN, K. E., SCHNEIDER, R. S. & ULLMAN, E. F. (1972) 'Homogeneous' enzyme immunoassay. A new immunochemical technique. *Biochem. Biophys. Res. Commun. 47*, 846–851

RYAN, J. J., PARKER, C. W. & WILLIAMS, R. C. (1972) Gamma globulin binding of morphine in heroin addicts. *J. Lab. Clin. Med. 80*, 155–164

SMITH, J. W., STEINER, A., NEWBERRY, W. M. & PARKER, C. W. (1969) The effect of dibutyryl cyclic adenosine 3′, 5′ monophosphate (dcAMP) on human lymphocyte stimulation by phytohemagglutinin (PHA). *Fed. Proc. 28*, 566

SPECTOR, S. & PARKER, C. W. (1970) Morphine: radioimmunoassay. *Science (Wash. D.C.) 168*, 1347–1348

SPECTOR, S., BERKOWITZ, B., FLYNN, E. J. & PESKAR, B. (1973) Antibodies to morphine, barbiturates and serotonin. *Pharmacol. Rev. 25*, 281–292

STEINER, A. L., KIPNIS, D. M., UTIGER, R. & PARKER, C. W. (1969) Radioimmunoassay for the measurement of adenosine 3′, 5′ cyclic monophosphate. *Proc. Natl. Acad. Sci. 64*, 367–373

STEINER, A. L., PARKER, C. W. & KIPNIS, D. M. (1972) Radioimmunoassay for cyclic nucleotides. I. Preparation of antibodies and iodinated cyclic nucleotides. *J. Biol. Chem. 247*, 1106–1113

STRYER, L. & GRIFFITH, O. H. (1965) A spin-labeled hapten. *Proc. Natl. Acad. Sci. 54*, 1785–1791

VAN VUNAKIS, H., WASSERMAN, E. & LEVINE, L. (1972) Specificities of antibodies to morphine. *J. Pharmacol. Exp. Ther. 180*, 514–521

VAN WEEMAN, B. K. & SCHUURS, A. H. (1972) Immunoassay using hapten-enzyme conjugates. *FEBS (Fed. Eur. Biochem. Soc.) Lett. 24*, 77–81

YALOW, R. S. & BERSON, S. A. (1960) Immunoassay of endogenous plasma insulin in man. *J. Clin. Invest. 39*, 1157

Discussion of the two preceding papers

Moffat: Earlier it was suggested that it would be useful to know whether patients had taken large amounts of drugs like digoxin, for which good methods exist for determining concentrations quickly. I am sure that doctors sometimes prescribe double the dose when the patients are really suffering from drug toxicity already.

Newton: It is useful to know digoxin levels but, in practice, I do not think that the clinician's judgement can be replaced. Proof of high levels is not necessary if the symptoms and signs of toxicity are present.

Sunshine: Radioimmunoassays have been designed which can be a useful extra tool for the clinician. They may not be essential for him, but I submit that they do have value.

Parker: I agree that digitalis can be given to the average cardiac patient with relatively little risk without routinely monitoring blood levels. I further agree that where multifocal ventricular premature contractions or paroxysmal auricular tachycardia with block are present the diagnosis of digitalis toxicity can be strongly suspected clinically. However, I would also point out that clinically it may be difficult to tell whether the patient has had too much digitalis or not enough (see p. 208). And during rapid changes in fluid balance (for example, if a patient is on haemodialysis for chronic renal disease), knowledge of the digitalis level may be critical for optimal management.

Leach: What do the very low levels of amphetamine you can detect mean, Dr Sunshine?

Sunshine: We can now detect 10 ng/ml and we think we can go lower. Thus we shall try to interpret the data obtained from hyperkinetic children treated with amphetamine.

Leach: We seem to be worrying about specificity, but surely a relatively non-specific radioimmunoassay or antibody–antigen reaction would be useful, allowing us to implicate or exclude vast groups of drugs at once? A great deal of effort seems to go into making specific antisera, and that may not be what would be of most use.

Sunshine: The greatest potential of immunoassays is perhaps their negative value.

Holmstedt: Lack of specificity is certainly what worries many of us. I cannot see how these immunoassay methods can be used unless they are checked against a chemically specific method of equal sensitivity. How much in an assay for opiates is due to heroin, monoacetylmorphine, morphine, codeine or morphine glucuronide? If someone has eaten bread or cake containing poppy seeds, the immunoassay will be positive, as Dr Sunshine told us—those seeds contain noscapine, an opium alkaloid.

Sunshine: A positive immunoassay reaction has to be confirmed by a method of comparable sensitivity.

Holmstedt: But are these methods being used for quantification and studies of pharmacokinetics of drugs?

Sunshine: We are thinking of venturing into this field, but I do not know that many others have done this yet.

Beckett: Couldn't we summarize by saying that immunoassay is a valuable screening test but should not be used quantitatively in a non-critical manner?

Curry: Do you mean that immunoassay shouldn't be used for the opiates or are you including digoxin there, Professor Beckett?

Beckett: Some digoxin metabolites will also interfere with the specificity of that assay.

Prescott: I am worried about the widespread introduction of drug assays of any kind for routine clinical use. Doctors do not think about drugs very much and if they are provided with a figure, their thinking will cease completely. The important thing in drug therapy is that doctors should think, and that they should give the patient the right dose to produce the desired response. The optimum plasma concentration in a given patient may not necessarily be the 'official' optimum level. Of course, this should not stop progress and the introduction of these methods but it would be most unfortunate if drug therapy consisted only of getting the 'right' figure back from a laboratory.

Sunshine: These assays can be of direct value to the patient. Neurologists treating patients with convulsive disorders are sometimes bewildered when the doses of phenytoin and phenobarbitone they prescribed do not control the convulsions. Our analyses sometimes show them that the patients have not been taking the drugs regularly or that therapeutic concentrations have not been reached because the prescribed dose was inadequate.

Prescott: I agree that the analyses may be useful, and the treatment of epilepsy has been greatly improved by monitoring of drug levels. But many clinicians do not think enough about drugs and the neurologists are particularly guilty! Do you ask the clinician at what time he took the sample in relation to the last dose, when the patient last had a meal, what other drugs the patient is taking, what the plasma proteins are like, and whether the patient has other diseases that might influence the relationship between the anticonvulsant concentration and the response? These are all important and it is not enough just to look at a figure and say 'Double the dose'.

Curry: Which drugs do you measure in blood, Dr Sunshine?

Sunshine: All our immunoassay work has been on urine, except that we use radioimmunoassay (RIA) for detecting opiates and barbiturates in serum. We are hoping to apply the amphetamine radioimmunoassay to serum. I understand that the group who developed the EMIT system have a project for the analysis of phenobarbitone and phenytoin in serum, and that this method is now available.

Curry: Are you using RIA to measure barbiturates other than phenobarbitone in serum?

Sunshine: Yes.

Goulding: Nowadays we have got to the stage when otherwise extremely competent cardiologists ask us whether their patients are taking the right dose. Since we began offering a service—although we do not test every patient in the hospital—we have been astonished how often the cardiologists guessed wrongly before we determined the level. I think we have kidded ourselves on our clinical acumen in the past.

Prescott: But how do you know whether the levels are wrong in a particular patient?

Goulding: Because patients get better when the dose is modified in response to the test.

Prescott: A level of 4 ng/ml two hours after a certain preparation of digoxin in a patient with a particular illness may be the optimum, whereas the correct level in another patient 10 hours after a dose of a different brand may be only 1 ng/ml.

Goulding: Assays help when a dose regime needs to be altered; they do not tell the clinician precisely what the dose should be.

Prescott: The correct dose is the dose that gives the required effect.

Curry: It is a clinical–chemical titration.

Parker: We have prospectively evaluated patients receiving digitoxin or digoxin and diagnosed toxicity on the basis of clinical criteria that everyone would accept. When we later correlated immunoassay levels with the clinical diagnosis of toxicity the correlations were surprisingly good. A number of other groups have made similar observations. It is this kind of information which leads to the impression that the assay is measuring something useful. Obviously factors other than the serum digitalis level, such as the concentration of potassium in the extracellular fluid, affect toxicity, and it may be that the best correlation will be obtained by considering serum electrolyte concentrations in combination with immunoassay values.

I would agree that for drugs which are rapidly metabolized to derivatives which cross-react poorly immunologically, the immunoassay may lose some of its quantitative value, unless the derivatives themselves are also measured. However, it may actually be the drug itself we want to measure rather than the metabolite, and for many drugs the level of degradation will be no more than 10–20%. In these circumstances we can get clinically useful information without ignoring the fact that metabolites may also be present.

Prescott: What I am against is clinicians prescribing even more by rote than they do at present. We must look at the patient, not at the laboratory result. It is the patient who counts, not what comes out of the laboratory. If there is agreement, that is fine, but this is not always the case. There may be very good reasons why this is so.

Parker: I am against people being treated blindly by physicians who arbitrarily change doses and do not recognize signs of toxicity. Those doctors will be better off knowing a level. There are many such physicians, just as there are many patients who fail to follow instructions on drug usage. And, particularly in patients with systemic disease affecting several organs, 'classical' manifestations of drug toxicity may be very difficult to recognize, even by an alert and skilful physician.

Prescott: The correct dose is not necessarily the one that gives the ideal textbook level in a given situation.

Parker: That will be true of some drugs in some situations but for digitalis the correlation between the serum level and the clinical state is surprisingly good. I suspect that the physician who ignores what is thought to be a toxic level and pushes the drug empirically, without a compelling reason for doing so, will be wrong more often than right.

Prescott: The correlation may be good in a group of 100 patients, but doctors have to make the right decision for individual patients. If you rely solely on the level, you may not be doing the best thing for that patient. You cannot ignore biological variation and the effects of disease on the response to drugs.

Parker: There are exceptions to almost every rule, such as the patient with rapid auricular flutter and incipient shock to whom further digitalis might justifiably be given despite an already elevated digitalis level.

Curry: There is a chemical correlation, but the clinician still keeps his freedom.

Goulding: The situation can be even worse than Dr Prescott implies. There are too many people giving 'the dose' of the drug and not looking at the patient either. It is time that some clinicians learned that there isn't 'a dose' of a drug but only a dose of a drug for that particular patient in that condition.

Beckett: A correct figure, correctly used, would be valuable. What would scare me would be incorrect figures being used in a manner which you indicate is a danger. With some of these assays that could well be the case. Also, one may determine the level of amphetamine correctly, but if the patient has taken ephedrine and norephedrine the figures for observed levels of amphetamines are useless for decision making.

Sunshine: In a controlled study where we know that hyperkinetic children are being treated only with amphetamine, the information may have some value.

Curry: That is an ideal situation, because you said you wanted to measure the children who are *not* taking the drug, and there the information would have a negative value.

Prescott: What is the evidence that any level is the 'correct' level? You must make objective clinical measurements of drug effects which can be correlated with laboratory results, and the clinical measurement is a very weak link. It may be all right for digoxin, where you can see an arrhythmia on the ECG, but what do you do about hyperkinetic children? In real life on hospital wards where doctors are working with acutely ill patients, some of whom are receiving 10 drugs simultaneously, things are not straightforward.

Scott: As a physical chemist, I find this an extraordinary discussion. The more information one can get on a problem, the better. One has to make one's own judgement. One may reject results from some assays that are known to have errors of $\pm$ 50%, but one does not reject results on the basis that one is not too sure one can use them properly. It is our job to find out if we can use them properly. We must use all the data we can get to solve any problems.

Parker: The first digitalis assay was described in 1968 and the first assay for morphine in 1970. These assays have only been around for a short time and their usefulness is still being evaluated.

Prescott: I am not saying they are not useful. But unless doctors are taught a lot more about drugs they will not be able to make proper use of the data.

Newton: It is helpful to have as much information as possible but one must consider what resources are available. In the National Health Service in Great Britain, where these facilities are not available, is it really important to push for them at the expense of some other facility?

Parker: Aren't we talking now about setting up newly developed immunoassays at a few major medical centres, where they will be done and interpreted properly as a first-level evaluation, and then we can see how and when they can be used and whether the information that comes out is useful? I agree that the extension of these assays to small laboratories may be premature and, if it occurs, careful attention to cost-effectiveness and quality control will be needed. But if we are ever going to find out what is useful and what is not, trained clinical investigators have to do this type of analysis and see what the correlations are. As far as physician education is concerned this is a major and continuing problem in the United States as well as in the United Kingdom, but I don't think we are any closer to solving it than we were 10 years ago. There is a great deal that a responsible practising physician needs to know but up to now the renewal and updating of medical knowledge has been largely a matter of individual effort, often less well sustained as one gets older.

Drug analysis in the overdosed patient

B. WIDDOP

Poisons Unit, Guy's Hospital, London

Abstract 'Drug overdosage' is coming to mean overdosage with several drugs rather than just one. Rapid and comprehensive screening procedures are therefore needed. At the Poisons Unit of Guy's Hospital a screening method based on colour tests, solvent extraction and thin-layer chromatography is used for samples of urine or gastric juices, and a wide range of drugs can be detected. Where appropriate, drug concentrations in blood are also measured. Cases of drug overdosage are described where treatment would have been discontinued prematurely if analyses had not been performed.

An efficient and useful toxicological service must be organized in such a way that a close working relationship is possible between the clinician in charge of the patient and the medical staff at the laboratory; the latter must filter all requests for help and discuss the results with the clinician.

The Hill Report (1968) predicted that the trend in drug overdosage would be towards multiple drug ingestion and away from the familiar pattern of barbiturates or salicylates. This prompted the Poisons Unit of Guy's Hospital to develop and assess rapid, simple and economical procedures for the detection of a wide range of commonly prescribed drugs in urine samples from overdosed patients. The criteria of speed, simplicity and economy have been emphasized here since the object has been to fashion a system which would fall within the scope of the average chemical pathology laboratory.

THE SCREENING METHOD

The screening method we use (Berry & Grove 1973) is based on a combination of colour tests, solvent extraction and simple thin-layer chromatographic techniques. Urine (50 ml) is the sample of choice for toxicological screening, but in its absence gastric specimens can prove an adequate substitute.

Solvent extraction

Two screw-topped bottles (McCartney bottles, capacity 28 ml) are half-filled with urine (or gastric fluid), one is acidified with dilute sulphuric acid and the other made alkaline with dilute sodium hydroxide. Both are filled with chloroform, polypropylene lids are screwed on and the bottles are shaken for two or three minutes. After centrifugation the aqueous phases are aspirated and the chloroform extracts are poured through moisture-absorbent filter paper to dry them. These extracts are evaporated to dryness in narrow conical tubes under a stream of air or nitrogen and the residue is redissolved in chloroform (0.1 ml). Thus a rapid separation and purification of acidic drugs, e.g. the barbiturates, and basic drugs, e.g. the tricyclic antidepressants, is achieved. Neutral drugs such as methaqualone will be present in both extracts.

Thin-layer chromatography

The acidic fraction is chromatographed on silica-gel plates in chloroform–acetone (9:1 v/v) and the basic fraction in methanol–12M-ammonium hydroxide (100:1.5). Since R_f values are not accurately reproducible under routine conditions, authentic samples of drugs are chromatographed alongside the extracts. Fig. 1 shows the most usual lay-out of the acidic and basic plates. Sample extracts are interspersed with pure specimens of representatives of the barbiturate, tricyclic antidepressant and carbamate drug groups. Methaqualone can be detected on both plates and since this is prescribed in the main in combination

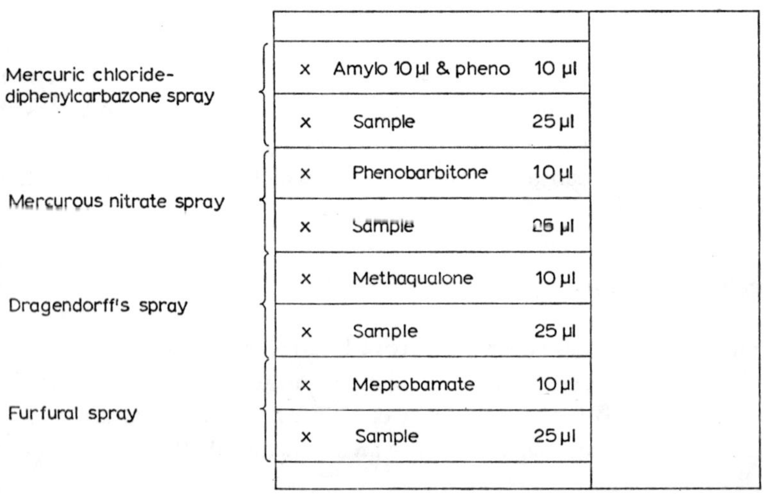

FIG. 1*a*

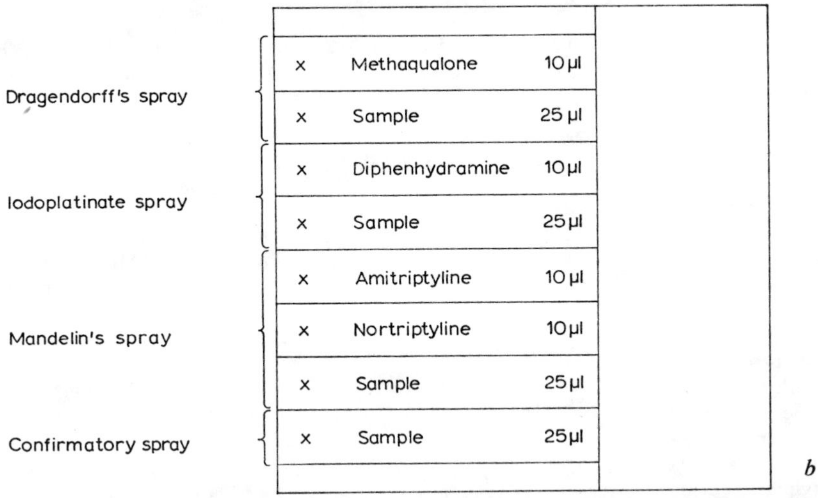

FIG. 1. The arrangement of the spots on a thin-layer chromatography (TLC) plate for (*a*) the acidic extract and (*b*) the alkaline extract. (Reproduced, with permission, from Berry & Grove 1973.)

TABLE 1

Colour reactions and R_f values of some acidic and neutral drugs in chloroform-acetone (9:1 v/v) (reproduced, with permission, from Berry & Grove 1973)

Drug	R_f *value**	*Mercuric chloride-diphenylcarbazone*	*Mercurous nitrate*	*Remarks*
Meprobamate	0.3	—	—	Lilac with furfural
Primidone	0.3	+	+	
Phenytoin	0.8	+	+	
Phenobarbitone	1.0	+	+	
Barbitone	1.0	+	+	
Cyclobarbitone	1.2	+	+	
Butobarbitone	1.3	+	+	
Heptabarbitone (heptabarb)	1.3	+	+	
Pentobarbitone	1.3	+	+	
Amylobarbitone	1.4	+	+	
Quinalbarbitone (secobarbital)	1.5	+	+	
Glutethimide	1.6	+	+	Weak reaction with Dragendorff's reagent
Methaqualone	1.6	—	—	Positive reaction with Dragendorff's reagent. Metabolites also react

* Relative to phenobarbitone

TABLE 2

Colour reactions and R_f values of some basic drugs in methanol–12M-ammonia (100:1.5 v/v) (reproduced, with permission from Berry & Grove 1973)

Drug	R_f *value**	*Dragendorff's reagent*	*Iodoplatinate reagent*	*Mandelin's reagent*	
				Daylight examination	*UV$_{254}$ examination*
Desipramine	0.43	+	+	Deep blue	—
Nortriptyline	0.57	+	+	Pale mauve	Mauve centre, yellow rim
Codeine	0.71	+	+	—	—
Morphine	0.71	+	+	—	—
N-Demethyl-orphenadrine	0.72	+	+	Pale yellow	Pale blue
Imipramine	0.86	+	+	Deep blue	—
Chlorpromazine	0.93	+	+	Red	—
Thioridazine	0.93	+	+	Blue	—
Amitriptyline	1.0	+	+	Pale mauve	Mauve centre, yellow rim
Diphenhydramine	1.0	+	+	Pale yellow	Pale yellow
Orphenadrine	1.07	+	+	Pale yellow	Pale blue
Quinine	1.14	+	+	—	Intense blue
Methaqualone	1.57	+	—	—	—

* Relative to amitriptyline.

with diphenhydramine (as Mandrax), the latter is included on the basic plate. If there is strong circumstantial evidence that a specific drug has been taken, an authentic sample of this is included in the system.

When sequential spraying is done as indicated in Fig. 1 there is a strong possibility that the unknown drug may be characterized, if not positively identified, on the basis of its colour reactions and reference to relative R_f values (Tables 1, 2).

In addition, certain drugs yield recognizable patterns of metabolites when urine extracts are chromatographed in this way, thus enabling a surer identification to be made. The benzodiazepine drugs are so extensively metabolized that the small amount of unchanged drug in the urine defies detection by conventional basic sprays such as the iodoplatinate and Dragendorff reagents. To overcome this, a third sample (10 ml) of urine is hydrolysed with 3 ml of concentrated hydrochloric acid, again in a screw-topped bottle which is placed in boiling water for 10–15 minutes. This converts the benzodiazepine drugs and their metabolites into the corresponding aminobenzophenones (primary amines) which are then extractable into light petroleum (b.p. 60–80 °C). After chromatography in toluene-glacial acetic acid (97:3), the aminobenzophenones are coupled with *N*-(1-naphthyl)ethylenediamine to form a purple azo dye (Bratton & Marshall 1939).

During the stages of extract evaporation and chromatogram development, the operator has time to perform simple direct colour tests on the remaining urine for salicylates, trichloro compounds, paracetamol and ethchlorvynol. By these inexpensive means, most of the drugs commonly encountered in overdosage can be detected or eliminated within two to three hours. Blood samples are spared from preliminary screening analysis since the need may arise to measure the concentration of drug(s) in this specimen. To this end, method evaluation and development has been applied over the past seven years and Table 3 lists the drugs which can be measured in the Poisons Unit, alongside the analytical techniques adopted.

TABLE 3

Drugs measured in biological fluids by the Poisons Unit and the analytical techniques used

Paracetamol	Colorimetry; Ultraviolet spectrophotometry
Salicylates	Colorimetry; Ultraviolet spectrophotometry
Nitrazepam	Colorimetry; Ultraviolet spectrophotometry
Imipramine	Spectrophotofluorometry
LSD (lysergide)	Spectrophotofluorometry
Chlordiazepoxide	Polarography
Diazepam	Polarography
Digoxin	Radioimmunoassay
Alcohol	Gas-liquid chromatography
Amitriptyline	Gas-liquid chromatography
Amphetamines	Gas-liquid chromatography
Barbiturates	Gas-liquid chromatography
Chloral (as trichloroethanol)	Gas-liquid chromatography
Fenfluramine	Gas-liquid chromatography
Glutethimide	Gas-liquid chromatography
Meprobamate	Gas-liquid chromatography
Methadone	Gas-liquid chromatography
Methaqualone	Gas-liquid chromatography
Methylamphetamine	Gas-liquid chromatography
Nortriptyline	Gas-liquid chromatography
Orphenadrine	Gas-liquid chromatography
Pethidine	Gas-liquid chromatography
Phenytoin	Gas-liquid chromatography
Primidone	Gas-liquid chromatography
Propoxyphene	Gas-liquid chromatography

ANALYSIS OF FINDINGS

Table 4 gives a breakdown in the data derived from urine analyses carried out

TABLE 4

The incidence of multiple drug detection in urine samples from suspected overdose patients analysed by the Poisons Unit in 1972

Total no. of urines analysed	=	268
No drug detected	=	37
Unidentified drug detected	=	24

No. of drugs detected	*No. of samples*
1	87
2	82
3	29
> 3	33

TABLE 5

The incidence of drugs and drug groups in urine samples from overdosed patients analysed by the Poisons Unit in 1972

Barbiturates	85	Methaqualone	17
Benzodiazepines	76	Paracetamol	16
Tricyclic antidepressants	65	Chloral hydrate	15
Phenothiazines	31	Glutethimide	9
Salicylates	19	Miscellaneous	49

in the Poisons Unit of 1972 using the procedure described above. In each case the analyses were performed at the urgent request of clinicians working in various hospitals in the south-east of England and further afield. In over 60% of these samples more than one drug was encountered. Table 5 depicts the incidence with which specific drug and drug groups were found. Two points to note here are the prominent position of benzodiazepines and tricyclic anti-depressants in the league table, and the surprisingly low figure for salicylates. This latter finding is probably explained by the fact that most hospital laboratories are capable of detecting salicylates in urine and furnishing a rapid measurement of its plasma level. Consequently, the vast majority of these incidents are not referred to the specialized unit. It might be argued that by the same token the barbiturate figure is also artificially low. This is debatable, for in our experience many hospital laboratories are unwilling or even unable to perform barbiturate analyses, because of staff shortage and lack of familiarity with the technique.

With this alarming incidence of multiple drug overdosage, the odds are heavily weighted against the clinician pin-pointing the exact combination of drugs ingested. Information derived from bottle labels and anxious relatives is notoriously unreliable. To substantiate this claim, Table 6 compares the prediction of clinicians with the eventual analytical findings in urine samples sub-

TABLE 6

Comparison of clinical predictions with analytical findings in urine samples from suspected overdose patients (October – December, 1973)

	Cases	*Percentage*
Prediction correct	24	22
Prediction partially correct (other drugs present)	39	36
Prediction incorrect (wrong drug suspected)	13	12
No prediction (drugs found)	15	14
No drugs detected	18	16

mitted to the unit over a period of three months. In only 24 of the referred cases were the evidence of the doctor and the analyses in complete agreement. Most predictions were partially correct in that at least one named drug was shown to be present. Incorrect predictions ranged from a request for barbiturate analysis in which methaqualone was the causative agent to a case where glutethimide was strongly suspected and the sample was shown to contain barbiturates, phenothiazines, orphenadrine, nitrazepam (Mogadon) and two other compounds which were not identified. It would be impertinent to assume that, in each of the 18 cases where no drugs were revealed, the doctor's diagnosis was in error, and this provides a continuing impetus to broaden our detection range in both selectivity and sensitivity.

To summarize, the Poisons Unit is capable of detecting, and sometimes positively identifying, a host of drugs in urine within two to three hours of samples reaching the laboratory. In addition, techniques are available which can measure with considerable accuracy the concentrations of many of these drugs in the blood. The crucial question in the context of the present meeting, however, is: what benefit is this service to the overdosed patient? Critics of the laboratory's role will argue, with some justification, that an experienced clinician can pilot a patient through an overdose syndrome in complete ignorance of which drugs are present. This argument is weakened when the many published accounts of adverse reactions are consulted (Palmer 1971; Prescott 1973), and it completely ignores the truism that to be forewarned is to be forearmed. To cite an example, the tricyclic antidepressants have anticholinergic properties which delay the absorption of drugs by decreasing intestinal mobility (Goodman & Gilman 1970). Patient S.S. (see Fig. 2) was admitted to hospital about 12 h after ingesting amitriptyline and amylobarbitone (amobarbital) and at this time the concentrations in plasma were 250 ng/ml and 18 μg/ml, respectively. Fourteen hours later these levels had almost doubled (amitriptyline, 375 ng/ml and amylobarbitone, 31 μg/ml). Six hours later, the patient died in cardiac arrest, 32 h after taking the drugs. In a second case (J. W., Fig. 3) the patient presented with an amitriptyline plasma level of 175 ng/ml and a pentobarbitone (pentobarbital) level of 16 μg/ml, the drugs having been taken at least 20 h before admission. Because of the experience with patient S.S., the clinicians were alerted to the possibility of delayed absorption and consequent deterioration in the condition of the patient.

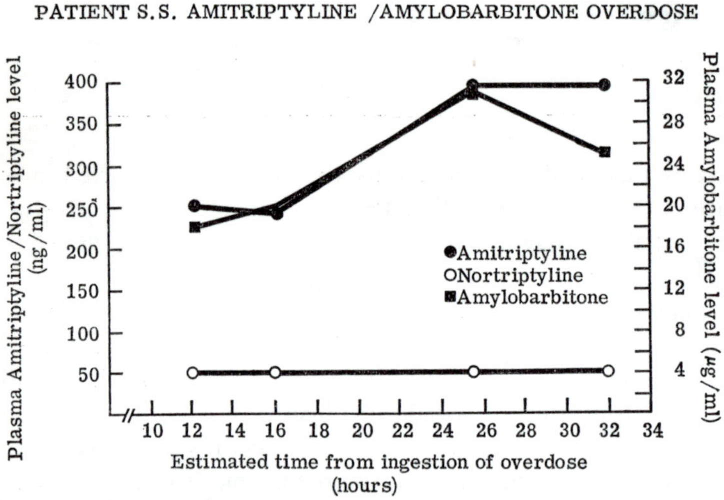

Fig. 2. Plasma drug-level profile of a patient (S.S.) who ingested amitriptyline and amylobarbitone (amobarbital).

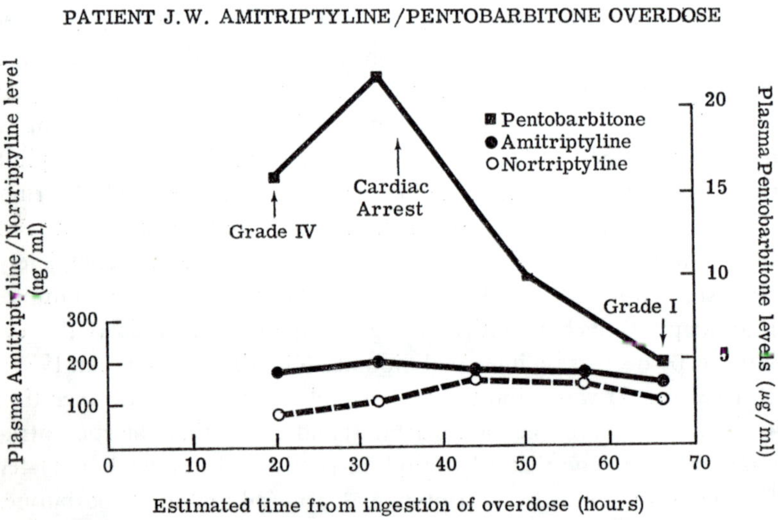

Fig. 3. Plasma drug-level profile of a patient (J.W.) who ingested amitriptyline and pentobarbitone (pentobarbital).

Measurements 10 h later in fact showed that the amitriptyline plasma level had risen to 200 ng/ml and the pentobarbitone plasma level to 24 μg/ml. Shortly afterwards, cardiac arrhythmias appeared and a subsequent cardiac arrest was successfully reversed. The patient recovered consciousness 60 h after overdosage without further complications.

Influence of laboratory analyses on treatment

It has been frequently stated (Goulding 1971; Matthew 1971) that active elimination procedures such as forced diuresis, peritoneal dialysis and haemodialysis are only effective for poisoning by salicylates, long-acting barbiturates such as phenobarbitone (phenobarbital), alcohol, bromides and amphetamines. These contentions are firmly established on analytical data, however, and not on clinical judgement alone. Other workers have produced evidence to the contrary (e.g. Linton *et al.* 1967), but a closer inspection of the analytical techniques used often reveals great inadequacies in accuracy and specificity. Nevertheless, forced diuresis in particular is still widely applied in treatment, even though the pharmacokinetic characteristics of the drugs taken are opposed to removal by this means. The futility of this is readily shown up by careful analytical work as in the following example. Patient P.B. swallowed at least 30 tablets of ami-

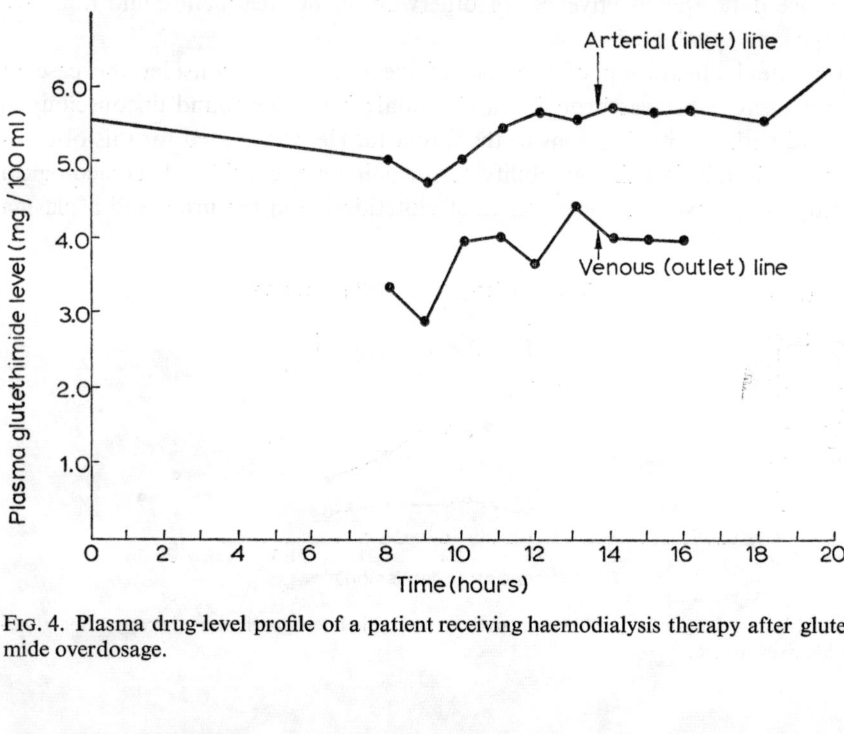

FIG. 4. Plasma drug-level profile of a patient receiving haemodialysis therapy after glutethimide overdosage.

triptyline (750 mg) and five hours later a diuresis was induced and maintained for nine hours. The urine collection (10 l) was subsequently analysed for amitriptyline and its active demethylated metabolite, nortriptyline, by a specific gas–liquid chromatographic method (Braithwaite & Widdop 1971). The total amitriptyline content was 14.3 mg and that of nortriptyline, 11.8 mg. Thus, forced diuresis had removed the equivalent of one amitriptyline tablet, or 3% of the ingested dose.

This means of evaluation can also be applied to haemodialysis, as it was for patient B.H. (Fig. 4) who took a large though unknown quantity of glutethimide and diazepam (Valium). She received intermittent haemodialysis for three days and the figure depicts analytical data derived during the first dialysis period of 10 h. Blood samples were withdrawn simultaneously from the arterial (inlet) lines of the dialysis membrane and the venous (outlet) lines and analysed for glutethimide and diazepam content, again by specific techniques. Calculation gave an average glutethimide clearance of 75 ml/min and the diazepam clearance was nil. The merits of haemodialysis in this case will be discussed elsewhere (A. J. Rees & B. Widdop, unpublished) but it is pertinent to say that in the absence of plasma glutethimide analyses, treatment would have been discontinued prematurely. Furthermore, had laboratory invigilation rested simply on measurement of the circulating plasma levels alone, and not on clearance data, the effectiveness or otherwise of the treatment could not have been properly evaluated.

As a final illustration of the role of the laboratory, consider the case of patient D. K. who was brought into hospital after being found unconscious in the road with severe abrasions to the forehead. He was treated for this obvious injury for 16 h before the possibility of poisoning was considered. Toxicological investigations revealed the presence of glutethimide in the urine and a plasma

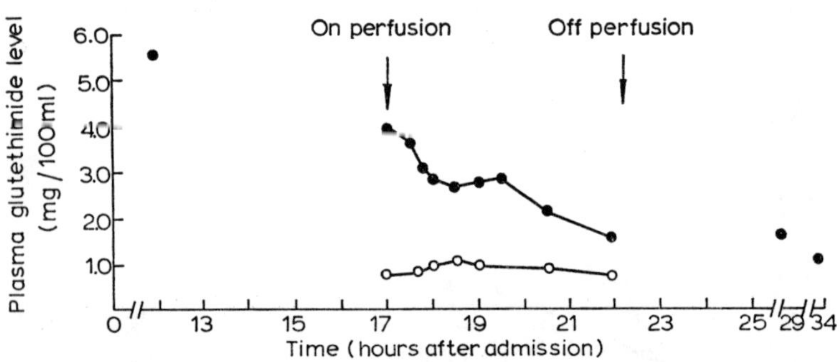

FIG. 5. Plasma drug-level profile of a patient receiving haemoperfusion therapy after glutethimide overdosage.

level for this drug of 55 μg/ml. The patient was successfully treated by a charcoal haemoperfusion technique and again the efficacy of the treatment was monitored and assessed by arterial (inlet) and venous (outlet) clearance measurements (Fig. 5).

CONCLUSIONS

It is imperative to underline the basic essentials in organizing an efficient and rewarding toxicological service. First, the service must be protected from abuse by those clinicians who regard all laboratories as impersonal machines into which samples may be dropped for processing and analysis in conveyor-belt fashion and who therefore feel no obligation to assess either the urgency or the necessity of their demands. This protection can be achieved by providing a medical filter (the chemical pathologist, laboratory director or their appointed deputies) between the laboratory staff and the doctor who requests assistance. By mutual discussion between these medical counterparts, most requests may be either forestalled and dealt with at leisure or dispensed with altogether, only those which warrant a concentrated and sustained analytical effort being allowed through the net. This clinical liaison serves a second purpose in that the doctor can be informed verbally of the type and volume of sample required and can be reminded to label each sample clearly with the patient's full name and the date and time of collection. Last, but not least, the doctor can be prevailed upon to see that the samples are correctly addressed and delivered with due haste to the laboratory. When the analyses have been completed the director or his deputy should convey the results to the physician in charge of the patient, discuss the significance of the findings and decide on the need or otherwise for further laboratory aid. Without this close working relationship on the clinical side, the toxicological service becomes futile and inoperable.

References

BERRY, D. J. & GROVE, J. (1973) Emergency toxicological screening for drugs commonly taken in overdose. *J. Chromatogr. 80*, 205

BRAITHWAITE, R. & WIDDOP, B. (1971) A specific gas-chromatographic method for the measurement of 'steady-state' plasma levels of amitriptyline and nortriptyline in patients. *Clin. Chim. Acta 35*, 461

BRATTON, A. C. & MARSHALL, E. K. (1939) A new coupling component for sulphanilamide determination. *J. Biol. Chem. 128*, 537

GOODMAN, L. S. & GILMAN, A. (1970) *The Pharmacological Basis of Therapeutics*, 4th edn., Macmillan, London

GOULDING, R. (1971) Self-poisoning. *Br. J. Hosp. Med. 5*, 249

HILL REPORT (1968) *Hospital Treatment of Acute Poisoning*, Report of the Joint Sub-Com-

mittee of the Standing Medical Advisory Committees of the Central Health Services Council, H.M. Stationery Office, London
LINTON, A. L., LUKE, R. G. & BRIGGS, J. D. (1967) Methods of forced diuresis and its application in barbiturate poisoning. *Lancet 2*, 377
MATTHEW, H. (1971) Acute poisoning: some myths and misconceptions. *Br. Med. J. 1*, 519
PALMER, R. F. (1971) Drug interactions. *Med. Clin. North Am. 55*, 495
PRESCOTT, L. F. (1973) Clinically important drug interactions. *Drugs 5*, 161

Discussion

Sunshine: What was the incidence of ethanol in your series, Dr Widdop? We always test for ethanol, because clinicians often say they smelt alcohol on the patient's breath.

Widdop: Smelling the patient's breath for alcohol would seem the obvious way of detecting it. We measure the blood level only if asked to do so.

Sunshine: But 20 mg/100 ml can give the same odour as 240 mg/100 ml.

Goulding: For a time we screened all our overdose cases and less than 10% were positive for alcohol.

Patel: At the Glasgow Western Infirmary we have some accurate figures both for the type of drugs used and the alcohol levels. Table 1 (Patel) shows the various drugs used. In 1971 520 patients admitted had taken 645 drugs: 76% had taken only one drug, 16% two drugs, 4% three drugs and 4% more than four. In 1973 the figures changed a little but not much. Overdose with multiple drugs does not seem to be as common as it seems to be in London (Dr Widdop's figures).

TABLE 1 (Patel)

Drugs used for self-poisoning by patients admitted to Glasgow Western Infirmary in 1971 and 1973.

Total no. of admissions	520	706
Total no. of drugs	645	851
Hypnotics	%	%
Barbiturates	21	15
Methaqualone	11	6
Others	7	9
Benzodiazepines	16	20
Phenothiazines	4	5
Antidepressants	11	12
Salicylates	13	9
Paracetamol	3	4
Other specified drugs	14	17
Drugs, unspecified	0	3

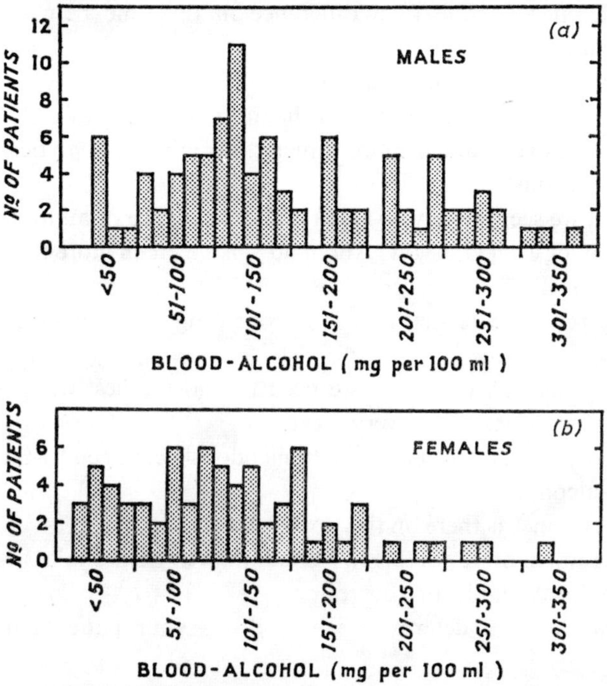

FIG. 1*a*, *b* (Patel). Association of alcohol intake with self-poisoning in 520 patients admitted to Glasgow Western Infirmary in 1971.

Amongst the 207 male patients admitted in 1971 heavy drinking preceded an overdose of drugs in about 70% of cases, and in them the mean blood-alcohol concentration on admission to hospital was 146 mg/100 ml (Fig. 1*a*). Of the 313 women about 40% had taken alcohol before the overdose, and their mean blood concentration was 102 mg/100 ml (Fig. 1*b*) (Patel *et al.* 1972). I agree with Dr Widdop that there is a clear opportunity for clinical pharmacologists to study the interaction of drugs with alcohol, but whether this helps the clinician to treat the patient, I don't know.

Widdop: I agree that this is an untapped field for the clinical pharmacologists. Most investigations into drug interactions have been carried out after therapeutic dosage, not after overdosage where the situation may not be entirely analogous.

Prescott: In Edinburgh we have much the same experience as Dr Patel in Glasgow. The selection of patients may partly explain the differences in alcohol consumption with self-poisoning between London and Scotland. The samples sent to Dr Goulding's laboratory may come from a much more restricted population, whereas we admit all patients who have taken an overdose.

Curry: Could the difference be due to a difference in the time between ingestion and taking the sample?

Goulding: Our samples might be taken a little later.

Curry: The clinician therefore has to make his diagnosis in terms of poly-pharmacology and it becomes very much more difficult. Aren't the analytical figures helpful in these conditions?

Prescott: I think so, but we seem to have a much higher incidence of multiple overdosage than in London or even Glasgow. About 40% have taken more than one drug, not counting alcohol.

Widdop: Our 1972 figures indicate that more than one drug had been taken in over 50% of the cases.

Beckett: With such high figures, obviously we need to find the best way to treat these patients. The interactions will be very great.

Curry: The rate of absorption of drugs must be tremendously changed by the simultaneous presence of alcohol.

Prescott: Why? What evidence is there on this point?

Curry: Many drugs are much more soluble in alcohol than in gastric juices—*a priori* they are more rapidly available for absorption.

Brown: Dr Patel, how did you determine which drugs your patients in Glasgow had taken?

Patel: When the patients were admitted we took accurate details about the drugs, from either the patients or relatives and friends. When there were doubts we sought the help of the chemist or the general practitioner, and even searched the homes of patients.

Brown: Laboratory investigations provide *objective* data on what patients have taken, but note that Dr Widdop was unable to identify 24 drugs out of a total of 268.

Prescott: Some patients state that they have not taken a particular drug yet it is identified in the plasma, and *vice versa.*

Newton: Where does the urine come from for all these tests? Patients who are severely poisoned and unconscious don't pass urine for a period of time. Those poisoned with tricyclic antidepressants retain urine because of the anti-cholinergic activity of these drugs. Catheters introduce infection and in Edinburgh we don't routinely use them. Is this practice routine in London?

Goulding: The patients are not all ours, but most of them are catheterized now. An odd spot that we often saw on the TLC plates turned out to be due to lignocaine (lidocaine) from the catheter lubricant.

Curry: If we want to correlate figures, we shall have to take into account different practices between different areas and laboratories.

Leach: The earliest and quickest sample to get is blood. It is often up to eight hours before we receive a urine sample although we ask for this in addition to blood and gastric contents. If any drug remains in the stomach contents it is easily identified.

In North Wales about 60–70% of poisoned patients have taken alcohol and we often find surprisingly high levels. An advantage of screening for alcohol is that, using gas chromatography, one occasionally picks up things like keto-acidosis quite easily. We also detect methanol, which otherwise would go unrecognized. Methanol is sometimes found when ordinary alcoholic drinks are not available and methanol, in the form of methylated spirits, is drunk with suicidal intent.

Sunshine: Were the drugs that you listed all confirmed in the laboratory, Dr Patel?

Patel: No.

Curry: It is difficult to compare figures when there are so many variables—regional distribution, effect of other drugs, alcohol, and different diagnostic criteria.

Sunshine: Often, because of the physical evidence, the clinician alleges that his patient has taken a particular drug, yet in many instances some other drug has been taken. It may be a similar chemical agent but they are seldom identical. Spare me hearsay evidence.

Goulding: That is why we won't accept requests to look for a particular drug; if we find that it isn't there we then have to proceed to a full screening.

Curry: It is a toxicological cliché that the drugs by the side of the bed are the ones the patient has *not* taken.

Scott: Before you dismiss the findings of Dr Patel, you must remember he has an awful lot of data. Therefore statistically he can be wrong quite a lot of times and right quite a lot of times.

Patel: In Glasgow we do not have difficulty in tracing the drugs involved; often the patients or relatives bring containers or unused pills. The Hill Report (1968) advised the Ambulance Services to ensure that any drug or poison containers, unused tablets, capsules etc., are also brought to the hospital; and in Glasgow they seem to do this.

Curry: Let us now ask why the chemists are doing the analyses. There is a clinical research area involving the laboratory; for example, people want to find out whether there is an increased rate of absorption and whether dialysis is effective. But why are we doing analyses for emergencies, where research doesn't matter very much until we can interpret the figures?

Beckett: Surely research on drug absorption or interactions wouldn't start with analyses from clinical practice, so maybe the research component is not very great.

Prescott: There is research and research: this is operational research, as distinct from intensive investigation of one drug or of one particular clinical problem.

Curry: Are we doing this solely for research, or do the clinicians feel it is of any value at all in treating the patient?

Goulding: Are we asking about qualitative detection?

Newton: At 3 a.m., we don't need help from the analysts.

Goulding: I don't agree. When we found a tricyclic antidepressant in a child with an arrhythmia and showing no other signs of drug overdose—as we did the other day—all the necessary help was mustered to look after that patient. It wasn't a serious arrhythmia at that early stage, but it became one shortly afterwards. One might say that the cardiologists could well look after an arrhythmia, but they took it a lot more seriously and in a rather different way when they knew it was due to the drug.

Curry: Some of these children are deliberately poisoned and the circumstances are covered up. In qualitative analysis as an emergency, special cases clearly exist.

Goulding: They are very special—we don't do every one. Dr Widdop told us about the patient found with head injuries who was taken into a surgical ward and was then found to have taken an enormous amount of a drug.

Curry: Dr Newton, would you accept that there are certain occasions when drug analysis at 3 a.m. may be useful?

Newton: I don't think we can be completely inflexible. We are not being critical of the laboratory in any way, but we have to take each case as it comes and for most cases we would not need emergency drug levels.

Goulding: I agree that most cases don't, but some do.

Bridges: In what percentage of cases was clinical treatment affected by identification of the drug?

Goulding: We don't know; we haven't always followed up what the clinicians did.

Newton: In Edinburgh clinical treatment is affected in less than 5% of cases.

Curry: Is the clinical situation the same in the United States?

Sunshine: Very few clinicians in the US have studied the care of the poisoned patient intensively. In most practices poisoned patients are rarely seen; when they appear, the clinician is looking for as much laboratory support as he can get. He may be asking the laboratory to hold his hand but he is looking for help in the treatment of his patients and we offer it to him when he asks for it. Like Dr Widdop we ask the clinician how urgent the case is. When he says a patient is comatose and he is not certain about the cause or whether it is drug-induced, we do the analysis very promptly.

Prescott: Laboratories should not be doing this work merely to reassure ignorant clinicians. This is absurd and quite unacceptable. Clinicians should be better educated about drugs. Students should be taught clinical toxicology in medical school. Their seniors should know something about the subject. But how much time is spent in teaching anything about drug overdosage, drug toxicity and pharmacokinetics in the average medical school? The answer is little or none. Other causes of coma are dealt with in detail but not drug overdosage. If doctors were adequately informed the laboratory could contribute usefully to patient care and the advancement of knowledge instead of reassuring doctors so that they can get a good night's sleep.

Curry: The question of whether laboratories are treating the patient or the clinician is one we will discuss again later. Now let us ask whether qualitative or quantitative tests are more necessary on these rare occasions. It seems to me that finding therapeutic levels by qualitative tests could mislead instead of help.

Dole: A striking qualitative difference between poisonings in London and New York is that here in London you hardly have any cases of heroin poisoning, while in New York an overdose usually means an overdose of heroin.

Machata: In Vienna we find barbiturates in 30% of autopsies and clinical cases, but in one lethal case we had to analyse for heroin.

Sunshine: What Dr Dole said is peculiar to New York City. Each region has its own drugs to which people are addicted. Cleveland, Ohio, has a population of two million, and we seldom see heroin overdosage as an acute problem in the emergency room or as a hospital admission. The cases we see are usually incidental to a homicide and are seldom a diagnostic problem in a hospital admission.

Bridges: I want to return to my question about how many times clinicians act on the results of an analysis. If there is a limited list of drugs for which such action can be taken, could we markedly restrict the analyses that need to be performed at 3 a.m.?

Curry: And do clinicians such as Dr Prescott and Dr Newton want a qualitative answer, a semiquantitative answer, or an answer accurate to 1%?

Prescott: There are perhaps half-a-dozen compounds which we really want to exclude or to know whether they are present in amounts corresponding to the clinical state of the patient.

Curry: Are barbiturates among those half dozen?

Prescott: It depends which barbiturates you mean. Forced diuresis may be indicated for phenobarbitone or barbitone intoxication but it is useless with short- or medium-acting barbiturates.

Sunshine: You must have both qualitative and quantitative data in that situation.

Prescott: There is usually no need for emergency estimations of short or medium-acting barbiturates unless a patient has taken them together with phenobarbitone, which is unusual.

The compounds we really want to know about are phenobarbitone, barbitone, salicylate, paracetamol, iron, lithium and perhaps meprobamate and ethchlorvynol. It is also sometimes helpful to know the carboxyhaemoglobin concentration in patients with carbon monoxide poisoning who may also have taken drugs.

Brown: Can we distinguish clearly whether you need *qualitative* or quantitative assays on urine or blood?

Prescott: Assays on urine are of no value in an acute situation and may be grossly misleading. The only exception is in poisoning with Paraquat. Assays may be useful later to see what has actually been taken.

Bridges: Do you need both qualitative and quantitative information for this restricted list?

Newton: At 3 a.m., we don't need to know a phenobarbitone level, or even whether phenobarbitone is the drug involved.

Patel: But you would want to know about a tricyclic antidepressant?

Newton: One would know that from clinical examination.

Goulding: The typical clinical picture with tricyclic antidepressants is not universal, especially if other drugs are present. I cannot share your confidence that when you see it you know it, Dr Newton.

Prescott: A diagnosis can usually be made with confidence on clinical examination if you know what to look for.

Curry: Can the laboratory provide any other information of use to the clinician in the therapeutic monitoring of drugs such as digitalis, anti-epileptic drugs and so on? Too small a dose may also poison the patient.

Prescott: Tricyclic antidepressants are ineffective if plasma concentrations are too low or too high, and high levels are associated with toxicity. I have been campaigning (unsuccessfully) for some time for routine monitoring of plasma concentrations of anti-arrhythmic drugs. Coronary care units are equipped with all sorts of expensive devices and ECG monitors, and intensive-care ambulances rush around the city with bells clanging. Patients with arrhythmias are given standard doses of lignocaine, and both therapeutic failure and toxicity are common. We know that patients with cardiac failure have an abnormally small volume of distribution and a decreased rate of lignocaine clearance, and therefore require much smaller maintenance doses by infusion. Patients may either be poisoned by the drug, or under certain conditions during the first few hours of infusion the concentrations may be sub-therapeutic. Clinicians look at their expensive ECG monitors and wonder why the arrhythmia has not been controlled. The answer may be that they have given an insufficient amount in the wrong way. It is also important to recognize that arrhythmias can be *caused* by too much anti-arrhythmic drug. The results of lithium therapy are also improved if concentrations are monitored regularly; the same applies to anticonvulsant therapy.

Gee: When we do a post-mortem on a known epileptic, we nearly always have an analysis done. Surprisingly often there is no trace of anti-epileptic drugs in the body.

Goulding: I am shattered to read papers in which the authors claim to do superb monitoring for anti-epileptic drugs, but in fact they measure only two drugs when the regimen includes three others. There seems to be no point in doing that.

Prescott: This goes back to the point I made earlier, that clinicians are not trained to interpret these results or to take account of the other relevant factors. The students in our medical school receive no formal instruction in pharmacokinetics or toxicology.

There are many other important factors to be considered. Patients who are seriously ill often have several drugs poured into them at the conventional rates yet their response to drugs may be exaggerated or they may not be able to eliminate the drug. They are at particular risk. Some patients with advanced liver disease may be almost completely unable to metabolize many drugs. And patients with renal disease may not be able to eliminate other drugs normally. The doses then have to be modified, and the only safe approach is to monitor plasma concentrations.

Curry: What value is normal clinical chemistry in assessing the poisoned patient? Serum enzyme values come in with paracetamol, for example.

Brown: I feel strongly that at 3 a.m. the clinical chemist can be doing more important things than Dr Widdop told us about. For the seriously poisoned patient (and the clinician of course must judge this), bread-and-butter clinical biochemistry, e.g. blood gases or plasma electrolytes, is likely to be more vital.

Goulding: This means a full 24-hour service. How many hospitals throughout the country have that? What are the clinical chemists doing about it?

Leach: Most hospitals provide this service. What worries me is that the chemist may get out of step with the clinician. Clinicians take blood and then commonly ask for sugar, urea and electrolyte levels. By the time these have been measured, the clinicians have poured several pints of fluid into the patient and the results are of little value. They themselves have changed the situation and the analysis is a pointless exercise.

Curry: What else besides electrolytes, acid-base balance and blood gases do clinicians need in treating a poisoned patient?

Leach: If you suspect liver damage, there is a good case for estimating liver enzymes such as γ-glutamyltranspeptidase and sorbitol dehydrogenase, which are sensitive and specific indicators of liver damage.

Prescott: One needs the same routine biochemical support as for any ill patient. The same things go wrong basically, and the same biochemical tests are required.

Curry: In a patient with a renal shut-down who is not metabolizing a drug, would any index other than blood warn you of this?

Prescott: We obviously watch the urine output. If this begins to fall off, we know that we had better start thinking about that problem.

Moffat: We haven't mentioned drugs like anticoagulants, which bring us to routine haematology. Patients on long-term anticoagulant therapy routinely have their prothrombin levels measured every six weeks or so, to make sure they are not being poisoned. There it is not the drug level that matters so much as what the drug is doing to the body, and it is the biochemistry that is being measured, obviously. Are there other examples of therapy being monitored by its biochemical effect?

Goulding: We are collecting information about this but it is too early to present our results. The value of monitoring plasma levels for patients on long-term therapy with various antidepressive drugs is well documented now (see, for example, Fry & Marks 1971; Braithwaite *et al.* 1972).

References

Braithwaite, R. A., Goulding, R., Theano, G., Bailey, J. & Coppen, A. (1972) Plasma concentration of amitriptyline and clinical response. *Lancet 1*, 1297–1300

Fry, D. E. & Marks, V. (1971) Value of plasma-lithium monitoring. *Lancet 1*, 886–888

Hill Report (1968) *Hospital Treatment of Acute Poisoning*, Report of the Sub-Committee of the Standing Medical Advisory Committee (Central Health Services Council, Scottish Health Services Council), Her Majesty's Stationery Office, London

Patel, A. R., Roy, M. & Wilson, G. M. (1972) Self poisoning and alcohol. *Lancet 2*, 1099

The morbid anatomist's role in drug detection

D. J. GEE

Department of Forensic Medicine, University of Leeds

Abstract In spite of the difficulties facing the morbid anatomist he has to try to select those cases in which death may be due to poison. The methods available to him are consideration of information from the police and relatives, examination of the scene of death, and the autopsy findings. The poison may produce characteristic external appearances of the body, or there may be distinctive internal findings, either to the naked eye or to the sense of smell. Microscopical examination may be too slow for detecting poisoning but may help in confirming a diagnosis.

Once poisoning is suspected, the pathologist has to select samples for analysis. Newer chemical techniques permit the use of new samples, but it is still uncertain to what extent the levels of poison found in tissues at autopsy truly reflect the distribution in the patient before death.

The pattern of poisoning is likely to change and simple chemical screening tests for new poisons, which can be used by the pathologist in the post-mortem room, will be needed. Histochemical techniques, especially of the macroscopic type, may hold promise for the detection of poisons.

I must make it clear at the outset that I have no new discoveries or particular techniques to proffer in the field of drug detection; indeed I am a man with problems rather than answers.

As a forensic pathologist, who as you know is a disreputable variety of morbid anatomist, my principal duty is to examine the bodies of persons who have either died suddenly, the cause of death being unknown, or who have died from obviously unnatural causes. Such persons die at home or in the street, and, unlike deaths in hospital, no one makes tests or keeps medical records during the hours or days before they die. In this respect I am usually at a great disadvantage compared to my colleague the hospital pathologist, who often possesses a lot of information when he makes an autopsy examination.

The forensic pathologist must depend on what information can be obtained for him by the Coroner's Officer, and what he can derive from his examination of the dead body. He has the added disadvantages, firstly of often being under pressure to reach a conclusion about the cause of death as quickly as possible, so that funeral arrangements will not be hindered; and secondly, of making his autopsy examinations predominantly on elderly persons, in whom degenerative changes have usually become sufficiently severe to be capable of causing death. Such readily available explanations for the deaths may give him a false sense of security in making the diagnoses, causing him to overlook the slender hints, in the autopsy findings, of the presence of poison (Gee & Dalley 1967).

Notwithstanding these difficulties, the principal role of the morbid anatomist in drug detection is to select, from the results of his autopsy examinations, those cases where death appears to have been, or could have been, from poisoning, and to ensure that the most suitable samples are passed to the analyst for further examination (Polson 1965). He has another role, which I regard as entirely separate, which is to investigate the actions of poisons by studying the morphological changes which they produce in the tissues of the organism. However, I shall not deal with this alternative function here.

Obviously, the principal method the morbid anatomist can use in detecting possible cases of poisoning is the autopsy examination; but before that, a consideration of what little history is available of the circumstances of the death or the past history of the deceased, or an examination of the scene of death, may alert him to such cases. In cases of deliberate self-poisoning, the history is often helpful. For instance, in a series of cases of barbiturate poisonings which we reported a year ago, out of 200 deaths 176 were clearly indicated as probable poisonings before the autopsy began, from a consideration of the history (Gee *et al.* 1974).

On the other hand, it is not uncommon for the history to be positively misleading. Thus on one occasion, an old man was described to me as having died sitting in an easy chair before the fire, while his son was in the room. The story sounded like a death from cerebral thrombosis. However, autopsy revealed that a large overdose of barbiturates had evidently been consumed surreptitiously by the old man while his son's attention was distracted.

And in accidental poisoning there is even more likelihood that the history may fail to suggest poisoning. In such circumstances a visit to the scene of death may be what alerts the pathologist. For instance, in cases of accidental carbon monoxide poisoning, the victim is sometimes found seated in front of a lit gas fire, having been dead for several days, and in an advanced state of decomposition. The appearance of the corpse and the fact that the fire is lit and burning normally is enough to persuade the lay observer that carbon monoxide may be discounted, yet the pathologist who has once met these circumstances will recognize the pattern. He will be able to detect pink discoloration somewhere on the body, and will realize that the flue, hidden behind the gas fire, has become blocked.

However, the pathologist is usually only called to the scene of death when, as in the type of case just described, a suspicion of 'foul' play arises. Otherwise the first time he sees the body is when it lies on the mortuary table. At this stage, for detecting poison, he depends on his eyes and nose. Whether he will become aware of the presence of poison depends on whether the poison produces any characteristic appearance of the body. If there are no such distinctive features, the autopsy may fail to reveal any explanation for the death and the pathologist will have to send samples away for analysis as part of a general search for the cause of death.

Some poisons, of course, are detectable even from examination of the exterior of the body. The pink post-mortem staining in carbon monoxide poisoning is well known, and the much less common but equally dramatic brown-grey hue of methaemoglobin—produced, for instance, by chlorate—is scarcely to be missed. On the rare occasions when corrosive poison has been ingested the burns are striking. Classically, in death after coma, as from barbiturate poisoning, blisters are to be found (Beveridge & Lawson 1965), though in my experience of people dying outside hospital, such blisters are rare.

The occasional drug addict, dying from overdose or infection, who has injected drugs intravenously should be unmistakable (Siegel *et al.* 1966), and of course once or twice in his lifetime the pathologist may see the skin pigmentation and hyperkeratosis of arsenical poisoning, or the dramatic hair loss caused by thallium.

When the pathologist examines the interior of the body the presence of poison may be obvious. Thus, signs of severe acute inflammation of the oesophagus and stomach suggest an irritant poison such as ammonia. Barbiturates may also produce irritation if present as sodium salts, and the strong dyes in the capsules will stain the mucosa. However, apart from barbiturates, most of the other commonly available and frequently consumed medicinal drugs produce less obvious signs. For instance, tricyclic antidepressant drugs will simply produce evidence of acute heart failure, which could be explained by any co-existent cardiac disease, although the intense pulmonary oedema and congestion can be highly suggestive. Mandrax (methaqualone plus diphenylhydramine), though it gives no distinctive colours, tends to produce pronounced haemorrhage in the tissues, especially of the lungs, and the stomach. I have seen a death certificate for one such case where an unwary doctor had made the diagnosis of haematemesis from a gastric ulcer.

If his eyes don't help the pathologist, then, if he is lucky, his nose may. A number of characteristic smells are associated with poisons such as cyanide, alcohol, halogenated hydrocarbons like carbon tetrachloride, and so on, as everyone knows; but not everyone can smell them. Indeed, although very sensitive, olfactory power is an unreliable tool: a cold or another strong body odour can mean that the pathologist fails to detect a fleeting smell, which may be the only indicator of the presence of a poison.

Then, of course, some drugs may produce obvious changes in organs, but only after an interval of several days. Thus paracetamol, if it does not cause rapid death, may produce liver necrosis which may prove fatal after several days (Davidson & Eastham 1966). In fact, hepatic damage must occur very rapidly: I have seen patches of focal necrosis scattered throughout a liver, even though the stomach still contained a white pasty mass of 36.7 g of paracetamol derived from Distalgesic (Dista Products).

In another case the dead man had been involved in a fight with a neighbour, about three weeks before death. He sustained minor though painful facial injuries, and he returned to hospital on a couple of occasions after the fight complaining of feeling unwell. The hospital could find nothing else wrong and analgesics were prescribed. Eventually he was found collapsed and he died soon after readmission to hospital, with bronchopneumonia. The police suspected manslaughter, but autopsy revealed jaundice due to gross liver necrosis. The possible connection between this and analgesics was suggested to the police, who visited the dead man's house and found the empty bottles which had contained the paracetamol prescribed by the hospital. Whether his death could be said to be indirectly the result of his injuries is an arguable point, but certainly the connection was not precise enough for a criminal charge to be made.

Apart from the gross autopsy, the morbid anatomist can also examine the tissues histologically. However, this usually takes much too long. By the time the slides are under the microscope important samples will probably have been destroyed or rendered useless for analysis. So this method is only of value when it can confirm a diagnosis which has already been made, or when, together with the gross autopsy findings, it can indicate the presence of natural disease which may modify the action of the drug, or account for unusually low levels of drug in tissue. However, the microscopic picture may be of value in indicating the precise physiological mode of death in a known case of poisoning, as in one instance of amphetamine poisoning associated with hyperpyrexia in which I saw generalized congestion of the organs; but histology demonstrated that the exact cause of death was a haemorrhage into the conducting tissue of the heart.

Other poisons may produce microscopical changes sufficiently distinctive to be diagnostic even if, due to the lapse of time, the causal agent cannot be detected by analysis. For instance, in acute hepatitis due to halothane, infiltration by eosinophils is said to be characteristic, distinguishing it from hepatitis due to an infective agent (Johnston & Mendelsohn 1971), though I have not had this experience. The pulmonary changes due to poisoning by Paraquat (dimethyl-bipyridinium dichloride) are not likely to be mistaken for any other condition (Kodagoda *et al.* 1973), and this may also be true with other substances such as cadmium (Anon. 1967). Then again the addict who injected his drugs intravenously may at autopsy have starch particles and granulomata (Siegel & Bloustein 1970; Cameron & Robinson 1973) in the pulmonary vessels and subcutaneous tissues, drawing attention to the circumstances of his death.

As a much later effect, prolonged therapeutic dosage of drugs can produce tissue changes only visible histologically, which may sometimes be sufficient to account for death. For instance peculiar changes in the small blood vessels of the heart, with damage to the cardiac muscle, have been associated with sudden and unexpected death in people taking high therapeutic doses of some phenothiazines for a long time (Richardson *et al.* 1966).

I have seen a couple of cases like this (Gee 1970) but have wondered whether such changes are really sufficient to account for death. However, the discovery of such changes during microscopic examination should prompt the pathologist to enquire about the deceased's past medication.

If, at the time of autopsy, it seems probable that death was due to poisoning, then another important part of the morbid anatomist's role is the selection and preservation of appropriate samples for later chemical analysis. Some exotic drugs require unusual specimens, for instance the acidified blood samples required for detection of isoprenaline, or bile for narcotic drugs, etc. (Curry 1969). Even the vitreous humour has been used (Felby & Olsen 1969).

Of course, with the advent of the gas chromatograph, the pathologist sometimes has to tie off a lung in a case of death from inhaled poison, so that the analyst can sample the gases in the airways (Kade & Abernethy 1961). However, for most conventional poisons the standard blood, urine, stomach contents, brain and liver suffice. Or do they?

Although these samples may allow the toxic substance to be identified, do they truly reflect the quantity of the drug in the body, or the amount circulating? Thus it is beginning to be appreciated that the concentration of drug to be found in different parts of a single organ may vary. And my colleagues and I are at present interested in the different levels of drugs to be found in samples of blood taken from different parts of the body. In a series of barbiturate poisonings we reported substantial differences in the amounts of barbiturate in samples of heart blood and of peripheral blood from leg veins. Thus in a single case the difference can be as much as 6.0 mg/100 ml (Gee *et al.* 1974). Other workers have drawn attention to the differences between drug concentrations in peripheral blood and liver blood (Robinson 1967).

Most people dying from barbiturate poisoning outside hospital have levels of about 2.0 mg/100 ml in the blood (Bonnischen *et al.* 1961). This is true for peripheral blood, almost irrespective of the levels in other organs, but not for heart blood, where the barbiturate level rises in proportion to higher levels in the liver and brain.

And we are finding the same results for other drugs. For instance, in one case of paracetamol poisoning the level in heart blood was 63 mg/100 ml but the level in a venous blood sample from each leg was 30 mg/100 ml.

So evidently the morbid anatomist should now always state precisely where he took his samples from, lest interpretations of the figures derived from analysis should be misleading. Moreover, I think it is important to consider why there should be this variation, and to ponder on the fact that post-mortem blood is not at all like the substance drawn from a living person's veins. Do we really know much at all, yet, about the true significance of the various tissue levels of drugs which can be measured by analysis of organs removed at autopsy? What relation do these levels bear to the distribution of the drug in the victim before death? There seems to me to be much scope for further research in this area.

Another pressing need is for simpler and speedy screening tests with which the morbid anatomist can detect, at the time of autopsy, the presence of drugs which would otherwise go unsuspected.

I have already mentioned some of the problems facing the pathologist who has to try to detect cases of poisoning by autopsy examination. We have a few simple chemical screens: for salicylate, carbon monoxide, alcohol, phenothiazine (Curry 1966; Clarke 1969) and a few other poisons; and a valuable one for barbiturates (Curry 1963). However, the number of deaths from barbiturate poisoning has fallen dramatically in the last couple of years, although the total number of suicides has not decreased. There are few simple screening tests for detecting the newer drugs likely to be taken instead of barbiturates.

On behalf of the morbid anatomist I would ask the analyst for more of these simple tests, specifically designed for chemical morons like me—paper strips, spot tests, and so forth, that we can apply to the ordinary body fluids available in the post-mortem room.

On our part I feel we must look perhaps to more sophisticated rapid histological techniques, perhaps to an extension of the few macro-enzyme techniques, like the method we use for demonstrating cardiac infarction (Knight 1965). Fairly elaborate histochemical methods are used of course as research tools, for instance in investigating monoamine oxidase inhibitors (Kesterson & Carlton 1971). If we modify such tests we may provide ourselves with valuable tools for the future.

ACKNOWLEDGEMENTS

I would like to acknowledge with gratitude the help of my colleagues in the Department of Forensic Medicine at the University of Leeds and of Her Majesty's Coroners in the County of Yorkshire, on whose behalf the examinations were made which form the basis of this paper.

References

ANONYMOUS (1967) Cadmium poisoning (leading article) *Br. Med. J. 2*, 392–393

BEVERIDGE, G. W. & LAWSON, A. A. H. (1965) Occurrence of bullous lesions in acute barbiturate intoxication. *Br. Med. J. 1*, 835–837

BONNISCHEN, R., MAEHLY, A. G. & FRANK, A. (1961) Barbiturate analysis: method and statistical survey. *J. Forensic Sci. 6*, 411–443

CAMERON, J. M. & ROBINSON, A. E. (1973) Pathology and toxicology of drug addiction: a Combined Approach. *Med. Sci. Law 13*, 272

CLARKE, E. G. C. (1969) *Isolation and Identification of Drugs*, Pharmaceutical Press, London

CURRY, A. S. (1963) Rapid method of screening for barbiturates. *Br. Med. J. 2*, 1040–1041

CURRY, A. S. (1966) Simple tests to detect poisoning, in *Broadsheet No. 52*, Association of Clinical Pathologists, London

CURRY, A. S. (1969) *Poison Detection in Human Organs*, 2nd edn., Thomas, Springfield, Ill.

DAVIDSON, D. G. D. & EASTHAM, W. N. (1966) Acute liver necrosis following overdose of paracetamol. *Br. Med. J. 2*, 497–499

FELBY, S. & OLSEN, J. (1969) Comparative studies of post-mortem barbiturate and meprobamate in vitreous humor, blood and liver. *J. Forensic Sci. 14*, 507–514

GEE, D. J. (1970) An iatrogenic cardiomyopathy. *Med. Sci. Law 10*, 266–267

GEE, D. J. & DALLEY, R. A. (1967) Unsuspected poisoning. *Med. Sci. Law 7*, 56–58

GEE, D. J., DALLEY, R. A., GREEN, M. A. & PERKINS, L. A. (1974) in *Forensic Toxicology* (Ballantyne, B., ed.), Wright, Bristol

JOHNSTON, C. I. & MENDELSOHN, F. (1971) Halothane hepatitis in a laboratory technician. *Aust. N.Z. J. Med. 2*, 171–173

KADE, H. & ABERNETHY, R. J. (1961) Identification of noxious gases in post mortem pulmonary air. *J. Forensic Sci. 6*, 125–133

KESTERSON, J. W. & CARLTON, W. W. (1971) Monoamine oxidase inhibition and the activity of other oxidative enzymes in the brains of mice fed cuprizone. *Toxicol. Appl. Pharmacol. 20*, 386–395

KNIGHT, B. (1965) The post mortem demonstration of early myocardial infarction. *Med. Sci. Law 5*, 31–34

KODAGODA, N., JAYEWARDENE, R. P. & ATTYGALLE, D. (1973) Poisoning with Paraquat. *Forensic Sci. 2*, 107–111

POLSON, C. J. (1965) The role of the pathologist in the investigation of fatal poisoning. *Med. Sci. Law 5*, 203–210

RICHARDSON, H. L., GRAUPNER, K. I. & RICHARDSON, M. E. (1966) Intramyocardial lesions in patients dying suddenly and unexpectedly. *J. Am. Med. Assoc. 195*, 254–260

ROBINSON, A. E. (1967) Critical survey of barbiturate and allied poisoning. *Med. Sci. Law 7*, 17–22

SIEGEL, H. & BLOUSTEIN, P. (1970) Continuing studies in the diagnosis and pathology of death from intravenous narcotism. *J. Forensic Sci. 15*, 179–184

SIEGEL, H., HELPERN, M. & EHRENREICH, T. (1966) Diagnosis of death from intravenous narcotism. *J. Forensic Sci. 11*, 1–16

Discussion

Brown: The Registrar-General's statistics for death by ingested poisons in England and Wales are most interesting. Table 1 (Brown) summarizes the data

TABLE 1 (Brown)

Registrar-General's statistics for deaths by poisoning, 1972 (data from Registrar-General 1974)

	Male (all ages)	*Female* (all ages)	*Total*	
Suicidal				
Amylobarbitone; quinalbarbitone	137	223	350	
Amylobarbitone sodium	42	79	121	
Pentobarbitone	36	69	106	
Barbiturate (not specified)	43	63	106	1011
Butobarbitone	33	65	98	
Amylobarbitone	36	52	88	
Quinalbarbitone	20	27	47	
Phenobarbitone	19	21	40	
Aspirin	44	47	91	146
Salicylate (not specified)	26	29	55	
Methaqualone	19	20	39	
Paracetamol	8	29	37	
Totals for 248 agents	714	1057	1771	
Accidental				
Amylobarbitone; quinalbarbitone	35	67	102	
Barbiturate (not specified)	24	29	53	
Pentobarbitone	17	18	35	257
Sodium amytal	13	14	27	
Butobarbitone	11	10	21	
Carbrital[a]	4	15	19	
Alcohol	29	14	43	
Aspirin	3	10	13	
Methaqualone	4	6	10	
Totals for 142 agents	263	305	568	
Intent undetermined				
Amylobarbitone; quinalbarbitone	38	78	116	
Barbiturate (not specified)	24	44	68	
Pentobarbitone	18	22	40	
Amylobarbitone sodium	16	20	36	313
Amylobarbitone	6	18	24	
Carbrital[a]	5	10	15	
Quinalbarbitone	3	11	14	
Amitriptyline	10	9	19	
Methaqualone	7	8	15	
Aspirin	4	10	14	
Totals for 120 agents	221	362	583	

[a] Pentobarbitone sodium plus carbromal

for 1972 and shows the named agents which head the lists for the three classifications of death—suicidal, accidental and intent undetermined. More than half of all suicides are attributed to barbiturates by the Registrar-General; aspirin and salicylate together form the next big category, followed by methaqualone and paracetamol. For death by accidental poisoning, a little less than half were due to barbiturates; alcohol and aspirin are then listed, and methaqualone appears as the next major lethal agent. The Registrar-General used the category 'intent undetermined' for the first time in 1972 and here again more than half the deaths were attributed to preparations of barbiturates. Professor Gee, in Leeds you are fortunate in having chemical confirmation, but how accurate do you think the official statistics are for England and Wales generally?

Gee: In Leeds we probably have a fairly accurate reflection of the barbiturate death rate because we have used Dr Curry's screening method (Curry 1963) on almost all our autopsy cases since 1966. Out of 200 cases of barbiturate poisoning about 10 had shown no visible evidence or history of poisoning before we screened them (Gee *et al.* 1974). We probably miss other poisons but not barbiturates. Nevertheless our known barbiturate poisonings over the last four years have dropped dramatically from 34 cases in 1970 to 11 cases in 1973. Our figures don't reflect the Registrar-General's figures, but we include 1973 and those in your Table 1 are for 1972.

Sunshine: The US Bureau of Vital Statistics, like the Registrar-General in England, accepts the physicians' diagnosis of the cause of death. Often this may be an intelligent guess and it is rarely substantiated either by autopsy or by chemical findings. I do not trust general figures from a national office, but where the reports from a local area are based on pathological and toxicological findings I think one can draw conclusions from the data. The prejudice that I have just expressed certainly reflects the situation in the States. I am not sure that it applies to the UK.

Gee: The Registrar-General's figures should be based on autopsy results, because most will be from coroner's reports. A few coroners have peculiar clairvoyant methods of assessing the cause of death, but on the whole it is rare in this country for a coroner to give the cause of death in a case of poisoning without a full investigation.

Goulding: The figures for the cause of death refer to just one drug, yet we know that it is not common for people to take an overdose of one drug. Barbiturates may be listed as common simply because they are the ones that can most easily be detected.

Gee: We looked for other common drugs in our cases of barbiturate poisoning. Out of the 200, only 16 took more than one drug.

Newton: These people were all dead so the figures are not strictly comparable to the Scottish figures Dr Patel showed (p. 230), where the patients were alive. The Registrar-General's figures for 1973 record that over 50 deaths were caused by nitrazepam (Mogadon), which I just do not believe. One case I know had an alcohol level of 360 mg/100 ml and another was reported by the laboratory as a death due to a barbiturate, yet both were recorded as deaths due to nitrazepam.

Patel: The distribution of the groups of drugs used in acute poisonings is certainly quite different from the Registrar-General's (England and Wales) statistics for suicide. The two groups of people are quite different from each other, though clearly there is an overlap: a self-poisoner may die and this would be called suicide. Barbiturates probably are still the commonest choice amongst the suicides but this is not so amongst self-poisoners.

Holmstedt: Professor Gee, you said that post-mortem blood had different properties according to whether you took it from the heart or from peripheral vessels. Can you also obtain cerebrospinal fluid (CSF) and determine, for example, centrally acting drugs.

Gee: A sample of CSF can be obtained.

Curry: In a small quantity of CSF the chance of finding all the drugs that we have to look for would be small.

Holmstedt: We can determine many compounds in 2 ml of CSF.

Curry: But not every laboratory has the equipment to do that.

Moffat: The question about post-mortem blood needs to be put into perspective. We estimate the levels of the drugs such as cardiac glycosides in plasma or serum. When we get post-mortem blood we spin it down until we get a fluid that we can work with. In some cases the erythrocyte: plasma ratio is 1:1, but with drugs like digitoxin, where the ratio is 1:9, what does the level in post-mortem blood mean compared with the level in a living patient? We have to start a whole range of new methods with post-mortem blood, since we do not really know what it consists of.

Gee: We are interested in post-mortem biochemistry in relation to diagnosing other causes of death, such as drowning. Electrolyte levels or haematological values alter rapidly after death. In 24 hours the specific gravity of serum goes way over 1.034 or something like that, and the haematocrit values for blood alter in about 24–48 hours. Some values change consistently and some quite inconsistently. This makes a terrific difference. Electrolyte levels in one leg tend to be comparable to those in the other leg, in the same way that drug levels are, but electrolyte levels in, for instance, a leg and an arm, or the right and left sides of the heart, may be totally different.

Curry: Alcohol levels in living patients may differ from leg veins to arm veins. David Blackmore (1970) published figures for the distribution of post-mortem carbon monoxide which physiologically he just could not understand.

Gee: Dr Ann E. Robinson (personal communication) has told me of observations of the same kind of thing.

Sunshine: I would like to stress that post-mortem blood is not blood but a fluid whose content vaguely resembles blood.

Curry: I would go further and say that post-mortem liver is not a liver. One has to be very careful in relating post-mortem figures to levels *in vivo*.

Gee: Many people do not appreciate this. For example, they may give elaborate conclusions based on calcium levels in post-mortem blood and then relate these to clinical findings.

Curry: You have pin-pointed the urgent need for studies of post-mortem chemistry.

Bridges: Could pathologists and clinicians be persuaded to standardize where they take blood from for testing drug levels?

Gee: Living blood is no problem. It is post-mortem blood that changes so much. Presumably we could standardize our techniques. For instance, because of the possibility of contamination most people take blood from a peripheral vein for alcohol determinations, although that is not now considered necessary by some workers. But different people take samples in different ways: some leave it to their technicians to take blood samples; others remember it long afterwards and gallop back to scoop up what is left in a cavity; and so on. One could try to specify how samples should be taken, but I think it is a question of education over a period of time.

Bridges: Would you be prepared to lay down standards?

Gee: Not until we know the significance of the result. I know which sample I trust when I need a barbiturate level now, but I think one needs a selection rather than one result only. If I send samples to one analyst in my area I get a full range of results for heart blood, peripheral blood, brain, liver, stomach contents, urine—anything I send. If I send exactly the same number of samples to another analyst, I get back a blood level, with no specification as to which of the samples he has analysed, and a liver level. If I send samples to a third analyst, outside my area, I get only a blood level.

Curry: In deaths from barbiturate poisoning, you said there were not necessarily any obvious pathological signs, yet we know that some people are walking around with the same concentrations of barbiturates in their bodies as those other people are supposed to have died from. On what basis do you assign such deaths to barbiturate poisoning?

Gee: I form my opinion from a number of different tissue levels: if a lot of barbiturate is unabsorbed in the stomach, or the tissue levels are not uniform, then I say death is due to barbiturates, but if all the levels are roughly equivalent I can't say that.

Curry: Figures from obvious poisoning cases need to be compared with analyses on people whose deaths were certainly not caused by drugs. There is a gap in the published work here.

Gee: If the laboratory could tell us by the next morning that seven out of eight autopsy samples were clear, and that one needed further examination, then we would be happy, as I said earlier.

Curry: This is very important, as otherwise you need 248 spot tests next year!

Sunshine: I do not think the toxicologist is prepared to do a complete toxicological examination encompassing all drugs in 24 hours on a biological specimen. If you could choose an incomplete toxicological examination, which substances would you include, and would immunoassay be useful? If you had seven antibodies that encompassed seven different types of drugs would that help?

Gee: It might. My list of drugs would be longer than Dr Prescott's (see p. 236) because the circumstances are somewhat different.

Newton: Does metabolism of drugs continue in the liver after death?

Gee: Algeri (1957) studied the effects of putrefaction on barbiturate determination in the liver. Post-mortem production of carbon monoxide, cyanide or alcohol, or the extinction of these things, certainly goes on, just as it does *in vitro*.

Gillette: The kind of drug is important. Obviously if the drug is metabolized by an oxidative reaction then its metabolism would stop soon after death because the liver rapidly becomes anaerobic. But if a drug is hydrolysed by an esterase, then its metabolism could easily continue long after death.

Newton: After death from an overdose, how many of your cases show pulmonary oedema of any extent? In patients who develop acute renal failure, despite our monitoring of the central venous pressure, it is possible to overload the circulation and produce pulmonary oedema which can result in death.

Gee: Nearly all our cases are people who died outside hospital. As a post-mortem artifact, most bodies develop some pulmonary oedema and the chance of having nice expanded dry lungs at post-mortem are remote, although obviously there are degrees of pulmonary oedema. A lot of our cases have massive pulmonary oedema. The most dramatic ones are the amitriptyline overdoses and we do not see many of those. A youngish person dying from an overdose of barbiturates or a young person dying from carbon monoxide poisoning will usually have quite gross pulmonary oedema, out of proportion to simple post-mortem change.

Newton: Our main problem with pulmonary oedema is during the initial treatment of Paraquat poisoning. We try to carry out a forced diuresis, assuming adequate renal function remains. At the last post-mortem that I attended after a death from Paraquat the patient had pulmonary oedema. I was reassured when the pathologist told me that the forced diuresis was not necessarily responsible for this finding.

Gee: Pulmonary oedema can develop in less than a minute in cases of mechanical asphyxia due to strangulation. It occurs both as an agonal phenomenon and to some degree as a post-mortem phenomenon. I don't assign much importance to it unless it is very gross indeed.

Curry: I am pleased to see that you still prefer glass jars and haven't gone over to plastic bottles, Professor Gee.

Gee: Unless someone leans very hard on the University Grants Committee the glass jars will go.

References

ALGERI, E. J. (1957) The determination of barbiturate after putrefaction. *J. Forensic Sci. 2*, 443–455

BLACKMORE, D. J. (1970) The determination of carbon monoxide in blood and tissue. *Analyst 95*, 439–458

CURRY, A. S. (1963) Rapid method of screening for barbiturates. *Br. Med. J. 2*, 1040

GEE, D. J., DALLEY, R. A., GREEN, M. A., & PERKINS, L. A. (1974) in *Forensic Toxicology* (Ballantyne, B., ed.), Wright, Bristol

REGISTRAR-GENERAL (1974) Public health: poisoning cases in 1972. *Pharm. J. 212*, 92–96

Drug-induced iatrogenic disease: the probability of its detection

HENRY LEACH

Group Laboratory, Caernarvon & Anglesey General Hospital and Department of Biochemistry, University College of North Wales, Bangor, Caernarvonshire

Abstract The problems arising from the growth in availability of very potent drugs have become so serious that facilities for analytical toxicology within hospitals are needed on a scale not envisaged ten years ago. As a result, the problems of detecting drug overdoses when samples are small and blood and urine levels of the drug are in the submicrogram range are now receiving more attention. Techniques sensitive enough to detect these low concentrations have been developed only recently and external evidence of the nature of the toxic agent may often still be necessary. A further aspect which has received little attention is that of iatrogenic disease. Most earlier studies have been epidemiological, based on recorded symptoms and related to drugs prescribed in the course of treatment. Some 5% of hospital beds are occupied by patients suffering from the effects of treatment and a high proportion of these illnesses are attributable to drugs.

Detection and identification of the causal agent in this type of disease is often very difficult. Only the use of new, highly sensitive methods of analysis and of indirect indicators of the possible presence of agents simulating organic disease will increase the probability of drug-induced disease being detected by laboratory methods.

Fifteen years ago the number of hospital laboratories providing any form of analytical toxicology service was very small. In the United Kingdom only about ten clinical chemistry departments were prepared to undertake more than the most rudimentary investigations. These were usually restricted to the determination of salicylates and the detection of barbiturates by simple chemical methods. Indeed, for many years there was a widely held belief that it was no part of the duty of a hospital laboratory to become involved in this work, and requests for toxicological analysis were either ignored or passed on to public analysts or the forensic science laboratories. This attitude persisted until the late 1960s and is not unknown today. The delays which resulted from sending the samples away only reinforced the conviction that toxicology was an unimportant luxury which should not be encouraged.

Those departments practising toxicology usually did so either because some elementary post-mortem toxicology was needed or because there was a local interest. As expertise grew, the facilities were extended to deal with clinical requirements in cases of poisoning and the challenge of a limited amount of sample and the need for speed stimulated interest in simple small-scale methods. For a long time, not only was there a shortage of experienced analysts, there was also the problem of lack of suitable equipment. Recording spectrophotometers were rare in the hospital laboratory and suitable chromatographic techniques were in their infancy. There were other difficulties: the analyst had often to devise his own methods, for many manufacturers of pharmaceuticals could only offer assay methods which needed far larger amounts of drug than would be found in body fluids. Detection methods were often totally unspecific; one method, for example, involved charring the residue with sulphuric acid. Quantitative methods involving dye complex formation or diazotization might be adequate for pharmacological studies but of limited value if more than one drug was present.

During the early 1960s it began to be appreciated that the problem of drug intoxication, whether deliberate or accidental, was unlikely to improve. And, when an unconscious patient was admitted to hospital, it was thought reasonable for clinicians to expect that laboratory help would be available in the same way as for a case of diabetic coma or cerebrovascular accident. In many cases a positive finding might be of little immediate value if treatment could only be symptomatic, but there were instances where laboratory confirmation could give reassurance and avoid the need for other diagnostic investigations.

The increasing use of ultraviolet spectrophotometry, particularly with recording instruments, and the use of chromatography for clinical chemistry generally, provided the analyst with the equipment needed for toxicological analysis. Simple screening schemes for the examination of samples from cases of poisoning had been published, for example the broadsheet by Curry (1966); but if even semiquantitative results were needed a more sophisticated approach was required. One of the major problems facing the analyst, that of identification and separation from interfering material, had been ameliorated by the use of paper chromatography and the introduction of thin-layer chromatography gave the speed and increased sensitivity that were essential for this kind of analysis. Gas chromatography introduced a new dimension, giving sensitivities several orders of magnitude greater than could be attained hitherto. For the first time identification and quantification of submicrogram amounts of drug became possible.

Partly due to these advances and also due to the use of labelled parent drugs for pharmacological studies, much more information became available on the metabolites of drugs. Although a considerable body of information about the analysis of biological materials for drugs had been built up, most of this referred to the unchanged drug; the likelihood that a major metabolite, possibly with different pharmacological properties, might not be distinguished by the method of analysis was seldom mentioned. Even today, a large number of published methods for the analysis of drugs in body fluids say nothing about the presence of metabolites or are reticent about their interference.

Analytical clinical toxicology is generally assumed to mean the analysis of samples, often under emergency conditions, from a poisoned patient admitted as an acute medical emergency. This was certainly true in the past and will probably remain in the next few years as the major role. But another facet of this subject which will continue to grow is the measurement of drug concentrations for therapeutic purposes. This may be necessary to ensure that patients do not default in treatment, to detect malabsorption or defective metabolism, or to maintain plasma levels below the toxicity threshold. Analyses of this kind are already done routinely by many hospital laboratories; digoxin, digitoxin and insulin determinations by radioimmunoassay methods are relatively commonplace. It would be unrealistic to assume that this kind of activity will fail to grow as rapidly as other clinical chemistry procedures. The scarcity and high cost of the antisera required for radioimmune methods has been the limiting factor in using radioimmunoassay for other drugs and steroids, but this situation is already changing rapidly as the range of commercially available material continues to expand.

There are thus two main areas where the laboratory is concerned with the poisoned patient. One is where death has occurred and the laboratory investigation can be regarded as a part of the post-mortem, and the second is where detection and determination of drugs are thought valuable by the clinician for providing or supporting a diagnosis or, rarely, for suggesting a line of treatment. The third role, that of estimating therapeutic drug levels, tends to be regarded either as an extension of other toxicological facilities or, often, as clinical biochemistry, albeit rather esoteric. In the living patient the laboratory will, of course, also be generating a considerable amount of conventional biochemical data.

There is a further situation where the laboratory might be expected to become involved with a poisoned patient. This is when the patient is poisoned not from an overdose of drug but by normal doses of drugs administered for therapeutic purposes; this may be by prescription or from self-medication. The size of the problem caused by adverse reactions to normal doses of drugs is not known with any accuracy but Dunlop (1969) suggested that 5% of general hospital beds were occupied by patients suffering from the effects of treatment and that even major reactions to drugs might go unrecognized. If the number of hospitalized patients is added to the number with ostensible organic disease attending outpatient departments or their own doctor, it is evident that this is a large and costly problem.

Most of the information on serious side-effects of drugs comes from reports by clinicians who have noted unusual effects after the administration of a drug and relief of these symptoms when the drug was withdrawn. Many reports of isolated instances or from small groups of cases appear in the literature and are summarized in the reports of the Committee on the Safety of Medicines. Recognition of the true cause of some symptoms depends on the knowledge that a drug is being administered; in self-medication or where records or exchanges of information are incomplete, the causal factor may not be apparent and the drug reaction may be unrecognized. In the worst type of case, attempts to treat a simulated organic disease could lead to the effects of drug interaction being superimposed, resulting in injury to the patient and perhaps his death. It is interesting to speculate on what proportion of reported serious reactions to a single drug are, in fact, the result of drug interaction where the other agent remains completely undetected.

A number of studies have appeared on the incidence of drug reactions in a controlled population such as a hospital or clinic. Hurwitz & Wade (1969) studied adverse reactions by monitoring drugs administered to patients in medical wards and recording their reactions. The logistics were formidable: patients were interviewed on admission and general practitioners' letters and hospital notes were scrutinized at the start of the period of surveillance. Drugs administered outside the wards in operating theatres or for radiology were not recorded. The incidence of drug reactions in this survey was about 10% for medical ward patients, a figure comparable to those reported in earlier surveys. It is interesting that in two surveys the reported incidence of adverse reactions was greater on the first or first and second days in hospital than on any other days, and although there are several possible reasons for this, interaction with drugs taken before admission and not revealed to the investigators is not unlikely.

At present the hospital laboratory does almost nothing to help in the detection of this type of intoxication with therapeutic drugs and, apart from those drugs which can be determined easily by radioimmunoassay or chromatography, plasma levels of drugs are monitored only in laboratories which have both the necessary equipment and—more important—the necessary experience and expertise.

For convenience it is better to exclude emergency analytical toxicology in considering the problems of detecting low levels of drug in the living patient, for although some of the available techniques are applicable to both emergency and non-acute cases, others are either unsuitable or unnecessary for the detection of poisons in cases of overdosage. Furthermore, in acute poisoning the presence of metabolites is less important and the concentration of parent drug is usually so much greater than that of the metabolites that they can be neglected. This is not always so but the proportion of acute poisonings where metabolic products are sought is very small.

If the investigation of drug levels as a guide to therapy or the application of laboratory methods to the detection of drugs responsible for adverse reactions —particularly drugs in combination—are to have any chance of success the analytical procedures must be designed with the importance of metabolites in mind. The ability to detect, identify and preferably quantify metabolites is a desirable attribute of any analytical system for the study of low drug levels. When metabolism is rapid, either because this is characteristic of the drug or because the rate of metabolism is enhanced by an increase in enzyme activity, the only means of detecting the drug may be by finding its metabolites.

When the pharmacological response to a dose is less than normally expected, the determination of plasma levels of the drug may provide an explanation. Lowered plasma concentrations may be due to poor absorption or destruction in the gut. A further possibility is that induction of hepatic microsomal enzyme activity has resulted from the previous or concurrent administration of another drug. Many drugs, including barbiturates, anti-inflammatory agents, sedatives, hypnotics, tranquillizers and some anaesthetics have been shown to induce hepatic enzyme activity in animals. Much less is known of the occurrence and significance of enzyme induction in man. The *British Medical Journal* was moved to editorial comment in 1972 on the lamentable lack of knowledge of the extent and significance of this effect (Anon. 1972).

Barbiturates lower the levels of tricyclic antidepressants and also enhance the metabolism of methyldopa. Organic disease can follow enzyme induction and, due to the increased metabolism of vitamin D, osteomalacia has been produced by anticonvulsants (Hunter *et al.* 1971). The effects of enzyme induction on the metabolism of warfarin has received considerable attention and Koch-Weser & Sellers (1971*a*, *b*) showed that a number of drugs were capable of modifying the action of warfarin, while Breckenridge & Orme (1971) found that both amylobarbitone (amobarbital) and quinalbarbitone (secobarbital) increased its metabolism in man.

Metabolic systems may be inhibited by drugs or by dietary constituents, and plasma levels of a drug may be increased if its metabolic pathway is blocked. The administration of neuroleptics like haloperidol and chlorpromazine has been shown to inhibit the metabolism of tricyclic antidepressants in man. Using nortriptyline, Gram & Overø (1972) found that total urinary excretion and plasma levels of metabolites decreased while plasma levels of unchanged drug increased after the administration of neuroleptics.

Plasma levels could also increase if renal excretion is impaired or if a tissue-bound or protein-bound drug is displaced by the later administration of a more strongly bound substance. Increased plasma levels of a drug, if its identity is unknown, only ease the task of the analyst slightly: at microgram and sub-microgram concentrations moderate increases give only marginal help in identification.

THE ROLE OF THE LABORATORY

If laboratory investigations are to assist in the diagnosis of iatrogenic disease from drugs the methods of analysis used at present for routine toxicology are not likely to be sufficiently sensitive. Refinements or improvements are necessary to give better sensitivity, or newer methods such as radioimmunoassay or mass spectrometry must be used.

It is unrealistic to think that any single technique will suffice and although a combination of chromatography and mass spectrometry is the most versatile and powerful technique now available to the toxicologist, there will continue to be circumstances where other methods will be valuable.

Another approach is to seek indirect evidence for the active presence of drugs by examining those biological systems which may be affected by drug administration.

REFINEMENTS IN EXISTING TECHNIQUES

Gas chromatography

The highly sensitive flame ionization detector already allows therapeutic levels of many drugs to be determined in small volumes of blood. The use of the electron capture detector, alone or in parallel with a flame ionization detector, can give useful additional sensitivity and selectivity if the drug contains electron capturing functional groups. Other drugs can be made to contain electron-capturing groups, in many instances, if suitable derivatives are formed. Unfortunately, the linear range of the electron capture detector is limited; when used for routine analysis it is subject to accidental contamination and may take many hours to recover from the resulting loss in response.

The nitrogen-selective detector or alkali flame ionization detector, a modified flame ionization detector with a caesium or rubidium salt annulus placed above the flame jet, is another highly sensitive and selective detector. The response to nitrogen-containing and phosphorus-containing compounds is enhanced and with a rubidium chloride annulus the response to nitrogen-containing compounds shows an increase in sensitivity of about 10^4 by comparison with that of the normal flame ionization detector. The alkali flame detector is more demanding than the ordinary flame detector, requiring more maintenance and stable gas supplies. It is also more noisy but improvements in design and electrode configuration should lead to the more widespread use of this detector. Its high sensitivity will allow it to be used with high resolution capillary columns. Although these columns would be of value for toxicological analysis the small amounts of sample they will tolerate limit their use unless a sensitive detector can be used. When Moffat *et al.* (1973) chromatographed 62 basic drugs on eight stationary phases in packed columns, only the SE-30 column successfully eluted all the drugs and more polar columns failed to give any significant aid in identification. The use of capillary columns of a low polarity phase such as SE-30, OV-1 or OV-17, together with a sensitive and selective detector, should prove advantageous in this type of analysis.

Spectroscopy

Although the ultraviolet scanning spectrophotometer is probably the most widely used of the laboratory instruments, its basic design has remained substantially unchanged for the last 15 years. With a few exceptions its sensitivity is low and even drugs with characteristic spectra cannot be detected if the concentration is below a few micrograms per millilitre. The use of micro-cells or scale expansion cannot offer a large improvement, for at low absorbancies noise interferes and the characteristic shape of the absorbance curve is no longer apparent. There is now no reason why these limitations should continue. Noise could be eliminated by repetitive scanning and electronic superimposition of a large number of scans. Since the signal change is constant at a given point, while noise is random, the noise cancels out and leaves an apparently noise-free signal. Repetitive rapid scans are not practical with the present instruments since the scan rate, usually several minutes, is dictated largely by the slow response of the recorder. If the recorder did not run in synchronism with the monochromator it would be possible to do a number of scans before presenting the composite scan to the recorder. Suitable electronic devices, the 'box-car integrator' and other signal averaging equipment, have been available for several years to abstract a wanted signal from a high background of noise. Now it can be done simply and inexpensively with a mini-computer; since these cost little and can be used for other jobs, this is an attractive way of dealing with the problem.

If the logarithm of absorbance is plotted instead of absorbance, the shape of the absorbance spectrum is largely independent of the concentration. Displaying the spectrum in this way eases the recognition of spectral curves. This is very useful at low concentrations where a characteristic spectrum is no longer recognizable. A logarithmic recorder can be used, but here also data capture by computer can provide a log absorbance scan with immediate conversion back to true absorbance.

Fluorescence spectroscopy is a more limited technique but is capable of detecting many drugs which fluoresce naturally or can be converted into fluorescent derivatives at submicrogram concentrations. Here, too, at high sensitivities noise is a serious limiting factor and the use of repetitive scanning with computer data capture for signal averaging would give useful increases in sensitivity. The signal could be presented to a recorder directly after averaging to give the conventional form of fluorescence and excitation scans, or it could be corrected for source variation and detector response to give corrected spectra. It is much cheaper to produce corrected spectra in this way from a standard spectrofluorometer than by the use of an instrument capable of producing corrected spectra by electronic and optical means.

NEWER METHODS OF ANALYSIS

Mass spectrometry

If a single technique of general application to the detection, identification and quantification of drugs were to be used, the mass spectrometer is the nearest approach to the ideal. When this is used in conjunction with a gas chromatograph, organic substances which are eluted from the column can be detected and identified in nanogram amounts. A substance not amenable to gas chromatography can be separated by some form of liquid chromatography and inserted directly into the instrument after the solvent has been evaporated. In high resolution studies undertaken to determine molecular formulae, expensive double-focusing instruments are needed to give the necessary resolution. For most routine analyses, instruments of more modest performance will suffice. Toxicological analysis seldom needs fundamental spectroscopic studies and identification is mostly done by comparing the spectrum of an unknown substance with a library of reference spectra of authentic drugs. For this kind of work an instrument with an upper mass limit of 600–1000 and a resolving power of 700–1500 is quite adequate.

The situation with mass spectrometry is not unlike that with infrared spectroscopy ten years ago when most instruments were large and expensive, designed for the spectroscopist undertaking fundamental studies. The experience gained in producing such instruments was then used to produce low-cost infrared spectrophotometers for routine work, and the performance of many of these cheap instruments was soon as good as that of their larger predecessors.

A number of small single-focusing magnetic deflection instruments and quadrupole mass spectrometers are now available, most with provision for an integral gas chromatograph. The need for high sensitivity has led to the total ion current being monitored, so the mass spectrometer functions as a gas chromatograph detector; usually the sensitivity is several orders of magnitude better than with a flame ionization detector. This allows a conventional gas chromatogram to be produced and suitable peaks can then be selected for mass analysis. The ability of these instruments to monitor a number of preselected ion fragments (mass fragmentography) is valuable for the detection of metabolites and other trace substances.

Conventional mass spectra produced by ion impact are usually very complex, for the ion beam energy is usually much greater than is required to ionize the molecule and the excess energy is dissipated in breaking intramolecular bonds, giving many ionized fragments. Often the molecular ion cannot be seen in the spectrum and a valuable parameter in identification is lost. If the molecule is bombarded with an ionized gas, the MH^+ion will be formed with an $m/e\ M + 1$ peak, where M is the molecular weight. This ion is usually the most prominent if chemical ionization is used; much simpler spectra are produced and can help in identification. Milne *et al.* (1971) described the use of chemical ionization with isobutane and direct insertion of crude extracts without any prior chromatographic separation.

Radioimmunoassay

Originally used for the determination of steroids and hormones, radioimmunoassay is also used for measuring trace amounts of drugs. The problems associated with producing labelled material of reasonable stability have been largely overcome and many drugs labelled with ^{14}C and ^{3}H are readily available. Material labelled with iodine isotopes is obtainable for use with γ-counting equipment but stability is less than with the less active isotopes.

The main difficulty has arisen from obtaining suitable antisera, and for several years investigators had to prepare their own. A number of antisera for digoxin, digitoxin, insulin, phenobarbitone, amphetamine, morphine and lysergide are now commercially available.

Sensitivity is high and drug concentrations in the nanogram and picogram range can be measured but, as would be expected, selectivity is sometimes poor and much cross-reaction occurs. Most morphine antisera will also react with codeine, and this is also the case with amphetamine and metamphetamine. Phenobarbitone antisera can be produced with high specificity but antisera to barbiturates without the phenyl substituents cross-react. Much effort is being expended in producing specific antisera and there will undoubtedly be much improvement as the use of this technique increases. Even for routine toxicology, and particularly in screening procedures for detecting the ingestion of drugs, there is a place for antisera of poor specificity for a single drug but capable of detecting a group of related substances. Although suited to pharmacological studies and specific toxicological problems, this method of analysis is not very practical for general toxicology since it requires antiserum and labelled material for each drug and the reagents are both expensive and unstable.

INDIRECT METHODS

Biochemical tests for enzyme induction

It is generally impracticable to examine the changes in liver microsomal activity directly but some indication of the changes which may occur can be obtained by measuring the normal biogenic products of this activity in the urine. Conney *et al.* (1965) postulated that changes in the excretion of 6β-hydroxycortisol, a polar metabolite of cortisol (hydrocortisone), was related to changes in the enzyme activity of liver cells. Determination of this steroid has been used to assess hepatic microsomal activity after administration of benzodiazepines (Orme *et al.* 1972) and dichloralphenazone (Breckenridge *et al.* 1971). D-Glucaric acid is a product of glucuronate conjugation in the liver and can be determined by heating urine to form the lactone. Glucurolactone strongly inhibits the enzyme β-glucuronidase (March 1963) and the inhibitory effect is proportional to the concentration of D-glucaric acid. Hunter *et al.* (1971) used this method to study the induction of liver microsomal enzymes by anticonvulsant drugs.

When monoamine oxidase inhibitors are administered, concentrations of 5-hydroxyindoleacetic acid (5-HIAA) in urine and blood fall because the conversion of 5-hydroxytryptamine to 5-HIAA is blocked. Catecholamine deamination is also prevented but metabolism via the catechol *O*-methyltransferase pathway continues. The result is an increase in metadrenaline and the excretion of tyramine, phenylethylamine and other biogenic amines is increased.

Although determination of 5-HIAA, 5-hydroxytryptamine, metadrenalines and biogenic amines may suggest monoamine oxidase blockade, the results generally are disappointing due to the difficulty of distinguishing changes caused by drugs from those which are physiological or occur in pathological conditions.

Cyclic AMP

In recent years there has been great interest in the role of adenosine 3′, 5′-cyclic phosphate (cyclic AMP) in mediating the action of many different hormones. It is now thought to act as a second messenger and is concerned with membrane transport at the cellular level. Cyclic AMP is formed from adenosine triphosphate by the action of adenyl cyclase and it is broken down by a phosphodiesterase. Changes in tissue levels and the excretion of cyclic AMP may be due to changes in the activity of the two enzymes, and caffeine and other methylxanthines have been found to inhibit phosphodiesterase. Abdulla & Hamadah (1970) and Hamadah *et al.* (1973) have shown that the low cyclic AMP levels found in depressive states can be reversed by tricyclic antidepressant drugs and this effect is probably due to the inhibition of phosphodiesterase by these substances. The sulphonylureas, glibenclamide and tolbutamide have been shown to inhibit phosphodiesterase and Sams & Montague (1973) suggest that the mechanism of action involves cyclic AMP.

It seems probable that the target action of many drugs involves cyclic AMP and only further studies will determine whether there are changes sufficiently significant and distinguishable for urine and blood concentrations of cyclic AMP to provide a general indication of the involvement of drugs. At present the situation is not too hopeful, for physiological and pathological changes cannot be clearly defined. Although cyclic AMP has occupied the most prominent place the other cyclic nucleotide, guanine 3′, 5′-cyclic phosphate (cyclic GMP), which has been shown to have a biological function has also been studied (Hardman 1971). The role of cyclic GMP is still obscure but it appears to be less affected by the action of hormones, and the preponderant interest in cyclic AMP should not allow this related nucleotide to be overlooked as a possible mediator of the action of drugs.

CYTOCHEMICAL TECHNIQUES

Although biologically active compounds act at the cellular level, limitations in techniques have prevented cellular studies being employed generally, except with some histochemical methods. Advances in cellular biochemistry have led to the development of sensitive methods for the assay of hormones. In many cases the high sensitivity of radioimmunoassay has been insufficient for the measurement of the very low circulating levels.

Chayen (1974) has shown that cellular biochemistry can provide extremely sensitive, specific and precise methods of assay for some hormones. If a specific intracellular biochemical process can be detected which is dependent on hormone concentration, it can be used for an assay. The sensitivity is far greater than has hitherto been possible and concentrations of a few femtograms per millilitre can be detected. ACTH can be detected down to 5 fg/ml, using guinea pig adrenal sections (Alagharad-Sadeh 1974), and similar assays for luteinizing hormone, thyrotropin and gastrin have also been produced.

This is of great importance for, if experience with immunoassay methods is a guide, it will be possible to use these techniques for other biologically active substances. There seems no reason why the principles of these assays should not be extended to the detection and study of the action of drugs that act intracellularly. Even if specificity was not high the ability to detect subpicogram amounts of members of groups of related drugs would provide the analyst with a powerful aid and stimulate the investigation of drug action in the cell. By this means the interaction of drugs may be detectable at the cellular level and allow the probability of undesirable reactions to be predicted.

THE PROBABILITY OF SUCCESS

At present the probability with which drugs responsible for iatrogenic disease can be detected depends on many factors. Even in overt cases of drug overdosage the analyst may fail to detect the causal agent in blood and success is often achieved only with great difficulty. The use of potent drugs effective in small doses and the possibility that the action may continue after plasma levels have fallen below the limit of detection complicates the problem. Even when the drug is known, the difficulties may be formidable, and when this information is lacking the difficulties may be immense. If the probability of detection is not particularly good there is no doubt that ignoring the problem will do nothing to improve the situation. The difficulties stem mainly from lack of knowledge and expertise and it is only by the continuing investigation of toxicological conundrums that the necessary information and experience will be gained.

Although the present probability of detection is low, the prospects for future work are distinctly brighter. The use of mass spectrometry, immunoreactive methods and cytochemical techniques, together with current routine high-sensitivity methods, will permit us to detect drugs at the submicrogram level. It is inconceivable that the middle seventies will not see the same advances as appeared during the middle sixties.

The problems associated with the administration of drugs are significant; if their true magnitude were realized I suspect that most of us would be appalled. Certainly this is a fruitful and useful field of endeavour and one in which the first timid and tentative steps are only now being taken. Efforts to increase the probability that iatrogenic disease can be detected by laboratory methods will benefit not only the patient but toxicology as a whole.

References

ABDULLA, Y. H. & HAMADAH, K. (1970) 3′, 5′ cyclic AMP in depression and mania. *Lancet 1*, 378–381

ALAGHARAD-SADEH, J. (1974) Development of a section bio-assay for the routine assay of corticotrophin. *Ann. Clin. Biochem.* in press

ANONYMOUS (1972) (Editorial) *Br. Med. J. 3*, 490

BRECKENRIDGE, A. & ORME, M. (1971) Clinical implications of enzyme induction. *Ann. N. Y. Acad. Sci. 179*, 421

BRECKENRIDGE, A., ORME, M., THORGEIRSSON, S., DAVIES, D. S. & BROOKE, R. V. (1971) Drug interactions with warfarin: studies with dichloralphenazone, chloral hydrate and phenazone. *Clin. Sci. 40*, 351–364

CHAYEN, J. (1974) General introduction to cytochemical hormone assay. *Clin. Endocrinol. 3*, 303–309

CONNEY, A. H., JACOBSON, M., SCHNEIDMAN, K. & KUNTZMAN, R. (1965) Induction of liver microsomal cortisol 6-hydroxylase by diphenylhydantoin and phenobarbital. *Life Sci. 4*, 1091–1098

CURRY, A. S. (1966) Simple tests to detect poisoning, in *Broadsheet No. 52*, Association of Clinical Pathologists, London

DUNLOP, D. (1969) (Book review) *Br. Med. J. 2*, 622

GRAM, L. F. & OVERØ, K. F. (1972) Drug interaction: inhibitory effects of neuroleptics on metabolism of tricyclic antidepressants in man. *Br. Med. J. 1*, 463–465

HAMADAH, K., HOLMES, H., HARTMAN, G. C. & PARKE, D. V. (1973) Diurnal variation of urinary cyclic AMP content in depressive illness. *Biochem. Soc. Trans. 2*, 81–82

HARDMAN, J. G. (1971) in *Cyclic AMP* (Robison, G. A., Butcher, R. W. & Sutherland, E. W., eds.), pp. 400–421, Academic Press, New York & London

HUNTER, J., MAXWELL, J. D., STEWART, D. A., PARSONS, V. & WILLIAMS, R. (1971) Altered calcium metabolism in epileptic children on anticonvulsants. *Br. Med. J. 4*, 202–204

HURWITZ, N. & WADE, O. L. (1969) Intensive hospital monitoring of adverse reactions to drugs. *Br. Med. J. 1*, 531–540

KOCH-WESER, J. & SELLERS, E. M. (1971*a*) Drug interactions with coumarin anticoagulants. *N. Engl. J. Med. 285*, 487–498

KOCH-WESER, J. & SELLERS, E. M. (1971*b*) Drug interactions with coumarin anticoagulants (second of two parts). *N. Engl. J. Med. 285*, 547–557

MARCH, C. A. (1963) Metabolism of D-glucuronolactone in mammalian systems. *Biochem. J. 86*, 77–86

MILNE, G. W. A., FALES, H. M. & AXENROD, T. (1971) Identification of dangerous drugs by chemical ionisation mass spectrometry. *Anal. Chem. 43*, 1815–1820

MOFFAT, A. C., STEAD, A. H. & SMALLDON, K. W. (1973) *Home Office Research Establishment Report No. 101*

ORME, M., BRECKENRIDGE, A. & BROOKS, R. V. (1972) Interaction of benzodiazepines with warfarin. *Br. Med. J. 3*, 611–614

SAMS, D. J. & MONTAGUE, W. (1973) Possible involvement of adenosine 3′, 5′-cyclic monophosphate in mechanisms of action of sulphonylureas on insulin secretion from islets of Langerhans. *Biochem. Soc. Trans. 2*, 33–34

Discussion

Curry: Mr Leach has told us that iatrogenic effects are due to a defect in our knowledge of drug interactions in normal biochemistry. We have touched on the fringes of this and here is a chance for us to consider it in detail.

Gillette: Drug induction of enzyme systems should be put into a better perspective than it is at present. It is evident that most drugs have a relatively wide safety margin and thus they seldom evoke adverse reactions, even though the rate of metabolism of a given drug may vary as much as 10–50-fold in different individuals. Since most inducers seldom increase the rate of metabolism more than twofold, the steady-state plasma level after induction will usually remain within the normal range. Thus, with most drugs induction is not a very important aspect of drug toxicity or drug resistance. Indeed, induction should really be considered important only for drugs such as digitalis, warfarin and diphenylhydantoin (phenytoin), that are fundamentally quite toxic and have a relatively small therapeutic index. I also believe that the various tests used to determine induction should be interpreted with caution. It should be pointed out that inducers do not always increase urinary 6-hydroxycortisol or D-glucaric acid. Indeed, increases in these substances may occur only with a relatively few inducers, such as the barbiturates.

Leach: Children given antiepileptics can develop rickets because they are metabolizing cholecalciferol. This is a pure iatrogenic disease. It is unrelated clinically to the drug that has been given. I am thinking about this sort of case, in addition to the others.

Goulding: In the ward, or in the outpatient department, if we think from the prescription chart that so-called iatrogenic disease is a possibility we then need to find out whether the patient is really taking the prescribed drugs. When we tried to do a qualitative survey of this kind in the outpatient department the results were so bizarre that we gave up in horror. In the ward we also found an enormous discrepancy between the drugs we thought the patient was having and what they were in fact taking. It is no good saying that a particular reaction is due to a particular drug until we have our facts right.

Leach: I agree about the measurement of drugs which are allegedly being taken. Information about possible drug usage in the general population might be useful here. We know absolutely nothing about this. In a sample of 100 people off the street, in how many of them would we find something we would call a drug?

Patel: We have largely overcome the discrepancies between what is prescribed in the ward and what is dispensed by using the Aberdeen system of prescribing and dispensing in the hospitals (HMSO 1973).

Goulding: Urine samples have not been examined to see whether that system really works. It is a great step forward, but I am not sure that it is the total answer.

Parker: The phenomenon of slow and fast acetylation brings us to another area of drug metabolism that is influenced by genetic factors. It has recently been recognized that diseases such as rheumatoid arthritis, psoriasis and chronic infective hepatitis are frequently associated with specified histocompatibility (HL-A) types (McDevitt & Bodmer 1974). Determination of HL-A phenotypes may well be of diagnostic value in these diseases. It will be important to attempt to correlate drug metabolism patterns with HL-A phenotypes as a possible means of prospectively identifying an individual who is likely to metabolize a drug abnormally. Whether significant correlations will be found is problematical, since the genes which specify drug-metabolizing enzymes and histocompatibility antigens are likely to be on different chromosomes. A better approach may be to give a test dose of the drug in question or to develop *in vitro* assays which measure relevant serum, leucocyte, erythrocyte or platelet enzymes.

Gillette: Isoniazid-induced hepatitis may result from metabolism of the drug. Mitchell & Jollow (1974) did a retrospective study of patients who suffered from hepatitis due to isoniazid and found that they were mainly fast acetylators, contrary to our expectations. Mitchell & Jollow suggest that acetylated isoniazid is hydrolysed to acetyl hydrazide, which in turn forms a chemically reactive metabolite that causes the liver damage. In accord with this view, acetyl hydrazide and acetyl isoniazid produce marked hepatic necrosis in phenobarbitone pretreated but not in untreated animals.

Gee: We need to know a great deal more about iatrogenic disease from the point of view of the forensic autopsy, Somebody may die with a natural disease but they may have had some medication that might also be the cause of death. People taking propranolol, for example, may die suddenly. Death may appear to be due to coronary atheroma, yet the coronary arteries must have been in the same state for years. We don't know much about this. I would be far too cowardly at present to say that a person's death was due to something like a side effect of a therapeutic dose of a drug, yet I am sure this is often the case.

Beckett: We lack information about the rates of metabolism by different routes in man. In our laboratories, we have tried to deal with this by looking at two basic processes, namely *N*-oxidation and *N*-dealkylation. In man we have not found great intersubject variations in these rate processes or in carbonyl reduction, but I accept that there are intersubject variations in some other routes. It is important that we establish where there are intersubject differences in metabolism and where there are none.

Newton: Analgesic abuse is probably one of the greatest problems in iatrogenic disease at present. Some asthmatic patients would not be so affected if they weren't taking aspirin day after day. Similarly, much severe renal disease is caused by analgesic abuse. It is difficult to know in practice which patients are doing this and it would be useful if a simple screening test were available.

Leach: We tend to speak of the state of the art and perhaps we should look forward to what may be possible in the future. Some of the methods I mentioned are very blunt instruments indeed and leave much room for improvement. Unless we actively look for better methods and perhaps borrow from other disciplines we will never succeed in finding techniques with the sort of sensitivity and specificity needed to detect possible drug-induced disease. How many of the cases of hypersensitivity reactions that follow a single dose of a drug are, in fact, the result of interaction with another drug taken previously?

Curry: Are all isoenzymes inhibited by monoamine oxidase (MAO) inhibitors?

Leach: They are inhibited selectively and this depends on the drug. Iproniazid can behave as a substrate for the enzymic reduction of tetrazolium salts to the formazan. It should be possible to use this histochemically. Other examples of this would appear if we looked for them.

Moffat: We are looking at biochemical changes in the brain in response to MAO inhibitors. It is difficult when we can only use post-mortem material. In people taking therapeutic doses of MAO inhibitors the levels are apparently very low compared with the published normal values. People taking therapeutic doses may not be distinguishable from people who have taken large overdoses. We are now looking at some of the brain amines, such as noradrenaline and 5-hydroxytryptamine, which act as substrates for the enzyme.

Dole: Recently Dr G. C. Cotzias (personal communication) has found that MAO inhibitors facilitate the penetration of MAO substrates into the brain, so there is a much greater input from potentially toxic amines.

Beckett: Can we address ourselves to finding a broad test for various types of agents? Could we find selective electrodes for all bases where there is a big difference in lipid solubility between the ionized and un-ionized species? Those foreign compounds will be present in amounts completely different to those of the endogenous amines of the body; a simple test at two different pH values should therefore show whether such an organic base was present. The same approach could be used for acids. The selective electrodes are available.

References

HMSO (1973) *Standardisation of Hospital Medical Records* (report of the working party set up by the Scottish Home and Health Department), Her Majesty's Stationery Office, Edinburgh

McDevitt, H. O. & Bodmer, W. F. (1974) HL–A, immune-response genes, and disease. *Lancet 1*, 1269–1275

Mitchell, J. R. & Jollow, D. J. (1974) Activation of drugs to toxic substances. *Gastroenterology*, in press

Limitations of haemodialysis and forced diuresis

L. F. PRESCOTT

The Regional Poisoning Treatment Centre and University Department of Therapeutics, The Royal Infirmary, Edinburgh

Abstract Poisoned patients are often subjected to unnecessary and potentially harmful haemodialysis and forced diuresis, but much of the information on which claims for efficacy have been based is either inadequate or invalid. Identification and estimation of plasma concentrations of drugs is an essential preliminary to haemodialysis and diuresis, since there are so few indications for these forms of treatment. Because the volumes of distribution of polar drug metabolites (which are often inactive) are smaller than those of the parent drug, and the plasma concentrations are often much greater, the amount of drug claimed to have been removed by haemodialysis and forced diuresis may be overestimated by as much as 100-fold unless highly specific analytical methods are used.

Poisoned patients are often subjected to unnecessary and potentially harmful haemodialysis and forced diuresis. Unfortunately, there are few instances in which these measures have clearly been shown to reduce morbidity and mortality, and much of the information on which claims for efficacy have been based is either inadequate or invalid. Most poisoned patients recover with intensive supportive therapy, good nursing care and a minimum of meddlesome medical interference (Matthew & Lawson 1970). This is overlooked by many clinicians, and the misguided enthusiasm of some nephrologists for indiscriminate haemodialysis in poisoned patients may have done more harm than good. Similarly, many doctors hold the naive belief that drugs can be 'washed out' of the body by a good diuresis. Clinicians seem to have an irresistible urge to carry out some form of 'treatment' on their patients, and this is particularly so for an unconscious patient whose relatives may be clamouring for something to be done. In practice, there are few indications for the use of haemodialysis and forced diuresis to accelerate the removal of drugs in poisoned patients. For example, Matthew *et al.* (1969) found it necessary to resort to haemodialysis for drug removal in only one of 1067 patients admitted to the Edinburgh

Regional Poisoning Treatment Centre in 1968. The mortality rate in this series was 0.7 %, and only three deaths could be directly attributed to drug overdosage.

GENERAL CONSIDERATIONS

Even without reliable clinical data to support the use of haemodialysis and forced diuresis, it should be possible to predict their efficacy according to well-established physicochemical, pharmacokinetic and toxicological principles. These measures are obviously useless for poisoning with irreversibly acting drugs (e.g. organophosphorus cholinesterase inhibitors) or rapidly acting metabolic poisons such as cyanide. They are also contraindicated if specific pharmacological or biochemical antagonists are available, as for example with narcotic analgesics (Evans *et al.* 1973) or paracetamol (Prescott *et al.* 1974), or in cases of overdosage with 'safe' drugs such as the benzodiazepines.

Contrary to popular belief, an impressive value for dialysance or clearance means nothing unless the plasma concentration of the drug is high enough to ensure that enough is removed to influence the clinical course favourably. The amount of drug removed is directly proportional to the clearance and the plasma concentration; the latter in turn depends on the dose absorbed and the apparent volume of distribution. Haemodialysis is generally of no value for the treatment of overdosage with drugs which have very large volumes of distribution (e.g. cardiac glycosides and weak organic bases), since the plasma contains only a very small proportion of the total amount of drug in the body, and the rate of transfer from tissues to plasma may be very slow. Thus, after distribution of a therapeutic dose of haloperidol, the plasma contains only about 0.25 % of the total amount of drug in the body. Finally, the rate of removal by haemodialysis or forced diuresis must be realistic in comparison with the spontaneous rates of elimination by metabolism or renal excretion.

HAEMODIALYSIS

The literature is replete with glowing accounts of 'successful treatment' of intoxication with many drugs by haemodialysis. Such treatment is often claimed to be 'life-saving', but evidence to support these claims is rarely to be found. Little publicity is given to the failures, and reports of controlled studies which fail to demonstrate any benefit from haemodialysis are largely ignored. Patients may still die or suffer permanent sequelae despite the use of haemodialysis (Proudfoot *et al.* 1968; Hawkins & Dorken 1969; Hartitzsch *et al.* 1972). In other words, *the treatment was successful but the patient died.* Chazan & Cohen (1969) compared the results of haemodialysis (five patients) and conservative management (12 patients) in glutethimide overdosage. Haemodialysis did not shorten the duration of coma (41 h with dialysis, 36 h without), it did not reduce the incidence of respiratory complications, and it did not improve survival since two patients died and both had been subjected to haemodialysis. Although Schreiner & Teehan (1972) admit that the clinical results with haemodialysis in glutethimide poisoning are 'frequently disappointing' they still advocate its use. Nephrologists probably see the most severely ill patients, some of whom are likely to have been grossly mismanaged, with pulmonary oedema or electrolyte problems after attempts at forced diuresis. Nevertheless, their enthusiasm for indiscriminate haemodialysis is totally unacceptable.

Some authorities have published lists of drugs which are said to be 'dialysable'. The important question, however, is 'at what rate?' According to Schreiner & Teehan (1972), drugs with molecular weights above about 350 permeate most currently available membranes very poorly, and dialysance is not significantly increased if the flow rate is increased above 200 ml/min. Notwithstanding these limitations, these authors state that many drugs with molecular weights exceeding 350 (e.g. digoxin) are dialysable. Many other drugs in these lists could not possibly be removed effectively because they have such large volumes of distribution (e.g. amphetamines and tricyclic antidepressants). Haemodialysis has even been carried out for heroin poisoning (Schreiner & Teehan 1972). This is utterly ridiculous since not only would negligible amounts be removed, but intoxication can be reversed immediately by antagonists such as nalorphine and naloxone.

Recovery from drug overdosage after haemodialysis can never be interpreted as sole evidence of efficacy since patients usually recover without such 'treatment'. Similarly, the plasma concentrations of hypnotic drugs are no certain guide to prognosis, and patients with high levels may recover without haemodialysis, especially if they have previously been taking these drugs regularly (Matthew 1971; Prescott *et al.* 1973). A rapid decline in plasma concentrations during haemodialysis means only that the drug is being removed rapidly from the plasma. It gives no indication whatsoever of the amount of drug being removed from the tissues, which is after all what counts. Few investigators draw attention to the rise in plasma concentrations of drug which may occur as a result of redistribution when dialysis is discontinued. An example of the rebound in serum concentrations of lithium after haemodialysis is shown in Fig. 1. Of particular importance is the fact that haemodialysis had no obvious effect on the cerebrospinal fluid concentrations of lithium. Nevertheless, a shortening of the half-life of the drug in plasma during dialysis is trotted out time and time again as evidence of efficacy (Maher 1972; Farid *et al.* 1972).

The drug history in poisoned patients is notoriously unreliable (Matthew

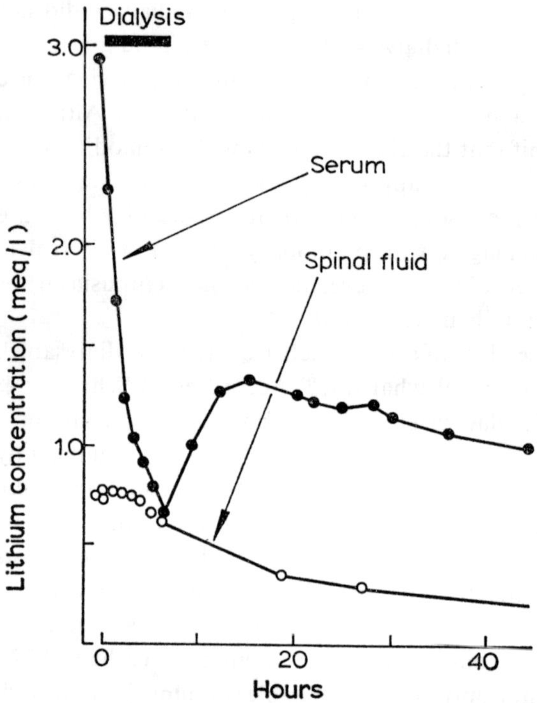

FIG. 1. Concentrations of lithium in serum (●) and cerebrospinal fluid (o) during and after haemodialysis. (Reproduced, with permission, from Amdisen & Skjoldborg 1969.)

1971), but in many reports extolling the virtues of haemodialysis there is no chemical evidence that the drug named was ever taken, let alone removed by the procedure. Thus Schreiner & Teehan (1972) state that tranylcypromine is 'dialysable', but in the report to which they refer (Matter *et al.* 1965), no attempt was made to identify the drug or to document its removal. Again, Schreiner states that phenacetin is 'dialysable'. However, haemodialysis could never remove significant amounts in a poisoned patient because this highly lipid-soluble drug has a very large volume of distribution and is rapidly dealkylated to paracetamol. In the report quoted as evidence (Fennelly & Lasker 1964), the patient had taken aspirin, phenacetin and caffeine, but haemodialysis was not carried out until 48 h after admission, at which time all the phenacetin would surely have been metabolized! Not surprisingly, no evidence was provided to show that there was phenacetin in the blood or that any had been removed. In other reports purporting to demonstrate the efficacy of haemodialysis, inspection of the data and a few simple calculations may show that dialysis had been carried out in patients who had less than therapeutic plasma concentrations of drug, or that amounts equivalent to little more than one tablet had been removed (Prescott 1972*a*).

These examples are typical of many of the reports supporting the alleged value of haemodialysis in the treatment of poisoned patients. Many others could be cited. It is clear that much more work has to be done to establish the true place of haemodialysis. On theoretical grounds it is unlikely to be effective unless the drug in question has a small volume of distribution. Compounds which come into this category include salicylate, phenylbutazone and other non-steroid acidic antiinflammatory agents, phenobarbitone, sulphonamides, sulphonylureas, some antibiotics, *d*-tubocurarine, gallamine, methanol and ethylene glycol. The toxicity of the last two compounds is caused by metabolites which are presumably also readily dialysable. Haemodialysis may also be indicated in severely intoxicated patients unable to eliminate drugs normally because of cardiac, hepatic or renal failure.

Emergency haemodialysis is not without risk, and the hazards include haemorrhage, air embolism, infection, circulatory overload or depletion, loss of a peripheral artery, and the dangers associated with the transfer of a deeply unconscious patient to a dialysis centre. Loss of platelets and clotting factors during prolonged haemodialysis may increase the risk of haemorrhage, and there is always the possibility that a genuinely suicidal patient might disconnect the shunt and exsanguinate.

FORCED DIURESIS

Forced diuresis has a limited application in the management of drug overdosage as few drugs are excreted to a significant extent unchanged in urine (Prescott 1972*b*). Most drugs are lipid-soluble in the un-ionized state and are passively reabsorbed as the concentration rises due to the progressive reabsorption of water during passage down the nephron. The concentration gradient between the tubular fluid and the medullary blood vessels is reduced during diuresis, less drug is reabsorbed, and the renal clearance is increased. A moment's thought will show that diuresis cannot increase the clearance of compounds which are not reabsorbed. It is therefore unlikely to be of value in the treatment of poisoning with poorly lipid-soluble substances. In keeping with this hypothesis, the renal clearance of polar conjugates of paracetamol is not influenced by changes in the urine flow rate and there is only a modest effect on the clearance of the sparingly lipid-soluble parent drug (Table 1). The overall elimination rate of paracetamol is not significantly increased by forced diuresis (Prescott & Wright 1973). On the other hand, the clearance of drugs such as barbiturates, which are extensively reabsorbed, is related to the urine flow rate. But even if such a rela-

TABLE 1

Ineffectiveness of forced diuresis in paracetamol poisoning

	Number of patients	*Urine flow (ml/min)*	*Renal clearance of paracetamol*	
			Unchanged (ml/min)	*Conjugated (ml/min)*
Control	5	1.6 ± 0.3	12.3 ± 1.6	132 ± 15
Forced diuresis	4	13.7 ± 2.1	23.9 ± 2.3	146 ± 15

From Prescott & Wright (1973). Figures given are means ± S.E.

tionship can be demonstrated it does not follow that diuresis will necessarily be of value, since the renal excretion of unchanged drug may still be insignificant in comparison with removal by hepatic metabolism. This is the case with all the commonly used barbiturates except barbitone, phenobarbitone and possibly butobarbitone (Bloomer 1965, 1966; Mawer & Lee 1968; Raeburn *et al.* 1969).

Manipulation of the urine pH is believed to influence the renal clearance of weak organic acids and bases with pK_a values in the ranges of 3.0–7.5 and 7.5–10.5 respectively (Milne 1965). The ionization of weak acids is increased (and lipid solubility decreased) in alkaline solution and clearance is increased because less drug is reabsorbed. The converse applies to basic drugs. Since pH is a logarithmic function, a small change in urine pH could theoretically have a disproportionate effect on clearance, especially with drugs which have pK_a values close to blood pH.

Unfortunately, forced diuresis has been shown to be of value in the treatment of overdosage with very few drugs. Only patients with moderate to severe salicylate, barbitone and phenobarbitone intoxication are treated routinely by forced alkaline diuresis at the Edinburgh Regional Poisoning Treatment Centre. Forced acid diuresis has been used for poisoning with basic drugs such as amphetamine, quinine and fenfluramine, but symptomatic treatment is usually adequate and is probably much safer. Forced diuresis is useless for poisoning with most other drugs, including short- to medium-acting barbiturates, diphenylhydantoin (phenytoin), glutethimide, methaqualone, phenothiazines, tricyclic antidepressants, paracetamol and ethchlorvynol. Many clinicians seem to think that it is indicated for overdosage of the short–medium-acting barbiturates, despite unequivocal evidence of ineffectiveness in a recent controlled trial (Hadden *et al.* 1969). In some cases forced *alkaline* diuresis has even been carried out (presumably on a spinal reflex basis) in vain attempts to enhance the elimination of basic drugs!

The 'cocktail' forced alkaline diuresis described by Lawson *et al.* (1969) is remarkably effective in relieving the symptoms of salicylism after aspirin overdosage, but this cannot be attributed solely to removal of salicylate since the average urinary excretion of the drug by those patients in 6 h was little more than 400 mg/h. Haemodilution and changes in the distribution of salicylate may be contributing factors.

Although Bloomer (1966) and Mawer & Lee (1968) have shown that the renal *clearance* of phenobarbitone is significantly increased by forced alkaline diuresis, no one seems to have looked to see how much unchanged drug can actually be removed in this way in practice. Using the forced alkaline diuresis

TABLE 2

Effect of forced alkaline diuresis on the renal clearance of phenobarbitone in 3 patients with overdosage

Hours after overdosage	*Plasma concentration (µg/ml)* [b]	*Urine flow (ml/h)*	*Urine pH*	*Renal clearance (ml/min)*	*Excretion rate (mg/h)*	*Ratio U/P* [c]
Patient 1 (28 yr, F)						
6– 30[a]	250	482	8.1	6.6	99.2	0.82
30– 54[a]	170	520	8.1	8.1	82.3	0.93
54–104	127	146	6.7	1.7	13.3	0.72
104–127	104	99	7.6	1.4	8.3	0.86
127–135	94	33	6.4	0.6	3.7	1.17
135–159	95	104	6.8	1.6	9.1	0.92
159–183	84	68	6.7	1.0	5.0	0.88
Patient 2 (29 yr, F)						
22– 44	127	20	5.3	0.3	2.1	0.83
44– 68[a]	115	379	7.7	7.4	51.0	1.17
70– 94	83	79	8.1	2.4	11.8	1.79
94–118	76	58	6.5	1.2	5.4	1.23
118–142	52	47	6.8	0.9	2.8	1.17
Patient 3 (21 yr, F)						
40– 64	126	76	—	1.7	12.8	1.34
64– 89	97	78	—	2.6	15.8	1.98
89– 92	97	150	—	3.3	19.0	1.31
92– 96[a]	94	650	7.3	13.4	75.4	1.23
96–100[a]	77	440	7.6	16.9	77.8	2.30
100–102[a]	65	885	8.0	31.1	121.2	2.11
102–108[a]	59	233	8.2	7.0	24.9	1.81
108–112[a]	55	625	8.2	18.0	59.0	1.72
112–116[a]	45	537	7.9	16.5	44.6	1.84
116–140	36	125	—	3.6	7.9	1.78
140–164	32	83	—	2.3	4.4	1.66

[a] Forced alkaline diuresis was carried out in these periods.
[b] Plasma concentrations at mid-points of urine collections.
[c] Ratio of phenobarbitone concentrations in urine and plasma.
Patients 1 and 3 took phenobarbitone and diphenylhydantoin (phenytoin) in overdosage.

regimen of Matthew & Lawson (1970), we have recently carried out such a study in three patients with phenobarbitone intoxication. Phenobarbitone in plasma and urine was estimated by direct gas liquid chromatography of chloroform extracts on SE-52 columns prepared according to Street (1970). The results are shown in Table 2. The mean clearance of phenobarbitone rose from a control value of 1.8 to 14 ml/min during the diuresis and the maximum excretion rate achieved was 121.2 mg/h. The recovery of phenobarbitone during four separate 24-h periods of diuresis in the three patients was 2.38, 1.98, 1.23 and 1.42 g compared with maximum excretion rates of 0.32, 0.28 and 0.36 g in 24 h without diuresis.

As expected, the clearance of phenobarbitone was directly related to the urine flow rate ($r = 0.96$) (Fig. 2). However, contrary to traditional teaching, changes in urine pH seemed to have little effect on the tubular reabsorption of the drug, as shown by the ratio of urine to plasma concentrations (Fig. 3). This is particularly obvious when the data points for individual patients are considered. Some patients have a consistently higher ratio than others, irrespective of the urine pH. According to Bloomer (1966), the renal clearance of phenobarbitone rises sharply as the urine pH exceeds 7.5. However, his data correspond closely to those shown in Fig. 3, but the individual values for each patient were not identified. The major discrepancies between the theoretical and observed urine-to-plasma ratios at pH values below 7.5 in the data of Bloomer confirm also that phenobarbitone clearance in poisoned patients is not dependent on urine pH to the extent claimed by the experts. In practice there would seem to be little point in making the urine alkaline.

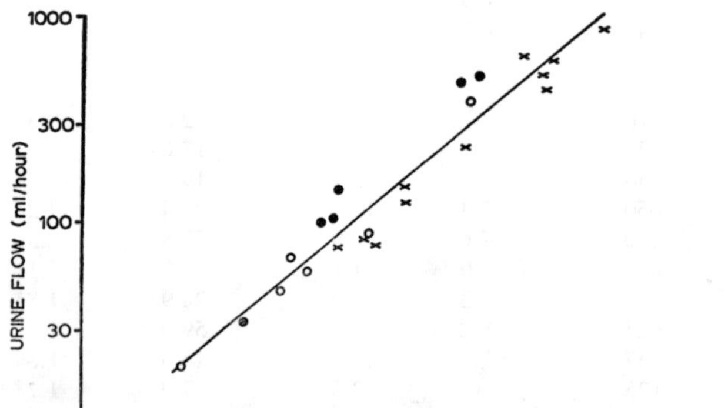

FIG. 2. Relationship between urine flow and phenobarbitone clearance after overdosage. Data from patients 1, 2 and 3 in Table 2 are represented as ●, o and x, respectively.

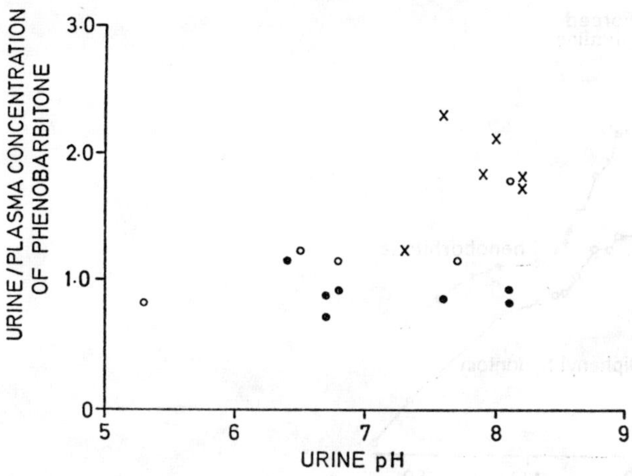

FIG. 3. Lack of correlation between ratio of urine to plasma concentration of phenobarbitone and urine pH. Data from patients 1, 2 and 3 (Table 2) are represented as ●, o and x, respectively.

As with haemodialysis, there are many reports extolling the benefits of forced diuresis in the treatment of drug overdosage. Most studies have been completely uncontrolled, and the urinary recovery of drug has often been grossly overestimated through the use of non-specific analytical methods which also measure inactive metabolites present in the urine in very high concentrations.

Contrary to popular belief, a reduction in the plasma half-life of a drug during diuresis cannot be interpreted as sole evidence of efficacy. The plasma concentration of drug may fall more rapidly because of haemodilution or pH-induced changes in distribution. There may also be a 'rebound' effect when diuresis is discontinued, but this is rarely seen because few investigators bother to monitor drug concentrations in this period. This phenomenon is shown in Fig. 4. The patient (No. 3 in Table 2) had taken phenobarbitone and diphenylhydantoin and it might be thought that the latter drug was removed by the diuresis. However, the apparent increase in the rate of elimination could be explained by distribution changes or dose-dependent metabolism since diuresis has little effect on the overall elimination of diphenylhydantoin (Bochner *et al.* 1973).

The response to diuresis could be predicted to some extent if the pharmacokinetic characteristics, metabolism, mechanisms of renal excretion and pK_a values of drugs were known. It is a pity that the drug industry cannot provide such information for clinicians instead of subjecting them to a constant barrage of banal uninformative promotional 'literature'.

Forced diuresis should never be undertaken lightly. It is potentially lethal in

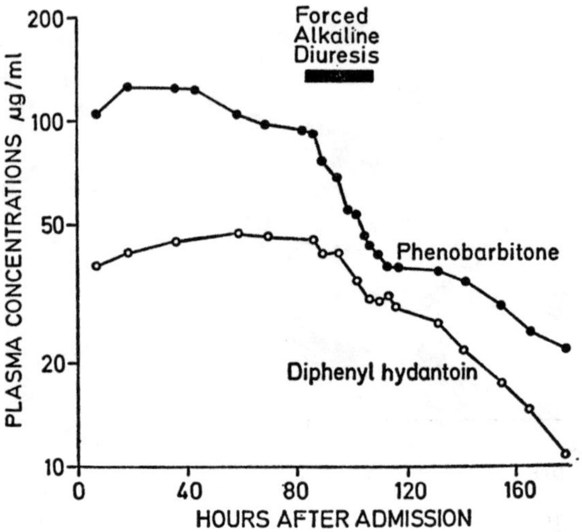

FIG. 4. Plasma concentrations of phenobarbitone and diphenylhydantoin (phenytoin) before, during and after forced alkaline diuresis (patient 3).

the old and in patients with cardiac and renal disease. There is no doubt that many patients have died with pulmonary oedema after attempts at forced diuresis. Other complications include electrolyte and acid-base disturbances, water intoxication and cerebral oedema.

THE ROLE OF THE LABORATORY

The laboratory plays a crucial role in the management of patients subjected to haemodialysis or forced diuresis. Before these measures are undertaken it is essential to identify the drug or drugs taken and to determine the plasma concentrations. Indeed, this is the most important direct contribution of the toxicology laboratory to the management of patients. The efficacy of treatment should also be documented by serial determination of plasma concentrations and of drug recovery in dialysate and urine. For such work the analytical methods used must be sensitive and highly specific. Unfortunately, the enthusiasm of clinicians for dialysis and diuresis has greatly outstripped the ability of most hospital laboratories to carry out rapid, precise and specific drug analysis. The days of simple colour tests and direct spectrophotometric assays are all but past. It is now almost always necessary to employ some form of chromatographic separation to avoid interference by metabolites and other drugs.

Gas-liquid chromatography is probably the best available general purpose technique. Very few drugs of toxicological importance cannot be measured by this method, and identification is reasonably certain with columns of different polarity and the use of on-column derivative formation (Street 1969). Unfortunately, most hospital laboratories rely on obsolete optical methods and the results obtained by inexperienced staff in emergency situations may leave much to be desired. The use of combined gas chromatography–mass spectrometry with computer matching of spectra would be an ideal approach, but is obviously far beyond the resources of the National Health Service for routine purposes in the UK.

Unbelievable confusion has been caused and is still being caused by the use of non-specific methods. Many drug metabolites have ultraviolet absorption spectra similar to or identical with those of their parent drugs, and as a general rule the major polar metabolites have little or no pharmacological activity. In spite of the low solubility of such metabolites in organic solvents, they can still interfere with the analysis, especially if short cuts are taken. Furthermore, these metabolites usually have a much smaller volume of distribution than the parent drug and their concentrations in plasma may be much higher. In this way it is possible to obtain spuriously high values for 'drug' clearance and urinary recovery.

This effect can readily be shown by the comparison of true drug concentrations with total radioactivity after administration of isotope-labelled compounds. Thus the plasma concentrations of [^{3}H]haloperidol declined normally over a period of 48 h in healthy subjects after intravenous injection of a 2 mg dose when a specific thin-layer chromatographic assay was used. However, when the 'drug' was measured as total plasma radioactivity, there was a progressive *increase* in apparent plasma concentrations over a period of 96 h (Cressman *et al.* 1972)!

Many clinical examples of erroneous results obtained by the use of non-specific methods could be cited. Matthew (1971) has already drawn attention to a dangerously misleading article which recommends the use of peritoneal dialysis and forced diuresis for the treatment of tricyclic antidepressant poisoning (Royds & Knight 1970). Impressive (but impossible) values are quoted for plasma concentrations and urinary recovery but unfortunately the hopelessly non-specific methyl orange method was used. Not only could this have included inactive tricyclic metabolites, but also the chlorpromazine, lignocaine (lidocaine), diazepam, *d*-tubocurare and unspecified antibiotics given to the patients in hospital. The fiasco was completed by the suggestion that hyperglycaemia (produced in these patients by the glucose in the dialysis fluid) might be a valuable screening test for overdosage with tricyclic antidepressants. It is a sad commentary that the authors of this paper felt that they had received advice of 'immense value' from the Poison Reference Service of a London hospital. In another report, patients with glutethimide intoxication were said to have regained consciousness with *higher* blood glutethimide concentrations than those measured when they were admitted to hospital in deep coma (Chazan & Garella 1971). It has been suggested that this was an artifact caused by interference by metabolites in the non-specific assay used (Prescott *et al.* 1973). Interpretation of some reports claiming to show the remarkable effect of diuresis and dialysis is impossible because no mention is made of the analytical methods used (Kennedy *et al.* 1969).

Some idea of the magnitude of the errors which may be introduced can be seen in Table 3. These data were selected from a report by Gibson & Wright (1972) in which ethchlorvynol in blood, haemodialysate and urine from a poisoned patient was estimated by a non-specific spectrophotometric method (Wallace *et al.* 1964) and by gas–liquid chromatography. With the method of Wallace, blood and urine concentrations of ethchlorvynol and recovery in dialysate and urine were over-estimated by factors of 22.5, 140, 7 and 82 respectively! Bloomer (1965) has shown that estimation of pentobarbitone in ether extracts of urine by spectrophotometry may yield values 10 times higher than the true concentrations as measured by gas chromatography, and similar discrepancies have been observed with the spectrophotometric assay of methaqualone in blood (Bonnichsen *et al.* 1972). In another study, only 167 mg of unchanged butobarbitone (i.e. less than two tablets) was recovered in the urine of a poisoned patient in 72 h, while the excretion of metabolites amounted to 2.86 g. Even with barbitone, a drug thought to be excreted in the urine virtually unchanged, the 72 h urinary recovery of unchanged drug and metabolites during diuresis in another patient was 11.53 and 5.38 g respectively (Raeburn *et al.* 1969).

Finally, those who perform haemodialysis must be taken to task for their *ex cathedra* statements that haemodialysis is indicated if plasma concentrations of the drug exceed a certain value. Schreiner & Teehan (1972), for example, persistently claim that plasma barbiturate concentrations above 35 μg/ml

TABLE 3

Results of ethchlorvynol assay in a poisoned patient, using a non-specific spectrophotometric method (Wallace *et al.* 1964) (A) and gas-liquid chromatography (B)

	Wallace (A)	*GLC (B)*	*Ratio A/B*
Blood concentration (μg/ml)	45	2.0	22.5
Recovery in dialysate (g)	2.1	0.3	7.0
Recovery in urine (g)	0.7	0.005	140
Concentration in urine (μg/ml)	2.61	0.032	82

Extreme values taken from data of Gibson & Wright (1972)

(short–medium-acting) and 80 μg/ml (long-acting) are potentially fatal and an indication for haemodialysis. This simply is not true. Thus barbiturate addicts and epileptics on chronic anticonvulsant therapy may be fully conscious or even ambulant at these concentrations (Matthew 1971; Prescott *et al.* 1973). The interpretation of data on plasma concentrations of drugs and the correlation with toxicity have recently been reviewed (Prescott 1973; Prescott *et al.* 1973).

References

AMDISEN, A. & SKJOLDBORG, H. (1969) Haemodialysis for lithium poisoning. *Lancet 2*, 213

BLOOMER, H. A. (1965) Limited usefulness of alkaline diuresis and peritoneal dialysis in pentobarbital intoxication. *N. Engl. J. Med. 272*, 1309–1313

BLOOMER, H. A. (1966) A critical evaluation of diuresis in the treatment of barbiturate intoxication. *J. Lab. Clin. Med. 67*, 898–905

BOCHNER, F., HOOPER, W. D., SUTHERLAND, J. M., EADIE, M. J. & TYRER, J. (1973) The renal handling of diphenylhydantoin and 5-(*p*-hydroxyphenyl)-5-phenylhydantoin. *Clin. Pharmacol. Ther. 14*, 791–796

BONNICHSEN, R., FRI, C-G., NEGOITA, C. & RYHAGE, R. (1972) Identification of methaqualone metabolites from urine extract by gas chromatography-mass spectrometry. *Clin. Chim. Acta 40*, 309–318

CHAZAN, J. A. & COHEN, J. J. (1969) Clinical spectrum of glutethimide intoxication. *J. Am. Med. Assoc. 208*, 837–839

CHAZAN, J. A. & GARELLA, S. (1971) Glutethimide intoxication. A prospective study of 70 patients treated conservatively without haemodialysis. *Arch. Intern. Med. 128*, 215–219

CRESSMAN, W. A., RENZI, N. L. & BARTHOLOMAY, A. C. (1972) Effect of volume of distribution on plasma levels of total radioactivity. *J. Pharm. Sci. 61*, 1170–1171

EVANS, L. E. J., ROSCOE, P., SWAINSON, C. P. & PRESCOTT, L. F. (1973) Treatment of drug overdosage with naloxone, a specific narcotic antagonist. *Lancet 1*, 452–455

FARID, N. R., GLYNN, J. P. & KERR, D. N. S. (1972) Haemodialysis in paracetamol self-poisoning. *Lancet 2*, 396–398

FENNELLY, J. J. & LASKER, N. (1964) Acute renal failure following acetophenetidin ingestion. *J. Med. Soc. New Jersey 61*, 115–117

GIBSON, P. F. & WRIGHT, N. (1972) Ethchlorvynol in biological fluids: specificity of assay methods. *J. Pharm. Sci. 61*, 169–171

HADDEN, J., JOHNSON, K., SMITH, S., PRICE, L. & GIARDINA, E. (1969) Acute barbiturate intoxication. *J. Am. Med. Assoc. 209*, 893–900

HARTITZSCH, B., HOENICH, N. A., LEIGH, R. J., WILKINSON, R., FROST, T. H., WEDDEL, A. & POSEN, G. A., (1972) Permanent neurological sequelae despite haemodialysis for lithium intoxication. *Br. Med. J. 4*, 757–759

HAWKINS, J. B. & DORKEN, P. R. (1969) Lithium. *Lancet 1*, 839–840

KENNEDY, A. C., LINDSAY, R. M., BRIGGS, J. D., LUKE, R. G., YOUNG, N. & CAMPBELL, D. (1969) Successful treatment of three cases of very severe barbiturate poisoning. *Lancet 1*, 995–998

LAWSON, A. A. H., PROUDFOOT, A. T., BROWN, S. S., MACDONALD, R. H., FRASER, A. G., CAMERON, J. C. & MATTHEW, H. (1969) Forced diuresis in the treatment of acute salicylate poisoning in adults. *Q. J. Med. 38*, 31–48

MAHER, J. F. (1972) Determinants of serum half-life of glutethimide in intoxicated patients. *J. Pharmacol. Exp. Ther. 174*, 450–455

MATTER, B. J., DONAT, P. E., BRILL, M. L. & GINN, H. E. (1965) Tranylcypromine sulphate poisoning. *Arch. Intern. Med. 116*, 18–20

MATTHEW, H. (1971) Acute poisoning: Some myths and misconceptions. *Br. Med. J. 1*, 519–522
MATTHEW, H. & LAWSON, A. A. H. (1970) *Treatment of Common Acute Poisonings*, Churchill Livingstone, Edinburgh
MATTHEW, H., PROUDFOOT, A. T., BROWN, S. S. & AITKEN, R. C. B. (1969) Acute poisoning: organization and work-load of a treatment centre. *Br. Med. J. 3*, 489–493
MAWER, G. E. & LEE, H. A. (1968) Value of forced diuresis in acute barbiturate poisoning. *Br. Med. J. 2*, 790–793
MILNE, M. D. (1965) Influence of acid-base balance on efficacy and toxicity of drugs. *Proc. R. Soc. Med. 58*, 961–963
PRESCOTT, L. F. (1972*a*) Haemodialysis in paracetamol self-poisoning. *Lancet 2*, 652
PRESCOTT, L. F. (1972*b*) Mechanisms of renal excretion of drugs (with special reference to drugs used by anaesthetists). *Br. J. Anaesth. 44*, 246–251
PRESCOTT, L. F. (1973) The measurement of drug concentrations in plasma—clinical applications, in *Symposium: Advances in Laboratory Medicine*, pp. 36–53; Royal College of Physicians, Edinburgh
PRESCOTT, L. F. & WRIGHT, N. (1973) The effects of hepatic and renal damage on paracetamol metabolism and excretion following overdosage. A pharmacokinetic study. *Br. J. Pharmacol. 49*, 602–613
PRESCOTT, L. F., ROSCOE, P. & FORREST, J. A. H. (1973) Plasma concentrations and drug toxicity in man, in *Biological Effects of Drugs in Relation to their Plasma Concentration* (Davies, D. S. & Prichard, B. N. C., eds.), pp. 51–81, Macmillan, London
PRESCOTT, L. F., NEWTON, R. W., SWAINSON, C. P., WRIGHT, N., FORREST, A. R. W. & MATTHEW, H. (1974) Successful treatment of severe paracetamol overdosage with cysteamine. *Lancet 1*, 588–592
PROUDFOOT, A. T., NOBLE, J., NIMMO, J., BROWN, S. S. & CAMERON, J. C. (1968) Peritoneal dialysis and haemodialysis in methaqualone (Mandrax) poisoning. *Scott. Med. J. 13*, 232–236
RAEBURN, J. A., CAMERON, J. C. & MATTHEW, H. (1969) Severe barbiturate poisoning. Contrasts in management. *Clin. Toxicol. 2*, 133–142
ROYDS, R. B. & KNIGHT, A. H. (1970) Tricyclic antidepressant poisoning. *Practitioner 204*, 282–286
SCHREINER, G. E. & TEEHAN, B. P. (1972) Dialysis of poisons and drugs—annual review. *Trans. Am. Soc. Artif. Intern. Organs 18*, 563–599
STREET, H. V. (1969) Gas-liquid chromatography of submicrogram amounts of drugs. IV. Identification of barbiturates, hydantoins, amides, imides, carbamates, phenylbutazone, carboxylic acids and hydrazine derivatives by direct derivative formation within the gas chromatograph. *J. Chromatogr. 41*, 358–366
STREET, H. V. (1970) The use of gas-liquid chromatography in clinical chemistry. *Adv. Clin. Chem. 12*, 217–307
WALLACE, J. E., WILSON, W. J. & DAHL, E. V. (1964) A rapid and specific method for determining ethchlorvynol. *J. Forensic Sci. 9*, 342–352

Discussion

Beckett: Why is diuresis used at all on scientific grounds? The rate of elimination can probably only be increased twofold, at the most, by diuresis. Why don't we just control pH for ionized drugs which are eliminated significantly in urine? This would do away with much of your criticism of forced diuresis.

Prescott: Patients are subjected to forced diuresis because doctors are naive enough to believe that as urine flow increases, more drug goes out, and that this will shorten the period of intoxication. I agree that we could make use of the pH effect, but this only applies to a few drugs and there are dangers in giving acidifying agents. How do you explain the situation with phenobarbitone, where pH has no effect on the renal clearance but the urine flow does?

Beckett: Was the excretion of 1.3–2.3 g/24 h (p. 276) by diuresis alone?

Prescott: That was with forced alkaline diuresis, which gave about a sevenfold increase in the renal excretion of phenobarbitone. Phenobarbitone clearance was directly related to urine flow, but increasing the urine pH had little or no effect. Amphetamine behaves differently.

Curry: What are the lipid solubilities of amphetamine and phenobarbitone?

Prescott: Amphetamine is much more lipid-soluble.

Beckett: In your follow-up studies, you correlated plasma levels with urinary excretion rates. If the drug is still being released from store, this correlation is not valid.

Prescott: No, it is all right because the clearance must be calculated from the plasma level. However, phenobarbitone has a pK_a of about 7.2, so a very small change in blood pH around that figure will alter the distribution between plasma and tissues greatly. There must also be haemodilution, and there is a lot more to it than just an increase in urinary excretion.

Beckett: If the pH is 7 and the pK_a is 7 a small change in pH is of no significance because we have to consider the *percentage* change of the un-ionized molecules. If it changes from 40 to 60 it is unimportant. If we are going to get rid of acids the pK_a values must be in the region of maybe 3. Then a small change in pH of the urine makes a big change in the percentage un-ionized. With bases we ought to be considering pK_a values of maybe 8.5 to 10. This is what we might recommend in terms of the drugs that will be susceptible to pH changes. General rules on these lines might be helpful.

Bridges: We can't talk about distribution volumes without rate constants. It would be wrong for a clinician to think that a particular distribution volume alone could serve as a determinant of whether dialysis should be attempted.

Goulding: I feel bound to defend the mass of clinicians who, you say, function at a spinal reflex level. There is remarkably little treatment of poisoning by haemodialysis in England at present, so perhaps the lesson has got through after all. Our follow-up is fairly intensive throughout the country and we find that the practice of diuresis is also ebbing fast!

Prescott: Don't you get patients referred from other hospitals in a parlous state after misguided attempts at forced diuresis?

Goulding: No. The urge to diurese is uncommon now.

Prescott: We don't see much ourselves either, but we hear stories.

Sunshine: Another type of therapy under evaluation is one which involves passing blood through a cylinder of charcoal. What is your opinion of that, Dr Prescott?

Prescott: The same general arguments apply. Probably the charcoal column is more efficient and produces a higher clearance of drug than haemodialysis.

Goulding: We wouldn't like to comment on that method yet. I think Dr Prescott's principles hold just the same. One needs a high volume of distribution, with enough drug in the plasma.

Scott: Carbon can contain anything from 20–30% ash, with phosphate, calcium and all sorts of things in it. Lampblack, for example, contains a significant proportion of carcinogenic hydrocarbons. If carbon is being used, I hope there is extremely rigorous control of its properties.

Goulding: There is.

Beckett: Suitable coating should prevent release from the surface of the charcoal.

Scott: Some of the techniques for determining the properties of carbon are very complicated and I doubt will be done at all.

Closer *rapport* between the clinical laboratory and the clinician is a highly attractive thought, because it can only lead to a vastly improved service to the patient, which is what we are all after.

Patel: I have conducted a retrospective study of 3500 admissions to Glasgow Western Infirmary with self-poisoning over 17 years (1954–1970) (Patel 1973). The use of forced diuresis is quite interesting. For example, there were 1136 cases of barbiturate poisoning during the decade 1962–1971 (average 113/yr, S.D. 20.57). The percentage of patients treated by forced diuresis rose suddenly in 1965 (Fig. 1*a*), coinciding with the arrival at our hospital of an enthusiast for this technique. The percentage dropped again when he left. A similar situation occurred for salicylate poisoning (Fig. 1*b*, Patel). If this can happen in one of the leading teaching hospitals in Scotland one wonders what happens in a peripheral hospital. I entirely agree with what Dr Prescott has said.

However, clinicians in the last decade have been confronted with this great increase in self-poisoning. It is the commonest cause of admission in the acute female medical ward and the second most common cause of admission in the acute male medical ward of the Glasgow Western Infirmary. One often gets the impression that physicians like to feel as if they are doing something for these patients. After all we have not forgotten the use of bemegride in the treatment of barbiturate poisoning. In spite of an excellent report from Denmark (Clemmesen & Nilsson 1961), it was a few years before we stopped the indiscriminate use of bemegride.

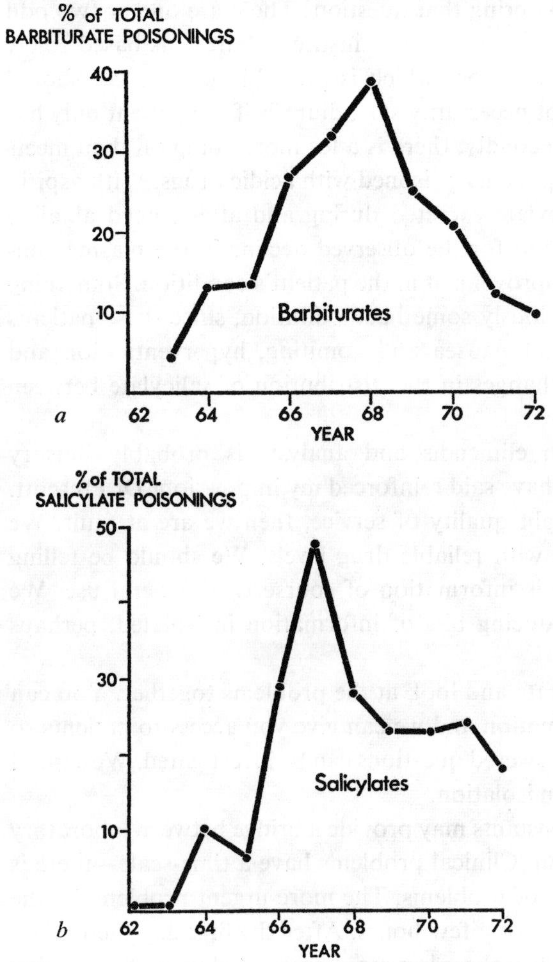

FIG. 1*a*, *b* (Patel). Effect of a change in staff on the percentage of patients who underwent forced diuresis in Glasgow Western Infirmary between 1962 and 1972 for (*a*) barbiturate poisoning and (*b*) salicylate poisoning.

Brown: Dr Prescott spoke about the demands on the laboratory in terms of drug levels. But obviously haemodialysis or forced diuresis should not be carried out without imposing a work-load of straight clinical chemistry on the laboratory. Haemodialysis, I am sure, is not done without clinical chemistry, but in smaller hospitals forced diuresis probably is, and this is a bad thing.

What actually is the mechanism of the therapeutic effect of forced alkaline diuresis in salicylate poisoning? Are you really seeking to remove the drug, or are you simply replacing the fluid deficit and correcting acidosis?

Prescott: You should be answering that question! There are one or two odd things about salicylate. Firstly, the decision to institute diuresis is based solely on the plasma salicylate concentration, which is probably wrong. We should also look at the patient, and not necessarily start diuresis if the patient only has signs of very mild salicylism. Secondly, there is a lot more going on than meets the eye when alkali is given to patients poisoned with acidic drugs. With aspirin poisoning the amount of salicylate excreted during and after forced alkaline diuresis couldn't possibly account for the observed decline in the plasma concentration or for the marked improvement in the patient's condition. Something else is happening. There is obviously some haemodilution, since these patients are often dehydrated because of nausea and vomiting, hyperventilation and sweating. There may also be changes in the distribution of salicylate between the plasma and the tissues.

Leach: The schism between clinicians and analysts is probably illusory rather than real, and what you have said reinforced my impression, Dr Prescott. If we are not providing the right quality of service, then we are at fault. We should be providing clinicians with reliable drug levels. We should be telling them about metabolites. All this information of course is of general use. We tend to think that we are producing bits of information in isolated, perhaps unique, instances.

Prescott: We have to cooperate and look at the problems together. You can provide us with valuable information and we can give you access to patients so that these many important unanswered questions can be investigated. We cannot remain independent and work in isolation.

Dole: The analysis of rate constants may provide a bridge between laboratory research and the clinical domain. Clinical problems have a time-scale—there is a kind of half-life for the decay of problems. The more urgent problems of the emergency ward have a duration of a few hours. After the first day the patient is either dead or has survived. Then there is a more protracted type of poisoning which involves metabolites and tissue-bound drugs. Thirdly, there are poisonings with a much longer time-scale, such as plutonium in the bones. It might be useful to classify clinical problems in this way because it relates to the kinetics of the metabolic processes, and also to the demands that the clinician brings to the analyst.

Our task here is to formulate clinical problems in terms that are meaningful for the laboratory. One conclusion from a study of drug kinetics is that dialysis and forced diuresis are of dubious value in treating any kind of poisoning. If these procedures have any use at all, it would certainly only be for water-soluble poisons of low potency. Diuresis in barbiturate poisoning is not likely to produce a clinically significant increase in the clearance of drug from the blood.

What the clinician needs most from the laboratory is the discovery of effective antidotes. My heart went out to Dr Widdop when he told us about getting up at 3 a.m. to shake out weak bases in chloroform, and then Professor Beckett told him that chemically this method is unreliable, while the clinicians said that the inaccuracy was really not important anyway since treatment in the emergency room is governed by symptoms rather than analytical results. Of course if antidotes were available, diagnosis would be critically important.

Gillette: Before people make decisions about dialysis or diuresis they also need to know more about the extraction ratios of drugs by liver. If 75% of the compound is really being extracted, diuresis is not going to help at all, because this would essentially represent a clearance of about 20–30% of the total cardiac output. The rate of blood flow from the various tissues really is the rate-limiting step in the elimination of some of these compounds. But the total volume of distribution really doesn't tell us what tissues bind the drugs and what the clearance of the drug from those tissues would be. We need to know whether the drugs are localized in highly perfused tissues or poorly perfused tissues, since the rate-limiting step of drug metabolism may be the mobilization of the drug from poorly perfused tissues.

Did you measure the concentration of un-ionized, unbound phenobarbitone in the plasma and in the urine, Dr Prescott? And is the plasma: urine ratio in equilibrium?

Prescott: It seems to average about 1:1. One possible explanation for the lack of effect of pH on phenobarbitone clearance is that phenobarbitone is rather slowly diffusible, and even though the pH favours reabsorption there may not be time for this to take place during diuresis because the drug is carried out of the nephron too quickly. According to the books and the experts, there ought to be a very much greater effect of pH on phenobarbitone clearance than we observed. I don't know the explanation.

Riess: Would you go so far as to discourage people who are trying to improve haemodialysis by using lipid phases and improving the properties of the membrane?

Prescott: It depends what intoxication they are trying to treat, and whether extraction of that drug can be improved. I am not against haemodialysis when it can remove useful amounts of drug, but I think that the number of such occasions is fairly small.

Riess: Many of our discussions have totally ignored the statistical aspects. Each specialist is working away on his own technique, and each supports his own findings—rightly, of course! But which national or international institute will collect all reported cases to evaluate them statistically and provide a feedback to the different clinics?

Brown: Many reports on poisoning are anecdotal and hardly worth the paper they are written on. A basic problem is the difficulty of achieving a controlled study; there are many circumstances in which one cannot ethically obtain 'controls'. I feel it is very important to set up regional poisoning treatment centres, or at least to centralize treatment, as the Scandinavians first did, so that eventually enough patients are available for meaningful statistics to be obtained.

Prescott: I agree. We have to look at this treatment in exactly the same way as at any other. We have to assess it by controlled studies, and show that we are doing something useful—if morbidity and mortality are reduced then the treatment should be accepted, irrespective of the mechanisms involved. But we can't really accept it completely until we have statistical validation. Anecdote is valueless. We need to get together and pool our resources.

Dole: Dr Van Slyke was mentioned earlier. He developed so many useful tests because he was a competent chemist faced with a variety of clinical problems in a small hospital. Today many of our best analytical chemists work in laboratories away from hospitals. This certainly contributes to the difficulty of doing rigorous clinical research.

Curry: A good example of iatrogenic disease occurred in people working with Dr Van Slyke when he was developing his mercury devices. They were heavily exposed to mercury.

Prescott: I would recommend forced alkaline diuresis for moderate and severe salicylate or phenobarbitone intoxication. Haemodialysis might be required for severe intoxication with salicylate and phenobarbitone, especially in the elderly or in patients with cardiac or renal failure. There may be a marginal benefit for very severe poisoning with glutethimide, meprobamate, ethchlorvynol and the short- and medium-acting barbiturates, but the evidence is not convincing.

Curry: What about barbitone?

Prescott: The quickest way to remove barbitone is by forced diuresis. The actual decision to institute these measures depends on many factors, such as the plasma concentration, the age of the patient, the severity of intoxication, other damage (e.g. aspiration pneumonia), the state of the cardiovascular system, and hepatic and renal function.

Curry: I was going on the physicochemical principles.

Prescott: Then for forced diuresis there are only two commonly used drugs, phenobarbitone and salicylate. Forced acid diuresis is not often used because ammonium chloride or arginine or lysine hydrochlorides have to be given intravenously. This is dangerous. If I had a patient with amphetamine intoxication, I might prefer to give diazepam rather than ammonium chloride intravenously. It would probably be safer and it would be immediately effective.

Curry: I think we have to recognize that there may be other views.

References

CLEMMESEN, C. & NILSSON, E. (1961) Therapeutic trends in the treatment of barbiturate poisonings: the Scandinavian method. *Clin. Pharmacol. Ther. 2*, 200

PATEL, A. R. (1973) The epidemic of self-poisoning. M. D. Thesis, University of Aberdeen Library

The poisoned patient: the clinician and the laboratory

ROY GOULDING

Poisons Unit, Guy's Hospital, London

Abstract After a brief survey of the earlier part of this symposium the place of the laboratory in relation to the treatment of poisoned patients is discussed. The Poisons Unit at Guy's Hospital, London, was set up in 1967 and its laboratory and information facilities are available to any hospital in the UK. The Unit's task of developing and evaluating appropriate analytical methods has been time-consuming and so far unimpressive in achievement. However, one of the lessons learned has been that laboratory findings must always be correlated with the clinical condition of the patients. Another lesson is that one of the contributions of the Poisons Unit has been in resolving diagnostic uncertainties. It is concluded that regional or supraregional centres of clinical pharmacology, of which clinical toxicology is a subspecialty, could be of increasing benefit in the National Health Service, although there is not necessarily sufficient scope or justification for separate departments of clinical toxicology.

At my advanced age I may perhaps be allowed to indulge first in historical recollection. In the years immediately after the Second World War electrocardiograms were becoming part of the equipment of numerous hospitals. Their use, however, was never routine; they were seldom to hand on an emergency basis. Often their interpretation in clinical terms was somewhat remote. At that stage a friend of mine, struggling with the clinical part of the MRCP examination and trying to master the enigma of a patient with heart disease, tried to invoke the ECG, only to have his renowned examiner tear up the tracing and disparagingly reject it with a remark about 'meaningless squiggles on a length of paper'. Yet today it would be a courageous cardiologist who would attempt to practise his specialty without such a crucial electronic aid. Possibly when the clinical toxicologist has similarly enjoyed some thirty years of a proper laboratory service, he too will appreciate its assistance.

If I may now comment on some of the contributions in this active three-day symposium, I will refer to *Dr Newton* first. I find his declaration of practical principles for managing poisoned patients, in the main, unassailable. May he not, at the same time, have slightly overstated his case? While I agree that precise identification of the drug taken in overdosage may not be essential in every instance, it is doubtful whether a doctor is even required for about 80% of patients so admitted. The patients' own physical resources will, with skilled nursing care, almost invariably allow them to recover. In the more problematic cases, though, there is no point in totally rejecting laboratory aid simply because in the past its methods have been unequal to the task. One might as well have condemned commercial air travel for ever in the 1920s because the machines then were neither adequate nor reliable.

Dr Dole's description of the mandatory application of chemical analysis to the urine of all drug-dependent patients and the subsequent exploitation of these findings for recriminatory measures was, to me, indeed alarming. In Britain no such system exists. Urine testing is at the selective behest of the physician looking after the patient, as a guide to treatment and rehabilitation, and to assist rather than to interfere with his *rapport* with the patient. In such circumstances it has proved—as I can assert from first-hand experience—invaluable, if only as a counter to self-delusion on the part of the physician.

However, in this connection 'second-rate laboratories', as Dr Dole emphasizes, can do more harm than good. In London we find it imperative to organize repeated 'quality control' testing of the laboratories participating in this work.

We are not only indebted to *Dr Gillette* but also filled with admiration for his elegant exposition of the manner in which fundamental research in the toxicology laboratory can form the foundation for clinical treatment in the hospital, notably for paracetamol overdoses and liver damage.

Next, *Professor Beckett's* almost iconoclastic disclosure of the foibles of most of the hallowed procedures commonly accepted in the laboratory was demoralizing enough to prompt all the chemists in the audience to commit hara-kiri on the spot. Surely, though, his condemnation has more implications for metabolic and pharmacokinetic studies than for patient management? At the same time it serves as a warning to us not to put too much emphasis at this stage on so-called 'pharmacokinetic principles' in fashioning our therapeutic and toxicological attitudes in the clinic.

Subsequently the beauties, the intricacies and the refinements to which *Professor Holmstedt*, *Dr Scott* and *Dr Riess* introduced us and with which they enthralled us in their descriptions of mass spectrometry and isotope techniques might well have indicated the 'shape of things to come', albeit in the not-too-distant future. Whether we are on the threshold of employing these undeniably expensive laboratory elaborations in the day-to-day service of clinical toxicology remains, to me at least, questionable. On the other hand, the immunological procedures which *Dr Parker* and *Professor Sunshine* described have already established a foothold in the hospital, notably in relation to the control of digoxin treatment and the avoidance of poisoning thereby.

The ignorance, to which *Professor Gee* drew attention, of the part possibly played by drugs in deaths being investigated by morbid anatomists is a feature we cannot ignore. Professor Gee's own discoveries about barbiturates, where the presence of these substances was not otherwise suspected, are arresting. It would be interesting to learn from him to what extent a virtually routine, yet comprehensive, toxicological analysis would be justified in his realm. This might uncover an incidence of 'drugged baby' incidents analogous to the 'battered baby' syndrome that has become increasingly recognized over recent years.

Finally, the comments made by *Mr Leach* and *Dr Prescott* are, surely, complementary. Until recently, laboratory instrumentation and manipulation had not kept pace with the clinicians' requirements. If and when they become suitably perfected then Dr Prescott's criticism may be substantially modified.

OBJECTS OF THE LABORATORY

Despite various suggestions, the place of the laboratory in relation to the treatment of the poisoned patient has never been well defined. Indeed that is why this symposium was held. Some practical steps have nevertheless been taken in an effort to clarify this issue and the unit for which I am responsible is probably a fair example of what has been done. A National Poisons Information Service was established in the UK in 1963. Four years later, and arising from that Service, a central toxicological laboratory was set up, with monies for both capital and recurrent expenditure granted from the Research and Development Fund of the Ministry of Health (Goulding 1971). Although administered as a department of Guy's Hospital, London, the facilities of this laboratory are used by any other hospitals in the country that choose to take advantage of the service. For reasons of transport and communications most demands come from the Greater London area and the south-eastern part of Britain, but they are by no means confined to those areas.

Looking back over the seven years of our operation, I must admit to some disappointment at what I regard as the limited progress that we have made. Not that I can complain of lack of either equipment or staff. But much time, energy, brain work and man-hours of technically qualified people have perforce been diverted to devising, developing and evaluating appropriate analytical methods. This task has been time-consuming and far from impressive in achievement, but on reflection quite a lot has been accomplished, even if our publications to date hardly reflect the advances we already accept in our day-to-day work.

Secondly, it is imperative that these laboratory exercises should not be conducted in isolation, but that the findings should be constantly referred to and correlated with the condition of the patients (or volunteers) from whom the samples have been derived. Many of the anomalies to which reference has been made at this meeting can probably be ascribed to failure to maintain this alignment between the ward and the bench.

As we have moved (as I hope) forward, we have been impressed with the different needs of, say, a highly specialized poisons unit like that at the Royal Infirmary, Edinburgh, and those of the district general hospital. In the latter, uncertainties of diagnosis are inevitable in emergency medicine, above all in the accident and emergency departments. This is no reflection on the competence of the physicians but is an illustration of the diversity of diagnostic possibilities encountered outside the exclusive type of poisons centre. During this symposium not only clinicians but also, somewhat to my astonishment, non-medical chemists and biochemists have asked: what does it matter what the patient has taken, for surely the management is virtually the same anyhow and will be altered not one iota by specific identification? May I reply that, to me, that is begging the question. In twelve months we have been called upon, as Dr Widdop has explained, to carry out upwards of 300 urgent analyses. Not all of these, I should add, present themselves at night. Yet, even though we accept none of the requests made to us as a routine and agree to carry out tests only when the physician responsible for the patient and his clinical counterpart in the unit consider that the laboratory may be of assistance, we have found that our principal contribution has been in resolving diagnostic uncertainties. For instance, a man was found unconscious in the road with obvious head injuries, but no fractures. Analysis then revealed a heavy overdose of methadone and barbiturates, without (as only subsequently became obvious) any traumatic damage to the brain at all. Conversely, two young people who were admitted semicomatose after a traffic accident, with their pockets loaded with tablets, capsules and so on, were found to be harbouring no drug at all in their body tissues. Their condition, indeed, was entirely traumatic in origin. Further, a young child was admitted to a children's ward with puzzling cardiac arrhythmias and although there was no history at all of contact with drugs, the laboratory demonstrated a massive overdose of tricyclic antidepressants. Corresponding examples could be catalogued at length. Maybe, with the superiority of hindsight, one could agree that this made no real difference to the outcome. I can only answer that, in the front line of emergency medicine, any illumination that the laboratory can cast on the dubious case can be enormously helpful, if only to offset further investigation, intervention and, possibly, unnecessary treatment.

Simply to promote the concluding general discussion, may I suggest, therefore, that the laboratory can unquestionably help the cause of the poisoned patient in the following ways:

(1) In emergency situations of the type I have instanced, when management can be more effectively and assuredly designed with a reliable check on the extent to which poisons may, or may not, be contributory;

(2) In the critical evaluation of allegedly improved schemes of management and treatment, for, when the overall mortality in hospital from poisoning is under 1%, statistically significant advances are difficult to demonstrate in terms of populations;

(3) For purposes of research, especially on pharmacokinetics;

(4) In experimental biochemical research aiming to elucidate toxicological mechanisms in order to formulate rational treatment in place of empirical management;

(5) In therapeutic monitoring of drugs, to avoid iatrogenic poisoning or—what may sometimes be just as dangerous for the patient—inadequate medication;

(6) By providing wider forensic support.

To bring all these needs together schematically I should emphasize that, although I cannot convince myself that there is sufficient scope or justification for clinical toxicology as yet another subspecialty in medicine—for any properly-trained and competent physician should be capable of caring for the poisoned patient largely according to the general supportive principles germane to all emergency medicine—, I feel sure that centres of clinical pharmacology (within the spectrum of which clinical toxicology reflects but one extreme) could be set up under the National Health Service with increasing benefit, on a regional or possibly a supraregional scale. Philosophically, as a doctor devoted to the greatest good for all concerned, I might then come to terms with that nagging question that troubles all of us preoccupied by poisoning—are we using too much of the limited expertise and funds of the health service for a limited section of the community that is intent, however misguidedly, on its own destruction?

Reference

GOULDING, R. (1971) in *Portfolio for Health* (McLachlan, G., ed.), pp. 137–142, Nuffield Provincial Hospitals Trust, London

General discussion II

PRECISE ANALYTICAL TECHNIQUES

Curry: Professor Goulding's survey will have reminded us of the general problems we have been discussing so far. The first question for this final discussion is: in view of the known limitations and pitfalls, particularly when we get down into trace determinations, do analytical procedures need to be more precise and accurate? Professor Beckett told us about some of the pitfalls and we know that great difficulties arise in the analysis of submicrogram amounts.

The differential results obtained with ultraviolet spectroscopy and gas chromatography illustrate what I was hoping would come out of the meeting, which is that analysts doing toxicology must know what they are measuring and that the minutiae of analyses must be emphasized. When the results are correlated with clinical effects, the analytical results must be right.

Sunshine: Editors who publish both the data and critical reviews must insist that authors provide explicit measurements.

Beckett: Meaningful levels, as distinct from gross overdosages, will become important for the clinical pharmacological laboratories and we need to prepare for this problem. But editors delete the sections of papers that refer to the pitfalls. Our discussions here will show up some of the basic pitfalls. Many laboratories use established methods and think everything is all right without realizing the many problems involved in separation techniques and analyses in biological fluids.

Curry: Professor Goulding emphasized how many man hours went into developing the techniques used in his laboratory.

Prescott: The laboratory should give the value and a standard deviation, which might be quite revealing.

Curry: The question is what has been measured, and the accuracy of the measurement.

Prescott: If the concentration of barbiturate is given as 15 μg/ml ± 4.5 μg or whatever the figure is, at least people might realize the problems facing the laboratory.

Beckett: But if the clinician doesn't know that the laboratory may be making mistakes, whatever they put in terms of the limits would be misleading.

Prescott: Clinicians accept laboratory reports with blind faith. If there is a discrepancy between the laboratory result and the clinical state, the clinician rarely first suspects the laboratory.

Goulding: I would like to support this. Typed laboratory reports and computer print-outs seem to acquire an undue righteousness and unassailability and we now have to check that our own clinical colleagues don't accept them without question.

Scott: It also depends on how the results are reported. If a value of 15.7 is given, the implication is that 0.7 has some significance, which it almost certainly doesn't. If a value of 15 is given, then 1 should have significance. Figures should be reported in units which are significant. Repeatability should also be known and determined, of course.

The idea of having standardized methods is not new. Many organizations or disciplines have standard methods and toxicologists need a body that will provide a textbook of standard methods that have to be used, just as British Standards are. This would need a lot of work and investment but it would allow both toxicologists and clinicians to know what was going on and how much confidence they could place on results.

Gillette: We must also remember that a method developed with plasma is not necessarily suitable for other tissues.

SIMPLE SCREENING TESTS

Curry: The next question is whether any more screening tests can be developed. At the nanogram level, is it technically possible to develop other methods?

Sunshine: I would say that radioimmunoassay is now at the nanogram per millilitre level. Specificity is a problem but in this context we are not concerned with specificity. We would rather have more immunoassays for more screening procedures. Lack of specificity for this application is no drawback so long as the positive results are confirmed by another technique.

Curry: But the clinicians are asking for a simple screening test which gives, say, a colour change, and at these low levels it is not possible to get a colour change.

Beckett: Doesn't it depend on whether we are really talking about the poisoned patient or about the drug that produces the effect, even though it may be a metabolite that is active? In general we don't want unduly sensitive tests but broad screens which will rule out the major possibilities.

There is a suitable test for barbiturates and another for basic drugs, so we can already deal with about 95% of poisoned patients. What we need to know is what other types of drugs are a major problem.

Curry: Do you mean that the immunological tests should be directed to these two groups?

Beckett: No. The barbiturate test is reasonable. Immunological tests should only be used for certain classes of drugs which are difficult to analyse by other methods.

Goulding: Our comprehensive screening is designed for the detection of just those drugs recognized as the most popular with patients taking an overdose. These drugs are the ones we look for. Of course, we have to watch out constantly for the new drugs. The next antidepressant released on the market is certainly going to give us cases of overdose within a week or two.

Leach: Methods developed for pharmacological studies are not necessarily suitable for this type of work. An investigator usually knows that a volunteer is taking only one drug so he doesn't need to worry about drug interactions at all. He can even restrict the diet if necessary. The temptation is to use a method that a pharmaceutical company has produced for laboratory research, but in many circumstances such a method is almost useless.

Goulding: Our experience of screening patients for what they have actually taken makes me agree with you.

Curry: A fundamental problem is that only one new screening test simple enough for bedside use has been introduced in the last 12 years—the one for Paraquat (dimethylbipyridinium dichloride) (Matthew *et al.* 1968*b*).

Leach: Nobody has mentioned the possibility of using latex agglutination tests for drugs. Radioimmunoassay is extremely sensitive, perhaps too sensitive, and a limit of detection of 1 μg/ml would be adequate for barbiturates, for example.

Gee: For my 'non-patient patients' we don't want a terribly sensitive test, which might give all sorts of trouble; we simply want to know whether a drug has been responsible for death. Iatrogenic disease is a different problem. We need to use most of the available screening tests because even when we think the cause of death is obvious, the person may have taken a drug overdose as well. The man who has a coronary thrombosis may have taken a barbiturate overdose because he couldn't stand the pain; but which really caused his death? In fact people who get run over should be screened, just as much as any others. I would like chemical analysis to be available for all autopsies, just as histology is.

Jackson: Until the poison is specified to the chemist, so that he knows the structure and has something to work on, 'poison' remains a biochemical concept. I don't think you can have a chemical test for a biochemical concept unless you are going to use a biochemical method. You need some form of life as a reagent.

Prescott: A patient who had a cerebral haemorrhage but who was also taking several drugs could provide a tricky problem. About a third of the adult population in the UK are taking drugs of some sort, and even with specific analytical methods and hard pharmacokinetic data, the problems would be immense. Professor Holmstedt has told us about the long half-life of methaqualone, and many other drugs probably also have unexpectedly prolonged disappearance curves if concentrations are followed for long enough. The plasma half-life may be much longer after chronic administration than after a single dose because of the slow release of drug from tissues. Many of the data on drug levels and half-lives in the literature have been obtained after administration of a single dose to healthy persons and must be interpreted with care.

RESEARCH AND ITS CONSEQUENCES

Curry: We are getting into what the biochemist can do in future research. There are two different aspects here. Is research inhibited because there is insufficient money, or insufficient understanding of what is going on? Cost affects what can be put into an emergency service. Is the cost of mass spectrometers coming down? Is Utopia imminent? We must now consider research and the consequences of research.

Goulding: Antidotes may not help much and so many people get better anyway. When we analysed the deaths from poisoning in our group of hospitals over six years, we found that half were physiologically irredeemable, even though they got to hospital alive. If we revise the mortality figures accordingly, the number of lives that might be saved becomes so small that expensive research in this field becomes difficult to justify.

Sunshine: Part of the answer here lies in the inadequate distribution of effort, which leads to inefficiency and poor results. I am essentially a centralist at heart and I envy the UK because it has the Central Research Establishment laboratories at Aldermaston, with all that has come out of there. It is a splendid effort. I understand that multipurpose regional units are under consideration, where research and service would be combined. I think we can get many answers in this way. Clinicians and chemists can work together in such units, to the benefit of the patient and the community.

Beckett: I don't think the search for new antidotes will solve our problems.

The cost of finding a new antidote would be prohibitive, relative to the profits from its sale.

Prescott: I disagree. In my view there *is* a great future in this approach. It is only if we understand the mechanisms of toxicity that rational and intelligent therapy can be applied to overcome the biochemical lesion. This is exemplified by the work of Dr Mitchell and Dr Gillette on paracetamol (Mitchell *et al.* 1973).

The mortality rate in self-poisoning in Edinburgh is much less than 1% and most deaths are unavoidable. Paracetamol and Paraquat are the drugs which have caused us most concern. We can now do something for paracetamol poisoning, but we are helpless against Paraquat. It is terrible to watch a patient die over a period of several weeks with progressive pulmonary lesions after accidental ingestion of Paraquat. We must use the best available techniques to establish the biochemical mechanisms of toxicity. We will never get anywhere otherwise.

Beckett: I accept that, provided that what you use is something already approved for use in man. If it has not been approved for use in man then I can repeat my question: who is going to pay for the cost of development? Even if you know the biochemistry, the cost will equal the cost of developing a new drug—about £4 million or £5 million.

Riess: Finding new antidotes would probably need the same effort as finding new drugs. We synthesize 7000 compounds before we find one therapeutic drug, and the cost of producing antidotes would be tremendous.

Prescott: I don't see any need for an antidote to go through the whole process for a new drug application. The Committee on Safety of Medicines in the UK and the Food and Drug Administration in the USA are political structures and there are ways of dealing with specific problems of this sort. There is nothing in law to stop me from giving beeswax in milk (or anything else) for the treatment of barbiturate poisoning if I judge this to be the right thing for my patient. It is also possible to give an unlicensed drug to a named patient. In any event the present system has not prevented the introduction of drugs such as naloxone—a specific narcotic analgesic antagonist.

Moffat: A very powerful medicine called a universal antidote is kept on the shelf in our laboratory for when we take poisons. It may be charcoal, but it may work!

Curry: In minor cases, if an antidote shortened the stay in hospital by a week, surely that is a benefit that weighs against the cost of the antidote?

Goulding: The average stay in hospital now is not very long. If we are really interested in cost–benefit and human welfare, we are looking at the wrong set of patients. There are about 5000 deaths every year from poisons in England and

Wales, over 4000 of which are entirely the concern of the forensic pathologists. They die before even reaching medical care. If we really want to salvage mankind we have to prevent these cases, not treat them. Most are deaths from barbiturate poisoning. It is my unfortunate experience to observe that patients seen by a psychiatrist after taking an overdose are not infrequently prescribed three or four different psychotropic drugs instead of perhaps the two that they were receiving before the event. Some people, I am told, make a living by taking in each other's washing. Clinical toxicologists and the psychiatrists seem to me to verge on a similar relationship.

Newton: We have good psychiatric support in Edinburgh; at the same time rarely do we see severe psychological illness in patients admitted to our ward. Most patients are making a manipulative gesture, and very few are psychiatrically ill enough to need further hospital therapy.

Prescott: You can't give drugs to cure the social ills which are the basis of most of the self-poisoning that we see.

Moffat: If radioimmunoassay methods like EMIT and FRAT are developed there is a possibility of using the antibodies for treatment. Dr Parker (p. 207) said that if a patient who had taken an overdose of digoxin had a theoretical level of 2–5 ng/ml, or up to 10 times the normal level, then 3–16 mg of antibody protein would mop up most of the digoxin. This is a possibility with some drugs given in very low doses, like digoxin, although perhaps not with barbiturates. Another way of preventing overdoses used to be to include ipecacuanha, which was supposed to make people sick before they could swallow too many pills.

Goulding: Ipecacuanha is too toxic to be used routinely in that way!

DRUG LEVELS AND INDIVIDUAL VARIATIONS

Curry: Are individual variations so great that they render the correlation between clinical features and blood levels useless in cases of poisoning?

Goulding: Many of the discrepancies that have been reported were probably due to the different analytical methods and techniques being used. I would like to see reliable blood level profiles for therapeutic doses of each of the common barbiturates in man—not in the rat, the guinea pig or any other animal species, for that matter.

Jackson: Parker *et al.* (1970) gave prisoners repeated large doses, supposedly therapeutic, of barbiturates and studied the blood and urine levels.

Prescott: Matthew *et al.* (1968*a*) studied the plasma concentrations of methaqualone, on admission to hospital, in relation to the grade of consciousness after overdoses of Mandrax (methaqualone plus diphenhydramine). Similar data are available for glutethimide and barbiturates (Matthew &

Lawson 1966; Wright & Roscoe 1970). There was a surprisingly poor correlation between the degree and duration of unconsciousness and the amount of drug measured in the blood.

Scott: You have two variables there—either the patient was different or the analysis was wrong. But the question was, do you as a clinician, irrespective of the value given, think that variability between individuals would render even accurate analyses useless?

Prescott: We are often faced with this problem in practice. Fortunately, we are well aware of the limitations of plasma concentration data in this situation. We rely on the clinical findings and not on the laboratory results for hypnotic drugs.

Scott: Forgetting about analyses, when you give a drug to different individuals with the same disease, how much does the dose vary from one individual to another if you are to get an effect?

Prescott: This can vary from the sublime to the ridiculous, depending on the circumstances.

Scott: So you are saying that however accurate the analyses are, the variability between individuals is too great for the results to be useful?

Prescott: It might well be in certain circumstances. To use the laboratory result intelligently we must understand the mechanisms responsible for individual variation in drug response.

Holmstedt: Dr Sjöqvist and associates showed that tricyclic antidepressants given in the same dose to different people can produce a 40-fold difference in plasma levels. This is probably due to genetically determined differences in metabolism (Sjöqvist *et al.* 1968).

In studies on nortriptyline Alexanderson (1973) found a fivefold range in the plasma half-lives and a twofold variation in the apparent volume of distribution of nortriptyline (assuming complete availability on oral administration). No correlation was found between the plasma half-life and the apparent volume of distribution. Analysis of variance showed that most of the interpersonal variations in plasma half-life, in apparent volume of distribution and in conjugation were genetically determined. The plasma half-life and apparent volume of distribution may contribute independently to the total variation in the 'steady-state' plasma level of nortriptyline.

Goulding: That is a good example to cite. Two factors must be taken into account. If you give the same dose of such a drug to a population of people you will find an enormous variation in the individual plasma levels, but when you study the clinical response, there is an extraordinarily close relationship with the plasma levels. Other groups of drugs have not been studied with the same thoroughness.

Holmstedt: We have two studies going on, with the technique I described in my paper (this volume, pp. 105–124). As many parameters as possible are monitored, including psychological reactions. One study is of methaqualone and the other, being done with Stig Agurell and his group, is on the effect of cannabis where tetrahydrocannabinol is monitored in the blood. The only way to do this is to study whatever one can, clinically and psychologically, in a number of individuals, and at the same time have an absolutely clear method for analysis. Our preliminary findings with methaqualone indicate that the effects we can record do not correspond at all to the blood curve except during the rising phase.

Prescott: In a series of patients who took short- to medium-acting barbiturates and no alcohol, consciousness was regained at plasma barbiturate levels (measured by GLC) ranging from 8 to 61 μg/ml (Table 1, Prescott). In another report (Haider 1971) the EEG was isoelectric (flat) in a patient with a blood butobarbitone level of only 19 μg/ml!

Curry: You cannot compare two different barbiturates.

Prescott: What is the relationship between the concentrations and pharma-

TABLE 1 (Prescott)

Plasma barbiturate concentrations and half-lives in 10 patients admitted in Grade IV coma following uncomplicated barbiturate overdosage (reproduced, with permission, from Prescott *et al.* 1973).

Patient	*Age & sex*	*Barbiturate*	*Maximum plasma level (μg/ml)*	*Duration of coma (h)*	*Plasma level on regaining consciousness (μg/ml)*	*Plasma drug half-life* (h)*
1A	44M	buto	118	16	61	12
1A	44M	buto	100	24	52	12
2R	74F	amylo	55	13V	32	13→6
3R	47F	quinal	67	42V	8	14→7
4	52F	amylo	66	40V	22	56→13
5	27F	amylo +	76	76V	11	46→12
		quinal	52		3.7	33→11
6	23F	amylo	47	30	26	15
7	33F	amylo	43	36V	14	13
8	24M	amylo +	17	38	5.2	32→12
		quinal	15		1.7	18→7
9	22F	amylo +	16	24	8.2	30→8
		quinal	13		4.9	35→8
10	27M	pento	28	24	13	26→17

A = Addicted to barbiturates, R = barbiturates used regularly as hypnotics, V = assisted ventilation. *The first and second figures represent initial and terminal plasma barbiturate half-life values respectively. There was no change in half-life in patients 1, 6 & 7.

cological actions of the commonly used short- to medium-acting barbiturates taken in overdosage in man?

Curry: There is a lot of published work on this (see, e.g., Curry 1969, 1972).

Sunshine: For four amylobarbitones in your table, Dr Prescott, the figures are 14, 22, 26 and 32 μg/ml (see Prescott *et al.* 1973). That is not a very big spread. For butobarbitone you show 61 and 52 μg/ml.

Prescott: The duration of coma in those cases was quite different, and the two values for butobarbitone were in the same patient admitted on two separate occasions.

Scott: Either the analytical procedure or the human patient may produce errors in those figures. You can't tell the difference. It would be much nicer if, as well as the analyses, you knew the actual dose given under clinical conditions. That would allow the correlation to be made.

Prescott: I am trying to show the actual variation we encounter in clinical practice. I am sorry that it does not agree with the textbooks, but we must face reality. The duration and severity of coma in patients poisoned with short- to medium-acting barbiturates, glutethimide and methaqualone bears little relation to the plasma concentrations. There are many possible explanations (Prescott *et al.* 1973). This problem will not go away just because we ignore it.

Sunshine: You have data on four or five experiments simultaneously recorded in that table, Dr Prescott. They have to be analysed individually. It is grievous to draw conclusions from a miscellany such as that chart represents.

Widdop: How sure were you that these patients had only taken one drug, Dr Prescott?

Prescott: A urine screening test was done on all patients, to exclude most of the commonly used drugs. Of course we can't exclude everything.

Dole: It is clear that clinically a given blood level, however exactly measured, can have different implications in terms of the biological effect. Tolerance is conspicuous with narcotics. With habitual use of barbiturates there is also a significant increase in cellular tolerance. The same burden in the body, measured by the plasma level or any other method, does not always have the same biological implications.

Goulding: What troubles me about addiction, or the continual taking of barbiturates, is that I thought this stepped up the metabolism and then a larger dose was needed to obtain the same plasma levels. I agree with you about narcotics, Dr Dole.

Beckett: Ruling out the problem of tolerance, surely there is still another variable: the fact that in very few cases indeed is the parent drug solely responsible for the activity seen. With all the antidepressants, for instance, the activity results from a mixture of many metabolites plus parent drug. Therefore I cannot see how we can expect a correlation between activity and the level of one component of a mixture of active compounds.

Leach: We often argue on insufficient data. We need a lot of data and a lot more work. We need to know the drug levels in members of the ordinary population who are not poisoned patients in the accepted sense, although in fact they may well be poisoned. They may be so near the edge of disaster that it would be very useful for us to know what the real situation is. What are the levels of parent drug and metabolites in the person who habitually takes barbiturates?

Brown: In clinical chemistry, many substances are measured relatively non-specifically, but there are also some that are measured highly specifically. It is now beginning to be possible to tackle the problem of temporal variation both between individuals and within individuals, and to set 'normal ranges' for age and sex for some of the more specifically measured components. It must be much more complicated to do this for substances that are not endogenous body constituents. We must look at this problem of the significance of drug levels in a statistical sense; I cannot believe that we will ever be able to interpret a 'one-off' drug level absolutely quantitatively.

Curry: I was afraid we had been denigrating measurements of blood levels of drugs here and I am glad we are now saying that quantification must make sense. We have some ideas and we are aiming for the day when we can interpret differences between individuals. Of course nobody's blood sugar levels are always the same. They vary with different individuals and between male and female. Genetic characteristics affect metabolic hydroxylation by microsomes, and several examples are coming along now. We need more information but we must not forget about blood levels.

Gillette: Blood levels should be related to the pharmacological response, not to a therapeutic response or to a toxic response. We frequently don't know the relationship between the pharmacology and the toxicity, or between the pharmacology and the therapeutic effectiveness of drugs. A good illustration of the distinction between these aspects was shown by Sjöqvist *et al.* (1968) for the antidepressants. Patients can become depressed by a variety of different mechanisms and not just by abnormal catecholamine metabolism. Those patients whose depression is not related to the abnormal catecholamine metabolism are not improved by amitriptyline.

Goulding: The term 'half-life' may be misleading in these circumstances. It is a perfectly good mathematical expression when one administers a single dose of a drug, say, by intravenous injection. But when patients take an overdose by mouth, absorption may be both inhibited and prolonged. The decline in plasma levels then reflects not elimination alone, but the product of continuing absorption and elimination.

Prescott: The half-life is often not constant.

Gillette: As a pharmacokinetic term it has significance only in the last phase of the plasma level curve, when all of the distribution phases, including absorption, are complete.

REPORTING THE EFFECTIVENESS OF TREATMENT

Curry: Procedures for reporting the adverse effects of drugs are already in existence. Could clinicians similarly record their successes and failures with treatment procedures in poisoning cases?

Prescott: It should be done. This has been put to the Committee on Safety of Medicines, but they do not seem interested in knowing about the morbidity and mortality of drug overdosage. They do not want the 'yellow cards' on which they asked doctors to report suspected adverse reactions to drugs.

Goulding: A few completed 'yellow cards' are sent to me. They are not very illuminating. Commonly the records of observation and management of poisoned patients who succumb are incomplete and uninformative. In two of the National Health Service regions we specifically followed up the deaths which took place in hospital from poisoning to find out exactly what had occurred. It proved very difficult to find the exact reasons for treatment failures.

Curry: The chemists are trying to get accurate and precise numbers but clinicians don't show the same inward-looking criticism. To judge efficiency you have to have numbers. Are we to go on with the idea of only reporting cases when we think they are successes?

Prescott: If doctors were paid for notifying adverse drug reactions, as they used to be for notifying infectious diseases, something might happen. But no one cares how many patients are killed by doctors or drugs. The whole emphasis is wrong. Infectious disease is not a very important cause of death now in this country, compared to death and morbidity caused by drugs taken for therapeutic reasons or in overdosage.

Patel: Table 2 (Patel) lists the sources from which patients in my 1971 survey (see p. 230) obtained their drugs. These figures have all been checked. Psychiatrists or hospital doctors prescribed only a small percentage. The patients who stole drugs or obtained them in a public bar were mostly abusers of drugs and they usually abused methaqualone or barbiturates with alcohol. We had no difficulties with the general practitioners. If we were in doubt about the source we contacted the chemist whose name appeared on the bottle, and occasionally we contacted the Scottish Pricing Bureau.

TABLE 2 (Patel)

Sources of drugs used for self-poisoning in Glasgow, 1971

	Men (207)		*Women (313)*	
General practitioner	146	54%	240	64%
Psychiat./hosp. doctor	11	4%	19	5%
Relative/friend	51	19%	60	16%
Bought (chemist/shop)	32	12%	49	13%
Stolen/public bar	30	11%	7	2%
Total No. of drugs	270	100%	375	100%

MULTIPLE DRUG ABUSE

Curry: That brings us to multiple drug abuse. Shouldn't multiple drug intake be assumed by the clinicians and the laboratory until proved otherwise? It might account for the present difficulties in diagnosis.

Goulding: Even if the patient has taken an overdose of three drugs, supportive management is usually sufficient. Often the combination is far from lethal. In the laboratory it is important not to be content with measuring just one blood level. First one needs to identify all of the drugs present and proceed to measure each of them. Only then will the figures be meaningful.

Newton: In practice it is usually the principal drug involved which produces the clinical syndrome, unless the other drugs involved have some particular action.

Gee: In our experience most people die from one drug.

Prescott: Sometimes the patient who takes more than one drug takes an antagonist, which is very convenient.

Goulding: I thought you were crying out for *more* screening, Professor Gee. Are you sure you are not missing other drugs?

Gee: I am reasonably sure we are not missing them. When a body is analysed, after screening or something else has shown the presence of barbiturates, other drugs are looked for too, and anything the dead person could have taken is checked.

SCREENING FOR INDUSTRIAL CHEMICALS

Gillette: What about screening for industrial chemicals to which people are normally exposed?

Goulding: We could well be accused of not looking for them and thereby missing them. We believe that this is not a major issue in this country at present.

Newton: We rarely see accidental poisonings in adult patients.

Sunshine: We seldom see anything other than medications as a serious cause of morbidity or mortality. There are occasional incidents involving household products but usually they are insignificant, except for the corrosives, of which we see maybe one or two a year.

Prescott: Do you get much poisoning with organophosphorus insecticides? I understood that they have become a problem in some agricultural areas in the USA since DDT was removed.

Goulding: This is not a problem in England, even in the agricultural areas.

Sunshine: Nor is it a problem in urban Cleveland. It is more of a problem in other areas. Faddism exists everywhere. Florida gets many cases of methaqualone and organic phosphate poisoning.

Leach: We should always consider the local conditions, because there are different patterns of prescribing in adjacent areas. We see strychnine poisoning in Bangor simply because we are in an agricultural area and there are a lot of moles.

Curry: We have a very difficult job in these last few minutes of the symposium. Differences in geography, people, and techniques have all been discussed but we still need to define what is needed, necessary and desirable, by clinicians and analysts, in three different sets of conditions. First there is emergency or 3 a.m. toxicology. Can the clinicians define this more precisely for us? Then perhaps analysts will tell us what is practicable now, and finally what they hope will be possible in the future.

EMERGENCY TOXICOLOGY: CLINICAL REQUIREMENTS

Goulding: I would modify your question slightly and ask what is needed in emergency *medicine*. The patients when first seen are not necessarily poisoned, but they are patients who might be poisoned. Treatment may then have to be tailored to this individual and to his condition rather than adopting a uniform management plan regardless.

Sunshine: When the clinician first sees the person he has to ask whether that person is poisoned. If he doesn't raise that question the laboratory can't help. But once the question has been raised, we can ask the clinician what he wants and indicate how long it will take to do the analyses.

Curry: The first question is about emergencies, and there are very few emergency tests. I am trying to get the chemists to tell us whether they can do any more than they are at the moment.

Prescott: The compounds for which we need analyses are salicylate, phenobarbitone, paracetamol, meprobamate, ethchlorvynol, lithium, iron, and perhaps bromide and Paraquat. These are not all needed on an emergency basis at 3 a.m.

Curry: No chemist would turn out to do that lot at 3 a.m. Do you want to know whether those drugs are there, or how much?

Prescott: If a patient says she has taken an overdose of ferrous sulphate we need to know whether this is true and how much she has absorbed. If the serum iron exceeds about 800 μg/100 ml, then she is in danger and we must start treatment immediately. We cannot wait until Monday morning.

Leach: Would you accept a level above which you can say that the patient is in danger, or are you interested in knowing whether the level is 500 or 550 μg/ml?

Prescott: We want to know if it is 300 or 800.

Leach: Then there is no problem.

Curry: There are two variables that we have not considered: blood and urine. We must also not leave the impression that we can measure meprobamate concentrations in blood easily; in addition we have learned that most poisoned patients don't pass urine for the first 12 hours or so.

Goulding: We can usually get enough urine for screening and, if not, we can usually obtain stomach contents.

Prescott: It is no use knowing what the level of iron is in the urine, or how much paracetamol there is in a gastric aspirate. Our assessments can only be based on what is in plasma or blood.

Widdop: But why do you need to know the actual level of iron in the blood? Why not use desferrioxamine (deferoxamine) on the basis of a positive test in gastric contents?

Prescott: Of every 50 patients who are admitted claiming to have taken iron, only two or three will have absorbed enough to give dangerously high serum levels which demand treatment. Without the level we might be treating 48 patients unnecessarily and this is very bad medicine.

Widdop: How detrimental is desferrioxamine when given to a patient who hasn't taken iron?

Prescott: It is a potentially toxic compound which should not be given without good cause. It is our duty not to harm our patients.

Goulding: Desferrioxamine is less harmful if it is given orally. Dr Prescott wants to know whether certain drugs are present, and then what the level is, and iron is one of those drugs.

Sunshine: That is just the point. We can ask the clinicians what they want, and then we can tell them what it would cost. If they feel a test is essential for patient care, we can provide that, if we have the tools. If we don't have the techniques then we should make it our business to find them.

Curry: The question about emergency toxicology can be summed up by saying that the first requirement is communication between the customer and the supplier. The needs cannot be matched by the supply: they have to be equated with what is possible in both areas. Requirements will also vary from district to district, environment to environment, hospital to hospital. Emergency toxicology has to be tailored to the needs of a particular situation.

WHAT THE LABORATORY CAN DO

Beckett: If enough people gave us their definitive lists, could we give attention to more rough and ready tests which might satisfy them now?

Curry: Facilities in different hospitals vary so greatly that to give an average of what is desirable would be grossly misleading.

Widdop: In our specialized unit, although the range of tests we can personally bring to bear is much wider than indicated in my paper (this volume, pp. 219–230), part of our remit has always been to furnish analytical schemes which fit in with the facilities available in the average hospital laboratory.

Leach: Another aspect that is easily overlooked is expertise. A good analyst will look for many more drugs and set his standards far higher than a less experienced one. He covers a far wider range with the same basic techniques. If the experience of the staff likely to be available at night varies much, you may well set your sights far too low. A good analyst using a different approach may do three times as much as a less experienced person in the same time.

Curry: A poor doctor will ask for more and a poor technician will do less.

Sunshine: George Lundberg (Lundberg *et al.* 1972, 1974) in Los Angeles addressed himself to this question. He too said that the first step is communication between the user and the supplier of the service. Once we can establish the need for that communication pathway, and encourage its development, there will be better liaison between the groups.

Clinical toxicology should be done either regionally or in some larger unit than a small hospital laboratory. You can support the necessary expertise if you have a broader base. It is easier to spend an hour sending a sample to a place where the analysis can be done better than it is to develop a whole series of small laboratory units that will never satisfy the needs of the local group.

Curry: Do the same considerations apply when the question asked is whether we are treating the patient or the clinician in providing the results of the analyses? That is, with the less urgent requests for analyses for diagnosis or the case file, do the same analytical constraints apply? What is desirable?

Newton: We routinely ask the laboratory for confirmation of the drugs taken in all grade 3 and grade 4 cases (Matthew & Lawson 1972). I certainly wouldn't think that information about levels was necessary until the morning after admission, at least.

Goulding: I would carry that further. If the patient is improving, then unless you are doing a fact-finding exercise simply to amplify the records, then forget the laboratory. It is a waste of time doing routine analyses and we will not undertake them.

Leach: If you carried this to extremes and everybody decided they had single drug overdoses, we would never see evidence of multiple drug overdosages. We might believe that these were all barbiturate poisonings.

Goulding: That comes under fact-finding, and so does measuring the comparative efficiency of different types of treatment. Blood levels and other measurements are then needed as another form of investigation.

OTHER WORK OF THE LABORATORY

Curry: Our third point brings in accurate measurement and the two areas of monitoring, that is, monitoring the drug addict and monitoring drugs as therapy.

Dole: Routine monitoring of people taking part in narcotics programmes is important for judging the efficacy of the programme. However, monitoring can be misused and actually be divisive in rehabilitation programmes. The solution is simple. If routine testing is done, results should go to a central place for statistical work, but not be used as a primary method of control. This obliges the therapist to look at the patient. I suspect that screening has got out of hand in the US and I am glad there is more common sense about this in the UK and in other areas. We are required by the Federal Government to do a vast number of tests. Clinicians and professional staff have become so accustomed to this that they have become dependent on laboratory reports, which is disastrous. There is no conceptual problem here, but there is a political issue.

Holmstedt: Does monitoring in these programmes mean deciding whether the drug is present in urine rather than how much of it is there?

Dole: Yes, we do quantitative analyses for research purposes, but not for the rehabilitation programmes. The routine monitoring that is required is the detection of opiates and other drugs of abuse, such as amphetamines, barbiturates and tranquillizers. The objective is only the discovery of illicit use of drugs by the patients.

Curry: Do clinicians need accurate quantitative methods in monitoring therapy?

Sunshine: As practice grows, the clinicians will be asking for more and more screening. This kind of service is closely related to the toxicology laboratory and rightfully becomes part of the unit, giving it a broad base on which to build.

Holmstedt: Complex and accurate determinations using either the molecular ion or some significant ion in the mass spectrum for quantification is expensive. About 50 tests a day can be done in this way. Our record is 172 in one day and half a night. I don't believe that this method will be routine anywhere except in large centres of population but I would like to stress again its extreme usefulness for calibrating other methods: you can find out how good other methods are and calibrate and check them. The less expensive methods can then be put to better use. This applies particularly to the immunoassays.

Curry: It is important to cross-check methods. Bioavailability of digoxin has been in the news recently, and we may get into the same sort of situation in the future for other drugs.

Goulding: I must here give a materialistic warning. I once calculated the cost of monitoring, without indulging in any fancy instrumentation, all the people taking tricyclic antidepressants. To make this exercise financially worth while for the country, prescribing of these antidepressants would have to be cut to one-third of the present rate.

Gillette: Specificity of methods can lead to another problem. Certain compounds can be converted to metabolites that are as effective as or more effective than the parent drug. So you should measure both compounds simultaneously. Non-specific methods may sometimes measure all the effective substances at once, which may be all the clinician initially needs to know.

Bridges: An analytical method may be good for one kind of sample but inappropriate for another.

Prescott: It is becoming increasingly obvious that many drugs have active metabolites. We should look to the drug industry for information concerning the relative and absolute activity of metabolites of new drugs. Only then can we know whether we should be measuring metabolites as well as the parent drug.

Holmstedt: How can the industry tell you that?

Prescott: They develop drugs and claim to know about them.

Holmstedt: They do animal screening.

Prescott: They also do studies in man. If a metabolite is active in animals it will probably be active in man.

Beckett: If we ask the drug companies for information on the pharmacology, in man, of each metabolite of a drug, then we shall be putting up the cost of developing a drug by two or three times.

Curry: We have discussed many types of patients, laboratories, techniques, and new areas of research. It seems obvious that what we need most is interdisciplinary cooperation and one hopes that this meeting has contributed to this to some extent.

References

ALEXANDERSON, B. (1973) Predictions of steady-state plasma levels of nortriptyline from single oral dose kinetics: A study in twins. *Eur. J. Clin. Pharmacol. 6*, 44–53

CURRY, A. S. (1969) in *Poison Detection in Human Organs*, pp. 65–66, 126–128, Thomas, Springfield, Ill.

CURRY, A. S. (1972) in *Advances in Forensic and Clinical Toxicology*, pp. 105–106, CRC Press, Cleveland, Ohio

HAIDER, I. (1971) The electroencephalogram in acute barbiturate poisoning, in *Acute Barbiturate Poisoning* (Matthew, H., ed.), pp. 147–174, Excerpta Medica, Amsterdam

LUNDBERG, G. D. & WALBERG, C. B. & GUPTA, R. C. (1972) The patient focused approach to clinical toxicology laboratory organization. *Lab. Med. 3*, 14

LUNDBERG, G. D., WALBERG, C. B. & PANTLIK, V. A. (1974) Frequency of clinical toxicology test-ordering (primarily overdose cases) and results in a large urban general hospital. *Clin. Chem. 20*, 121–125

MATTHEW, H. & LAWSON, A. A. H. (1966) Acute barbiturate poisoning—a review of 2 years' experience. *Q. J. Med. 35*, 539–552

MATTHEW, H. & LAWSON, A. A. H. (1972) *Treatment of Common Acute Poisonings*, 2nd edn, Churchill Livingstone, Edinburgh

MATTHEW, H., PROUDFOOT, A. T., BROWN, S. S. & SMITH, A. C. A. (1968*a*) Mandrax poisoning. Conservative management of 116 patients. *Br. Med. J. 2*, 101–102

MATTHEW, H., LOGAN, A., WOODRUFF, M. F. A. & HEARD, B. (1968*b*) Paraquat poisoning—lung transplantation. *Br. Med. J. 3*, 759–763

MITCHELL, J. R., JOLLOW, D. J., GILLETTE, J. R. & BRODIE, B. B. (1973) Drug metabolism as a cause of drug toxicity. *Drug Metab. Disposition 1*, 418–423

PARKER, K. D., ELLIOTT, H. W., WRIGHT, J. A., NOMOF, N. & HINE, C. H. (1970) Blood and urine concentrations of subjects receiving barbiturates, meprobamate, glutethimide or diphenylhydantoin. *Clin. Toxicol. 3*, 131–145

PRESCOTT, L. F., ROSCOE, P. & FORREST, J. A. H. (1973) Plasma concentrations and drug toxicity in man, in *Biological Effects of Drugs in Relation to their Plasma Concentration* (Davies, D. S. & Prichard, B. N. C., eds.) pp. 51–81, Macmillan, London

SJÖQVIST, F., HAMMER, W., IDESTRÖM, C.-M., LIND, M., TUCK, D. & ÅSBERG, M. (1968) Plasma level of monomethylated tricyclic antidepressants and side-effects in man, in *Toxicity and Side-Effects of Psychotropic Drugs* (*Proc. Eur. Soc. Study Drug. Toxicity*, vol. 9), pp. 246–257, ICS No. 145, Excerpta Medica, Amsterdam

WRIGHT, N. & ROSCOE, P. (1970) Acute glutethimide poisoning. Conservative management of 31 patients. *J. Am. Med. Assoc. 214*, 1704–1706

Index of contributors

Entries in **bold** *type refer to papers, other entries to contributions to discussions*

Indexes compiled by William Hill

Subject index